Psoriatic Arthritis

Editor

CHRISTOPHER T. RITCHLIN

RHEUMATIC DISEASE CLINICS OF NORTH AMERICA

www.rheumatic.theclinics.com

Consulting Editor
MICHAEL H. WEISMAN

November 2015 • Volume 41 • Number 4

ELSEVIER

1600 John F. Kennedy Boulevard • Suite 1800 • Philadelphia, Pennsylvania, 19103-2899
http://www.theclinics.com

RHEUMATIC DISEASE CLINICS OF NORTH AMERICA Volume 41, Number 4
November 2015 ISSN 0889-857X, ISBN 13: 978-0-323-41352-7

Editor: Jennifer Flynn-Briggs
Developmental Editor: Casey Jackson

Rheumatic Disease Clinics of North America (ISSN 0889-857X) is published quarterly by Elsevier Inc., 360 Park Avenue South, New York, NY 10010-1710. Months of issue are February, May, August, and November. Business and editorial offices: 1600 John F. Kennedy Boulevard, Suite 1800, Philadelphia, PA 19103-2899. Periodicals postage paid at New York, NY and additional mailing offices. Subscription prices are USD 335.00 per year for US individuals, USD 579.00 per year for US institutions, USD 165.00 per year for US students and residents, USD 395.00 per year for Canadian individuals, USD 722.00 per year for Canadian institutions, USD 465.00 per year for international individuals, USD 722.00 per year for international institutions, and USD 230.00 per year for Canadian and foreign students/residents. To receive student/resident rate, orders must be accompanied by name of affiliated institution, date of term, and the signature of program/residency coordinator on institution letterhead. Orders will be billed at individual rate until proof of status received. Foreign air speed delivery is included in all Clinics subscription prices. All prices are subject to change without notice. POSTMASTER: Send address changes to Rheumatic Disease Clinics of North America, Elsevier Health Sciences Division, Subscription Customer Service, 3251 Riverport Lane, Maryland Heights, MO 63043. Customer Service: 1-800-654-2452 (US and Canada). From outside of the US and Canada: 314-447-8871. Fax: 314-447-8029. For print support, e-mail: JournalsCustomerService-usa@elsevier.com. For online support, e-mail: JournalsOnline Support-usa@elsevier.com.

Reprints. For copies of 100 or more of articles in this publication, please contact the Commercial Reprints Department, Elsevier Inc., 360 Park Avenue South, New York, New York, 10010-1710; Tel.: +1-212-633-3874, Fax: +1-212-633-3820, and E-mail: reprints@elsevier.com.

Rheumatic Disease Clinics of North America is covered in MEDLINE/PubMed (Index Medicus), Current Contents/Clinical Medicine, Science Citation Index, ISI/BIOMED, and EMBASE/Excerpta Medica.

Contributors

CONSULTING EDITOR

MICHAEL H. WEISMAN, MD
Cedars-Sinai Chair in Rheumatology, Director, Division of Rheumatology, Professor of Medicine, Cedars-Sinai Medical Center, Distinguished Professor, David Geffen School of Medicine at UCLA, Los Angeles, California

EDITOR

CHRISTOPHER T. RITCHLIN, MD, MPH
Professor and Chief, Allergy, Immunology and Rheumatology Division, University of Rochester Medical Center, Rochester, New York

AUTHORS

JENNIFER L. BARNAS, MD, PhD
Allergy, Immunology and Rheumatology, University of Rochester Medical Center, Rochester, New York

WOLF-HENNING BOEHNCKE, MD
Professor, Department of Dermatology and Venereology, Geneva University Hospitals, Genève 14, Switzerland; Department of Pathology and Immunology, University of Geneva, Geneva, Switzerland

TRISTAN BOYD, MD
Assistant Professor of Medicine, Division of Rheumatology, Western University, Schulich School of Medicine; St. Joseph's Health Care London, London, Ontario

LAURA COATES, MBChB, MRCP, PhD
Leeds Musculoskeletal Biomedical Research Unit, Leeds Institute of Rheumatic and Musculoskeletal Medicine, University of Leeds, Leeds Teaching Hospitals Trust, United Kingdom; Division of Allergy, Immunology and Rheumatology, University of Rochester Medical Center, Rochester, New York

DAFNA D. GLADMAN, MD, FRCPC
Director, Psoriatic Arthritis Program, University Health Network; Senior Scientist, Toronto Western Research Institute; Professor of Medicine, University of Toronto, Toronto, Ontario, Canada

PHILIP S. HELLIWELL, MD
Leeds Institute of Rheumatic and Musculoskeletal Medicine, Chapel Allerton Hospital, Senior Lecturer in Rheumatology, University of Leeds, Leeds, United Kingdom

M. ELAINE HUSNI, MD, MPH
Vice Chair, Department of Rheumatic and Immunologic Diseases; Director, Clinical Outcomes Research; Director, Arthritis and Musculoskeletal Center, Cleveland Clinic, Cleveland, Ohio

ARTHUR KAVANAUGH, MD
Professor of Medicine, Division of Rheumatology, Allergy and Immunology, University of California, San Diego, School of Medicine, La Jolla, California

NEIL JOHN McHUGH, MBChB, MD, FRCP, FRCPath
Professor of Pharmacoepidemiology and Consultant Rheumatologist, Department of Pharmacy and Pharmacology, University of Bath, Bath, United Kingdom

PHILIP J. MEASE, MD
Clinical Rheumatology Research, Swedish Medical Center; University of Washington School of Medicine, Seattle, Washington

DARREN D. O'RIELLY, PhD
Senior Research Scientist, Faculty of Medicine, Health Sciences Centre, Memorial University of Newfoundland, St. John's, Newfoundland and Labrador, Canada

ALEXIS OGDIE, MD, MSCE
Assistant Professor of Medicine and Epidemiology, Division of Rheumatology, Center for Clinical Epidemiology and Biostatistics, Perelman School of Medicine, University of Pennsylvania, Philadelphia, Pennsylvania

MIKKEL ØSTERGAARD, MD, PhD, DMSc
Professor of Rheumatology, Copenhagen Center for Arthritis Research, Center for Rheumatology and Spine Diseases, Rigshospitalet - Glostrup; Department of Clinical Medicine, Faculty of Health and Medical Sciences, University of Copenhagen, Copenhagen, Denmark

RENÉ PANDURO POGGENBORG, MD, PhD
Copenhagen Center for Arthritis Research, Center for Rheumatology and Spine Diseases, Rigshospitalet - Glostrup; Department of Clinical Medicine, Faculty of Health and Medical Sciences, University of Copenhagen, Copenhagen, Denmark

PROTON RAHMAN, MD, MSc, FRCPC
St. Clare's Mercy Hospital, Professor of Medicine (Rheumatology), Memorial University of Newfoundland, St. John's, Newfoundland and Labrador, Canada

CHRISTOPHER T. RITCHLIN, MD, MPH
Professor and Chief, Allergy, Immunology and Rheumatology Division, University of Rochester Medical Center, Rochester, New York

ERIC M. RUDERMAN, MD
Professor of Medicine, Division of Rheumatology, Northwestern University Feinberg School of Medicine, Chicago, Illinois

ENRIQUE R. SORIANO, MD, MSc
Associate Professor, Rheumatology Unit, Internal Medical Services, Hospital Italiano de Buenos Aires, Instituto Universitario, y Fundcion PM. Catoggio, Buenos Aires, Argentina

LENE TERSLEV, MD, PhD
Consultant Rheumatologist, Copenhagen Center for Arthritis Research, Center for Rheumatology and Spine Diseases, Rigshospitalet - Glostrup; Department of Clinical Medicine, Faculty of Health and Medical Sciences, University of Copenhagen, Copenhagen, Denmark

PAMELA WEISS, MD, MSCE
Assistant Professor of Pediatrics, Division of Rheumatology, Children's Hospital of Philadelphia, Center for Clinical Epidemiology and Biostatistics, University of Pennsylvania, Philadelphia, Pennsylvania

Contents

> Psoriatic arthritis (PsA) is a chronic systemic inflammatory disorder characterized by joint and entheseal inflammation with a prevalence of 0.05% to 0.25% of the population and 6% to 41% of patients with psoriasis. PsA is a highly heterogeneous inflammatory arthritis. In this review, current knowledge is discussed regarding the epidemiology of PsA, including disease manifestations, classification criteria for adult and juvenile PsA, methods for recognizing early PsA, including use of screening tools and knowledge of risk factors for PsA, and medical comorbidities associated with PsA.

> Psoriatic arthritis is an inflammatory musculoskeletal disease affecting almost a third of patients with psoriasis. Clinical presentations are complex and varied and include peripheral arthritis, axial disease, dactylitis, and enthesitis, as well as skin and nail manifestations. We lack diagnostic biomarkers, but specific clinical and imaging features distinguish psoriatic arthritis from other forms of arthritis such as rheumatoid arthritis, gout, osteoarthritis, and other forms of spondyloarthritis.

> Although early reports suggested psoriatic arthritis was, with the exception of arthritis mutilans, a relatively mild arthritis, later studies have challenged this view. The burden of skin disease adds to disability and impaired quality of life. Patients in secondary care manifest increased morbidity and mortality, mainly owing to cardiovascular disease. A subset of patients, primarily men with oligoarticular disease, demonstrates low levels of joint involvement without disability. The socioeconomic impact of the disease is significant. We require more information on the impact of early diagnosis and treatment on outcome, according to phenotype, to guide policy.

Psoriatic arthritis (PsA) is an inflammatory joint disease characterized by arthritis and often enthesitis in patients with psoriasis, presenting a wide range of manifestations in various patterns. Imaging procedures are primarily conventional radiography, ultrasonography (US), and magnetic resonance imaging (MRI). Other modalities such as computed tomography are not used routinely. Imaging is an integral part of management of PsA. In this article, we provide an overview of the status, virtues, and limitations of imaging modalities in PsA, focusing on radiography, US, and MRI.

Skin psoriasis is a major risk factor for the development of psoriatic arthritis. Recent studies have shown that delayed diagnosis is associated with long-term adverse outcomes. Screening questionnaires have revealed a potential burden of undiagnosed disease. Lifestyle factors and genetic and soluble biomarkers have come under scrutiny as risk factors. Imaging modalities may have an important role in detecting early change. With more effective treatments, it may be possible to prevent significant joint damage and associated disability. However, the precise nature of accurate and cost-effective screening strategies remains to be determined.

There is a strong familial component to psoriatic disease as well as a complex array of genetic, immunologic, and environmental factors. The dominant genetic effect is located on chromosome 6p21.3 within the major histocompatibility complex region, accounting for one-third of genetic contribution. Genome-wide association studies (GWAS) identified additional genes, including skin barrier function, innate immune response, and adaptive immune response genes. To better understand disease susceptibility and progression requires replication in larger cohorts, fine-mapping efforts, new technologies, and functional studies of genetic variants, gene–gene interactions and gene–environmental interactions. New technologies available include next-generation sequencing, copy number variation analysis, and epigenetics.

The current model of psoriatic arthritis implicates both the IL-23/IL-17 axis and the tumor necrosis factor (TNF) pathways in disease pathogenesis. Although specific major histocompatibility complex class I molecules are associated with the psoriatic disease phenotype, no specific antigen or autoantibody has been identified. Instead, an array of genes may code for an autoinflammatory loop, potentially activated by mechanical stress and dysbiosis in the skin or gut. Danger signals released by innate immune cells activate a Th1 and Th17 response that leads to synovitis, enthesitis, axial inflammation, and altered bone homeostasis characterized by pathologic bone resorption and new bone formation.

Psoriasis is a common, chronic inflammatory skin disease most often appearing in the form of well-demarcated, scaly plaques. These lesions highlight the fundamental processes underlying its pathogenesis, namely, inflammation and epidermal hyperproliferation. Both phenomena are considered consequences of an intimate interplay between the innate and the adaptive immune system. This concept is supported by results of genetic studies, pointing toward the signaling pathways of nuclear factor-κB, interferon-γ, and interleukin (IL)-23 as well as antigen presentation as central axes of the psoriatic inflammation. Efficacy of biologics targeting tumor necrosis factor-α, IL-23, or IL-17 provides further evidence in favor of this model.

Epidemiologic studies have shown that, in patients with psoriatic arthritis (PsA), associated comorbidities may occur more frequently than expected. This article discusses related comorbidities in patients with PsA. Identifying these comorbidities may affect the management and treatment decisions for these patients to ensure an optimal clinical outcome. All health care providers caring for patients with PsA should be aware of the relevant comorbidities and should have an understanding of how these comorbidities affect management. The common comorbidities include cardiovascular disease, metabolic syndrome, obesity, diabetes, fatty liver disease, inflammatory bowel disease, ophthalmic disease, kidney disease, osteoporosis, depression, and anxiety.

In the last decade, there have been significant advances in outcome measure research in psoriatic arthritis (PsA). In this article, the outcome measures for disease activity in individual key domains of PsA are reviewed, followed by the key patient-reported outcome measures of function, quality of life, fatigue, and a new measure for disease impact, the psoriatic arthritis impact of disease. New research into composite measures of psoriatic disease is summarized, including response measures and proposed cutoff points for disease activity. Finally, the key future issues in outcome measurement in PsA are addressed.

Traditional disease-modifying antirheumatic drugs (DMARD) remain the first-line treatment of psoriatic arthritis (PsA), despite lack of randomized controlled trials, and with evidence based on observational studies. Anti-tumor necrosis factor agents remain a top choice for biologic treatment, complemented with new biologics with different targets (IL12-23 and IL17). Unmet needs have been identified for patients who do not respond to treatment. Among targeted small molecules Apremilast is approved for the treatment of PsA and Tofactitinib is under investigation. The drugs discussed herein have the potential to address unmet needs; however, additional research is required to identify more effective therapies for PsA.

Biologic medications, therapeutic proteins that inhibit or modulate proinflammatory immune cells and cytokines, have significantly altered clinicians' ability to effectively treat psoriatic arthritis (PsA). The first widely used biologics have been those targeting tumor necrosis factor alpha. Five agents (etanercept, infliximab, adalimumab, golimumab, and certolizumab) have shown significant benefit in all clinical domains of PsA as well as inhibiting progressive joint destruction. Treatment strategies such as treating PsA early in the disease course, treating to target and tight control, use of background methotrexate to reduce immunogenicity, and various cost-saving strategies are all being tested with biologic medicines for PsA.

The introduction of highly effective therapies and clearly defined targets has altered the treatment paradigm in psoriatic arthritis (PsA). Validated classification criteria and outcome measures specific to PsA have helped standardize a therapeutic approach to this heterogeneous disease that affects multiple clinical domains. This article discusses the importance of early intervention using a treat-to-target strategy, emerging evidence for tight control based on minimal disease activity criteria, disease considerations specific to PsA (prognostic markers, biomarkers, subclinical disease, comorbidities), and new treatment strategies to deal with refractory disease (eg, tumor necrosis factor inhibitor switching and use of novel disease-modifying therapies) and controlled disease (eg, tapering or discontinuing biologic therapy).

RHEUMATIC DISEASE CLINICS OF NORTH AMERICA

THE CLINICS ARE AVAILABLE ONLINE!
Access your subscription at:
www.theclinics.com

Foreword

Psoriatic Arthritis

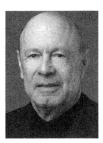

Michael H. Weisman, MD
Consulting Editor

Chris Ritchlin has done a remarkable job assembling the expertise necessary to put together a timely comprehensive review of Psoriatic Arthritis. We learn how many people have psoriatic arthritis and what the natural history of the disease is. Diagnostic considerations are displayed comprehensively, and management considerations are expressed in detail. But most importantly, Chris tells us the story, in a very detailed manner, about the current theories for the pathogenesis of the disease and why it is both similar and different from rheumatoid arthritis (RA). Clearly, there must be something very different (and special) about this disease phenotype that emerges as a consequence of its relationship to other spondyloarthritis conditions that occur in the same family, including inflammatory bowel diseases. Finally, why do the bone manifestations of this form of arthritis look so different from RA, and do we really know why disease management options might have unique effects on different skeletal tissues? This issue attempts to address these and many other important issues.

Michael H. Weisman, MD
Division of Rheumatology
Cedars-Sinai Medical Center
David Geffen School of Medicine at UCLA
8700 Beverly Boulevard
Los Angeles, CA 90048, USA

E-mail address:
Michael.Weisman@cshs.org

Rheum Dis Clin N Am 41 (2015) xi
http://dx.doi.org/10.1016/j.rdc.2015.09.002
0889-857X/15/$ – see front matter © 2015 Published by Elsevier Inc.

rheumatic.theclinics.com

Preface

Psoriatic Arthritis

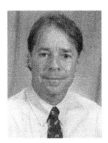

Christopher T. Ritchlin, MD, MPH
Editor

It is hard to believe that little more than 40 years have elapsed since psoriatic arthritis was first described as a separate entity, HLAB27 was linked to ankylosing spondylitis, and the spondyloarthritis concept was initially proposed. Following the elegant and comprehensive description of psoriatic arthritis by Moll and Wright in 1973, progress in our understanding of pathogenesis, diagnosis, and treatment of this disorder was slow with few major advances. Clinical studies were hampered by striking clinical heterogeneity and disease course coupled with the lack of a diagnostic marker, and investigations into disease mechanisms were rare compared with the prodigious efforts in rheumatoid arthritis.

A combination of events over the last 15 years, however, has transformed our understanding of disease mechanisms, clinical features, and treatment options for psoriatic arthritis. The development of the Classification of Psoriatic Arthritis Criteria (CASPAR) greatly improved selection of patients for clinical trials. Efforts by members of the Group for Research and Assessment of Psoriasis and Psoriatic Arthritis (GRAPPA) and Outcome Measures in Rheumatology (OMERACT) resulted in the development of validated and reliable outcome measures that included not only skin and joints but also enthesitis, and dactylitis, coupled with assessments of function and quality of life. These advances were triggered by the development of new biologic therapies with great efficacy for psoriasis and the many facets of psoriatic musculoskeletal inflammation. Over the last several years, new discoveries centered on key mechanisms that underlie skin and joint inflammations emerged and have proven to be quite distinct from pathways in rheumatoid arthritis. In parallel, new biologic agents and small molecules have been recently developed that show efficacy in psoriatic but not rheumatoid arthritis. These new findings have generated great excitement and expectations regarding the discovery of more effective and safer therapies for psoriatic arthritis.

This issue of *Rheumatic Disease Clinics of North America* addresses the landscape of advances, many of them recently described in psoriatic arthritis. The first three

Rheum Dis Clin N Am 41 (2015) xiii–xiv
http://dx.doi.org/10.1016/j.rdc.2015.09.001
0889-857X/15/$ – see front matter © 2015 Published by Elsevier Inc.

rheumatic.theclinics.com

articles present the epidemiology, clinical features, and natural history of psoriatic arthritis along with prognostic considerations. The next two articles outline imaging modalities important for diagnosis and monitoring in psoriatic arthritis and the critical elements important for early diagnosis and treatment. The next articles highlight genetic, epigenetic, and pharmacogenetic aspects and recent advances in our understanding of the cause and pathogenesis of psoriatic arthritis and psoriasis with emphasis on new disease paradigms that have unveiled new treatment targets. The next two articles discuss the critical importance of comorbidities in the diagnosis and management of psoriatic arthritis and the use of newly developed outcome measures in clinical trials and in the office setting. The next two articles provide an evidence-based review of disease management in psoriatic arthritis that includes traditional disease-modifying rheumatic agents, small molecules, and biologic agents. The concluding article provides a detailed overview of novel treatment concepts in psoriatic arthritis.

The authors who contributed articles to this volume are leaders in the field, and their contributions have advanced the science, diagnosis, and treatment of psoriatic arthritis over the last fifteen years. They have unique perspectives that provide a comprehensive overview of psoriatic arthritis. I want to express my sincere appreciation for their efforts.

Christopher T. Ritchlin, MD, MPH
Allergy Immunology
and Rheumatology Division
University of Rochester Medical Center
601 Elmwood Avenue, Box 695
Rochester, NY 14621, USA

E-mail address:
Christopher_ritchlin@urmc.rochester.edu

The Epidemiology of Psoriatic Arthritis

Alexis Ogdie, MD, MSCE[a],*, Pamela Weiss, MD, MSCE[b]

KEYWORDS

- Psoriatic arthritis • Juvenile psoriatic arthritis • Epidemiology • Classification criteria
- Screening tools • Risk factors • Comorbidity

KEY POINTS

- Psoriatic arthritis (PsA) is a clinically heterogeneous inflammatory arthritis that is common among patients with psoriasis.
- PsA remains underdiagnosed.
- Early identification of PsA is important in order to improve long-term outcomes.
- Knowledge of risk factors for PsA and use of screening tools may improve recognition of PsA among patients with psoriasis.

INTRODUCTION

Psoriatic arthritis (PsA) is a chronic, progressive inflammatory arthritis that is common among patients with psoriasis and may result in permanent joint damage and disability. PsA was once considered a relatively benign disease; however, research over the past 20 years has significantly changed this notion. It is now known that PsA is a systemic inflammatory disorder with health consequences beyond joint function, such as cardiovascular disease, and similar outcomes to rheumatoid arthritis (RA), including the prevalence of erosions and joint destruction.[1,2] In addition, it has been learned that patients with PsA have highly heterogeneous disease courses.[3] In this review, current knowledge is discussed about the epidemiology of PsA, including prevalence of disease characteristics, classification of adult and pediatric PsA, and the importance of early diagnosis of PsA, including methods for screening and knowledge regarding risk factors for the development of PsA. Finally, medical comorbidities associated with PsA are discussed.

Disclosure Statement: The authors have nothing to disclose.
[a] Division of Rheumatology, Center for Clinical Epidemiology and Biostatistics, Perelman School of Medicine, University of Pennsylvania, White Building, Room 5024, 3400 Spruce Street, Philadelphia, PA 19104, USA; [b] Division of Rheumatology, Children's Hospital of Philadelphia, Center for Clinical Epidemiology and Biostatistics, University of Pennsylvania, 3535 Market Street, Room 1526, Philadelphia, PA 19104, USA
* Corresponding author.
E-mail address: alexis.ogdie@uphs.upenn.edu

Rheum Dis Clin N Am 41 (2015) 545–568
http://dx.doi.org/10.1016/j.rdc.2015.07.001
0889-857X/15/$ – see front matter © 2015 Elsevier Inc. All rights reserved.

METHODS

The authors performed a systematic review by combining "psoriasis or psoriatic arthritis" with the following MeSH terms: epidemiology, classification, diagnosis, complications, mortality in Ovid Medline. This review resulted in 8936 citations. After limiting to English papers, humans, and 2006 to current, 3515 citations remained. Titles and abstracts were reviewed for these remaining papers. Papers were excluded if they did not refer to psoriasis or PsA (N = 288), were case reports (N = 644), reviews or editorials (N = 383), or focused on basic science or immunology topics (N = 210). Finally, 1698 papers were excluded because they focused on skin psoriasis exclusively or were not relevant to the topics of interest. The authors also included articles before 2006 if cited within articles retrieved by the Medline search and if they were considered highly relevant. Abstracts from meeting conferences were not included.

PREVALENCE AND INCIDENCE OF PSORIATIC ARTHRITIS IN THE POPULATION

Several studies have examined the prevalence of PsA in countries all over the world. Prevalence estimates in the United States range from 0.06% to 0.25% with the lowest estimate derived from a paper that used International Classification of Disease, ninth edition (ICD-9), codes to identify cases and the highest from articles using patient self-report of diagnosis of PsA.[4–6] Prevalence estimates in Europe range from 0.05% in Turkey[7] and the Czech Republic[8] to 0.21% in Sweden.[9–12] Only a few reports of the prevalence of PsA in South America and Asia exist and suggest that the prevalence is lower in these regions (0.07% in Buenos Aires and 0.02% in China).[13,14] The low prevalence of PsA in China may be due to underdiagnosis, as suggested in a study by Yang and colleagues.[15] Discrepancies in the prevalence of PsA among these studies is often related to differing definitions of PsA (eg, use of ICD-9 or medical codes vs use of clinical classification criteria). The incidence of PsA in the general population has been examined by relatively few studies. The reported incidence of PsA in recent publications ranges from 3.6 to 7.2 per 100,000 person-years.[8,13,16,17] However, publications in 2001 to 2003 reported a much wider incidence range (0.1–23.1).[18]

PREVALENCE AND INCIDENCE OF PSORIATIC ARTHRITIS AMONG PATIENTS WITH PSORIASIS

Although PsA has a low prevalence in the general population, it is common among patients with psoriasis. Again, prevalence estimates vary considerably (range 6%–41%) depending on the definitions used (ie, diagnostic codes, rheumatologist diagnosis, classification criteria, diagnostic codes, and the populations measured).[10,11,14,15,19–28] Wilson and colleagues examined the cumulative incidence of PsA over time in patients with psoriasis and reported 1.7%, 3.1%, and 5.1%, respectively, had developed PsA at 5, 10, and 20 years after their diagnosis of psoriasis.[17] Eder and colleagues[29] reported an annual incidence of 1.87% In a prospective cohort of 313 patients with psoriasis.

ALTERNATIVE DIAGNOSES, MISSED DIAGNOSES, AND MISCLASSIFICATION IN STUDIES OF PSORIATIC ARTHRITIS

Studying the epidemiology of PsA is challenging given the absence of definitive, gold-standard diagnostic tests for PsA and the heterogeneous manifestations of the disease. In addition, patients with psoriasis often have other common reasons for joint pain, such as osteoarthritis, gout, and fibromyalgia, which can easily be mistaken for PsA.[30–34] When using diagnosis codes to define PsA, there is often a concern for misclassification given that patients with psoriasis could have one of these alternate diagnoses. Unfortunately, without examination, this issue is difficult to resolve, and this is often a tradeoff for the large sample sizes and rich outcome data afforded by administrative and medical record data. Similarly, studies examining outcomes in patients with PsA compared with psoriasis alone, even within a clinic-based population, may suffer from misclassification of patients with psoriasis and undiagnosed PsA. Studies examining the prevalence of PsA among patients with psoriasis have found that underdiagnosis is common.[15,21,25] Mease and colleagues[25] found a prevalence of PsA of 30% among patients with psoriasis, and among the 285 patients with PsA, 117 (41%) were not previously diagnosed, suggesting a high prevalence of underdiagnosis.

DEFINING AND CLASSIFYING PSORIATIC ARTHRITIS

Classification criteria are designed to create more homogenous populations for research.[35] Several sets of classification criteria for PsA have been created since the original Moll and Wright criteria in 1973.[36] These criteria include the Amor criteria, European Spondylarthropathy Study Group criteria, Vasey and Espinoza criteria, and Classification of Psoriatic Arthritis (CASPAR) criteria.[3,37–42] There is a great deal of variability among the criteria components and test performance of each (sensitivity and specificity). Rheumatologist diagnosis is most commonly used as the reference standard.[43,44] The CASPAR criteria are the most widely used criteria, and their high sensitivity and specificity (both 90% or better in most studies but sensitivity as low as 77.3% in D'Angelo and colleagues[45]) have been demonstrated in many settings, including dermatology and rheumatology clinics, family practice clinics, and among early arthritis cohorts (despite early suggestions that CASPAR criteria were not ideal for early disease).[42,46–50] Most recently, the Assessment of SpondyloArthritis International Society (ASAS) developed peripheral and axial spondyloarthropathy (AxSpA) criteria. PsA could be classified under either of these criteria depending on whether axial involvement is present (**Table 1**).[51,52] In a recent study by Van den Berg and colleagues,[46] the peripheral spondyloarthropathy criteria were found to have much lower sensitivity for early PsA compared with CASPAR criteria using the diagnosis from the treating rheumatologist as the gold standard. It is unclear what role the new peripheral ASAS criteria will play in studies of PsA.[53]

PSORIATIC ARTHRITIS IS A HETEROGENEOUS DISEASE

PsA is a clinically heterogeneous disorder. Five subtypes of psoriatic arthritis were initially defined by Moll and Wright: monoarthritis or oligoarthritis, polyarthritis, distal interphalangeal (DIP) joint predominant disease, psoriatic spondylitis or sacroiliitis, and arthritis mutilans.[36] It is now recognized that patients can have any combination of the disease features: peripheral arthritis (monoarticular, oligoarticular, or polyarticular with or without DIP involvement), enthesitis, dactylitis, spondylitis or sacroiliitis, as well as psoriatic nail disease.[3] Peripheral arthritis (either oligoarticular or polyarticular depending on the cohort examined) is the most common disease manifestation. Arthritis mutilans, although one of the original 5 subtypes of PsA identified by Moll and Wright, is thought to be overall quite rare. However, the prevalence of arthritis mutilans is difficult to determine given the varied definitions.[54] As noted, the relative prevalence of the various manifestations varies considerably by site and study (**Fig. 1**).[10,15–17,28,55–60] This variation is in particular due to the highly varied definitions

Table 1
Commonly used classification criteria for psoriatic arthritis[a] and new Assessment of SpondyloArthritis International Society criteria for peripheral and axial SpA

Moll and Wright	CASPAR	Peripheral SpA	Axial SpA
All 3 of the following:	Inflammatory articular disease (joint, spine, or entheseal) with ≥3 points from the following 5 categories:	Arthritis or enthesitis or dactylitis plus either:	Sacroiliitis on imaging plus ≥1 SpA feature	HLA-B27 plus ≥2 SpA features

Moll and Wright	CASPAR	Peripheral SpA		Axial SpA
1. Inflammatory arthritis (peripheral arthritis or sacroiliitis or spondylitis)	1. Current psoriasis (2 pts), personal history of psoriasis or family history of psoriasis (1 pt)	≥1 SpA feature: Uveitis Psoriasis Crohn's/ulcerative colitis Preceding infection HLA-B27 Sacroiliitis on imaging	≥2 other SpA features: Arthritis Enthesitis Dactylitis Inflammatory back pain ever Family history of SpA	SpA features: Inflammatory back pain Arthritis Enthesitis Dactylitis Psoriasis Crohn's/ulcerative colitis Good response to nonsteroidal anti-inflammatory drugs Family history of SpA HLA-B27 Elevated CRP
2. Psoriasis	2. Psoriatic nail dystrophy (onycholysis, pitting, or hyperkeratosis) on exam (1 pt)			
3. Negative RF (usually)	3. Negative RF (1 pt)			
	4. Current dactylitis or history of dactylitis recorded by rheumatologist (1 pt)			
	5. Evidence of juxta-articular new bone formation (excluding osteophytes) on plain radiographs of the hand or foot (1 pt)			

[a] See Table 1 from Eder L, Gladman DD. Psoriatic arthritis: phenotypic variance and nosology. Curr Rheumatol Rep 2013;15:316 for comparison of additional classification criteria.

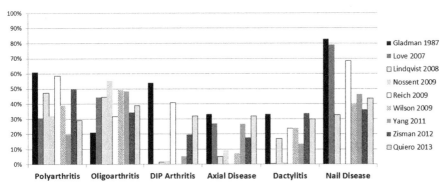

Fig. 1. Variability of disease characteristics by study. The prevalence of oligoarthritis, polyarthritis, axial disease, dactylitis, and nail disease in a handful of studies is shown. These manifestations of PsA, the definitions of the manifestations, and the populations included vary considerably by study. For example, Gladman, Lindqvist, and Love present data for patients at the first visit, whereas Wilson and Reich report data at incident diagnosis. Lindqvist represents a population of patients with early disease (<2 years' duration). Axial disease is particularly defined quite differently by study. Lindqvist used the original Moll and Wright subgroups to classify patients. Therefore, in that particular study, axial disease as represented here only refers to patients without peripheral arthritis (those patients are classified as oligoarthritis or polyarthritis). In Love and colleagues, axial disease represents patients with inflammatory back pain.

of subtypes (eg, allowing for more than one manifestation or exclusive classification) but also may reflect different subtypes in different populations, the duration of PsA in the population studied, the duration of psoriasis before PsA onset, or age and gender distribution of the population.[3,59,61] Recognizing the patient's disease features at onset and when selecting therapies may be important to understanding disease and treatment outcomes.[62] For example, polyarticular disease has been associated with more erosive disease,[63] and dactylitis may not respond as well to traditional oral disease-modifying antirheumatic drugs (DMARDs).[64]

Axial Spondyloarthropathy

Axial disease or psoriatic spondylitis is present in 7% to 32% of patients with PsA and may be asymptomatic.[10,15,58,65] Among patients with PsA without axial disease at presentation, nail dystrophy, number of radiographically damaged joints, periostitis, and elevated erythrocyte sedimentation rate increased the risk of developing AxSpA over time.[65] Among patients with psoriatic spondylitis, younger age of disease onset was associated with HLAB-27 positivity, family history of SpA, enthesitis, and an isolated axial pattern (without peripheral arthritis). Later, onset axial disease was more likely to be associated with polyarthritis and absence of inflammatory back pain. However, despite these differences, the 2 groups had similar patient-reported outcomes including the Bath Ankylosing Spondylitis Disease Activity Index, Bath Ankylosing Spondylitis Functional Index, Bath Ankylosing Spondylitis Metrology Index, and Bath Ankylosing Spondylitis Radiology Index.[66] Recognition of AxSpA is important given differing treatment approaches and prognosis.[67,68]

Enthesitis

Enthesitis, present in approximately half of patients, is hypothesized to be the site of disease initiation.[69] Enthesitis is generally more often found in the lower extremities with the Achilles and plantar aponeurosis the most commonly involved sites.[70] Unfortunately, examination of the entheses is often subjective; there is low interrater reliability even when standardized examination techniques are used, and tenderness on examination is often discordant with findings of inflammation on ultrasound or other imaging techniques.[71–73] Thus, enthesitis is difficult to follow in studies of therapy effectiveness. The Leeds Enthesitis Index (LEI) is the most commonly used index in studies of PsA, but others exist as well.[70,74] The LEI includes assessment of the lateral epicondyles, proximal Achilles, and medial femoral condyles.[74] Ultrasound and MRI examination of the enthesis have improved the understanding of enthesitis and may provide a more objective method to assess and quantify enthesitis.[75,76]

Dactylitis

Dactylitis is a common feature in PsA, present in approximately 40% of patients at some point in their disease course, and can occur in either the feet or the hands.[64,70,77] About half of the patients that have dactylitis have it in more than one digit.[70] MRI studies suggest that dactylitis is circumferential soft tissue edema in addition to synovitis and tenosynovitis.[78] However, in a recent radiographic and histologic evaluation of dactylitis in a child, radiographic features included enhanced signal at digital entheses in the absence of synovitis and tenosynovitis.[79] Histologically, there was increased vascularity of the tenosynovium and fibromyxoid expansion of fibrous tissue with perivascular lymphocytic inflammation.

Nail Disease

Features of nail psoriasis include pitting, onycholysis, oil spots, linear pitting, and splinter hemorrhages.[24,80–82] Nail psoriasis can be quite painful and result in decreased functional ability and quality of life.[83] The prevalence of nail disease among patients with PsA ranges from 41% to 93%. In fact, most studies have found that nail disease is more common in patients with PsA than patients with psoriasis alone. The prevalence of nail disease in PsO is around 15% to 50%.[10,80,82,84–87] Nail disease (pitting and onycholysis in particular) has been associated with inflammation at the enthesis where the extensor tendon connects to the nail unit[88] and is often correlated with DIP joint involvement.[89,90] Furthermore, thickening of the entheses of the extensor tendon on ultrasound was more common in patients with clinical nail changes.[91] Nail psoriasis is a risk factor for the development of PsA among patients with PsA, possibly because it is an early sign of entheseal inflammation.[17]

Imaging Features and Distinguishing Characteristics from Rheumatoid Arthritis

PsA is associated with both bone erosions and new bone formation (ie, juxta-articular bony proliferation). Erosions occur commonly and often very early in the disease course.[60,92] Kane and colleagues[92] found the prevalence of erosions was 27% within the first 5 months of disease onset and nearly 50% within 2 years of disease onset. Interestingly, Finzel and colleagues[2] reported the number of erosions were similar among patients with RA and PsA, although the shape and location of the erosions were different between the 2 groups. In this study, osteophytes were more commonly seen among patients with PsA than RA. The number of erosions in PsA was correlated with disease duration and the osteophyte count was correlated with age but not disease duration.[2] Juxta-articular bony proliferation (not including osteophytes) is among the most specific radiographic features of PsA (as are tuft osteolysis and interphalangeal bony ankylosis).[42,93] However, DIP erosions, periosteal new bone formation, and diffuse soft tissue swelling may help distinguish RA from PsA.[93] Studies using MRI[94,95] and ultrasound[96] examined differences among patients with RA and PsA. Findings from these studies have corroborated the differential locations of erosions between RA and PsA and the increased entheseal disease and periosteal involvement in PsA. In addition, imaging studies have demonstrated that there is more disease activity present on imaging than noted on physical examination (nearly 75% in one study by Freeston and colleagues[97]), although the clinical significance of this is not well understood.[91,98,99]

PSORIATIC ARTHRITIS IN CHILDREN

Psoriasis and PsA are not limited to adults. Juvenile psoriasis has a prevalence of approximately 0.7% increasing from 0.12% at age 1% to 1.2% at age 18.[100,101] Juvenile PsA (JPsA) accounts for approximately 6% to 8% of all cases of juvenile arthritis.[73,102,103] Unlike adult PsA, inflammatory arthritis precedes skin psoriasis in about half of children with JPsA,[104] often making the diagnosis and classification of JPsA quite challenging. Two sets of classification criteria for JPsA exist: the Vancouver criteria for PsA and the International League of Associations for Rheumatology (ILAR) criteria (**Table 2**). The ILAR criteria are the widely used criteria for classifying juvenile idiopathic arthritis (JIA) and include the following categories: oligoarticular, rheumatoid factor (RF)-positive polyarticular, RF-negative polyarticular, systemic, enthesitis-related arthritis (ERA), JPsA, and undifferentiated arthritis.[105,106] As shown in **Table 2**, the ILAR criteria include many restrictions on the diagnosis of JPsA, placing as many as 40% of children who meet Vancouver criteria into the undifferentiated category of JIA (children who meet criteria for more than 1 JIA category). Thus, there is some debate about how to best define JPsA.[104,107] An improved definition for JPsA

Table 2
Comparison of Vancouver criteria for juvenile psoriatic arthritis and International League of Associations for Rheumatology criteria for juvenile psoriatic arthritis

	Vancouver	ILAR
Inclusion	Arthritis plus psoriasis OR Arthritis plus at least 2 of the following: Dactylitis, nail pits, family history of first- or second-degree relative, psoriasis-like rash	Arthritis plus psoriasis OR Arthritis plus at least 2 of the following: Dactylitis, nail pits or onycholysis, family history of first-degree relative
Exclusion	None	Arthritis in HLA-B27 positive male ≥6-y-old AS, ERA, sacroiliitis with IBD, reactive arthritis, or acute anterior uveitis, OR history of one of these disorders in a first-degree relative Presence of IgM RF on at least 2 occasions at least 3 mo apart The presence of systemic JIA Arthritis fulfilling ≥2 JIA categories

Arthritis must be of unknown cause, begin before the 16th birthday, and persist for at least 6 weeks.

Under the Vancouver criteria, definite JPsA is arthritis plus psoriasis or arthritis plus 3 minor criteria. Presence of 2 minor criteria is considered probable JPsA.

Abbreviations: AS, ankylosing spondylitis; IBD, inflammatory bowel disease.

Adapted from Stoll M, Lio P, Sundel RP, et al. Comparison of Vancouver and International League of Associations for rheumatology classification criteria for juvenile psoriatic arthritis. Arthritis Rheum 2008;59(10):52; with permission.

may be important as long-term outcomes are potentially different among patients with JPsA compared with other forms of JIA. Among patients with JPsA, 33% still required DMARDs or biological DMARDs after 15 years of follow-up compared with 8% to 13% of patients in other JIA groups.[108]

Similar to adult PsA, JPsA is a highly heterogeneous disease.[109] The prevalence of nail disease and dactylitis (approximately 50% each) is similar to adult PsA, and enthesitis is also common (present in 27% in one study).[109] Forty percent to 88% have an affected first- or second-degree relative, and axial involvement affects 10% to 40%.[108,110] However, disease manifestations seem to differ by age. Stoll and colleagues[101,109,111] described 2 peaks in onset with the first in toddlers (1–2 years) and the second in early adolescence (age 8–12 years). Younger children (age <5) were more likely to be girls and to have dactylitis, small joint involvement, and a positive antinuclear antibody (ANA), whereas older children were more likely to have persistent oligoarthritis, spondylitis, and enthesitis. Development of asymptomatic anterior uveitis is associated with ANA positivity and younger age of disease onset.[112] Also, similar to adult psoriasis, juvenile psoriasis is associated with an increased prevalence of obesity and comorbidities (including hyperlipidemia, diabetes, hypertension, and Crohn disease).[100] This relationship has not been examined specifically in JPsA.

RECOGNITION OF EARLY PSORIATIC ARTHRITIS

Early PsA is generally considered within the first 2 years of symptom onset.[113] Increasing evidence supports the early diagnosis and treatment of PsA in order to improve long-term outcomes.[113–116] Gladman and colleagues[114] found patients presenting within 2 years of symptom onset had significantly less disease progression after adjusting for baseline characteristics, including start of DMARD therapy at the first visit. Treatment outcomes may also be different among patients with early PsA.[117] A cohort study within the Swedish Early Psoriatic Arthritis Register found that shorter symptom duration at diagnosis and start of therapy was a predictor of minimal disease activity at 5 years, again suggesting that the earlier disease is identified, the better the outcomes.[118] Sørensen and colleagues[119] recently reported an improvement in the delay from symptoms to diagnosis among patients with PsA and RA in Denmark. However, underdiagnosis still remains a significant problem.[25]

SUBCLINICAL DISEASE IN PATIENTS WITH PSORIASIS

Given that early initiation of therapy may decrease joint damage and improve long-term outcomes, how early should therapy be initiated? It has long been recognized that patients may not report symptoms of joint pain or may not be aware of joint inflammation. Several studies demonstrate that patients with psoriasis often have "subclinical" joint and entheseal inflammation.[120,121] The prevalence of subclinical synovitis and enthesopathy among patients with psoriasis ranges from 3% to 46% and 7% to 33%, respectively. In most studies, the frequency of these findings is significantly higher in patients with psoriasis than in healthy controls.[91,122–127] The meaning of subclinical joint inflammation remains unclear. However, some patients with subclinical inflammation go on to develop symptomatic PsA.[128]

IMPROVING DETECTION OF PSORIATIC ARTHRITIS AMONG PATIENTS WITH PSORIASIS

How can one better identify PsA? Understanding risk factors for PsA among patients with psoriasis could help identify patients with psoriasis who are more likely to develop the disease.[129] In addition, the use of screening tools for PsA in dermatology clinics could facilitate improved recognition of existing disease.

Risk Factors for Psoriatic Arthritis

A handful of studies have examined risk factors for PsA among patients with psoriasis (**Box 1**). Most of the risk factors identified have not been replicated in additional studies with the exception of obesity, family history of PsA, and injuries or trauma.[130,131] Smoking is generally considered to be a risk factor for psoriasis.[132–134] However, studies of smoking as a risk factor for PsA are mixed with one suggesting an inverse association and one suggesting a positive association.[133,135]

Screening for Psoriatic Arthritis

Screening for PsA can be as simple as asking about the presence of arthralgias or performed using validated screening tools.[145–147] Several groups have developed questionnaires to assist in the identification of psoriasis patients with PsA (**Table 3**). These questionnaires each have a cut-off value that suggests a high likelihood of having inflammatory arthritis, prompting subsequent rheumatology evaluation.[147] Screening tools generally should have high sensitivity,[148] but given the difficulty with access to rheumatology in many countries, screening for PsA should ideally also have high specificity. Most of the screening tools developed have relatively high sensitivity and specificity in the initial validation studies. However, subsequent studies have noted decreased sensitivity or specificity when applied in new populations.[23,149–151] No studies have examined the effectiveness of a screening tool versus usual care in capturing patients with PsA and the overall impact of screening on health care utilization.

Box 1
Potential risk factors for psoriatic arthritis

Nail dystrophy[17]

Injury/trauma/bone fracture[136,137]

Family history of psoriatic arthritis[138,139]

Obesity[140,141]

Elevated body mass index at age 18[142]

Smoking[133,135,137], *

Lifting cumulative loads of greater than 100 pounds/h[137]

Severe psoriasis[138]

Psoriasis location: scalp lesions, intergluteal/perianal lesions[17]

Corticosteroids in the 2 years before psoriasis onset (through PsA onset)[143]

Rubella vaccinations[136]

Recurrent oral ulcers[136]

Moving to a new house[136]

Infections requiring antibiotics[137]

Hypercholesterolemia[144]

* refers to conflicting studies on the association between smoking and PsA.

Table 3
Available screening tools

Screening Tool	Publication(s)	Description and Caveats	Validation Population	Test Characteristics in Initial Studies	Test Characteristics in Subsequent Studies
Psoriatic Arthritis Screening and Evaluation (PASE)	Husni 2007[152] Dominquez 2009[153] Ferreyra 2013[154]	Total of 15 questions with score range 15–75 Has been translated into Spanish. Captures disease activity so use of concomitant therapy may change results[155,156]	Patients with psoriasis, PsA before therapy, and osteoarthritis. The reference standard was rheumatologist's diagnosis and Moll and Wright criteria	Cut-off 47/75 Sensitivity 82% Specificity 73% Cut-off 44/75 Sensitivity 76% Specificity 76% Spanish version: Cut-off 34/75 Sensitivity 76% Specificity 74%	Haroon 2013: Sensitivity 24% Specificity 94% Coates 2013: Sensitivity 75% Specificity 39% Walsh 2013: Cut-off 44 Sensitivity 76% Specificity 41% Cut-off 47 Sensitivity 63% Specificity 52%
Toronto Psoriatic Arthritis Screen (ToPAS)	Gladman 2009[157]	12 questions This questionnaire is unique in its inclusion of photographs of inflamed joints and dactylitis	Patients with PsA, psoriasis, general dermatology, general rheumatology, and family medicine. The reference standard was a rheumatologist diagnosis of PsA	Cut-off 8/12 Psoriasis 89.1%, 86.3% dermatology 91.9%, 95.2% rheumatology 92.6%, 85.7% family medicine 90.4%, 100%	Mease 2014: Sensitivity 77% Specificity 72% Haroon 2013: Sensitivity 41% Specificity 90% Coates 2013: Sensitivity 77% Specificity 30% Walsh 2013: Sensitivity 60% Specificity 55%

Psoriasis Epidemiology Screening Tool (PEST)	Ibrahim 2009[158]	5 questions (swollen joints, history of arthritis, heel pain, nail pitting, dactylitis) and a manikin. The manikin does not add to the discriminative ability or scoring but may be helpful to the clinician	Patients with psoriasis identified by medical codes, mailed questionnaire, and 55% of the respondents were examined. The reference standard was a rheumatologist diagnosis	Cut-off 3/5 Sensitivity 92% Specificity 78%	Mease 2014: Sensitivity 84% Specificity 75% Haroon 2013: Sensitivity 28% Specificity 98% Coates 2013: Sensitivity 77% Specificity 37% Walsh 2013: Cutoff 44 Sensitivity 69% Specificity 47%
Electronic Psoriasis and Arthritis Screening Questionnaire (ePASQ)	Khraishi 2011[159]	Ten yes or no questions plus 2 follow-up questions with weighted scoring for each and a diagram to mark painful joints, which is also weighted	Patients with suspected early PsA. The reference standard was CASPAR criteria	Cut-off 7/15 Sensitivity 98% Specificity 75% Cut-off 8/15 Sensitivity 88% Specificity 75%	Mease 2014: Sensitivity 67% Specificity 64%
Early Arthritis for Psoriatic Patients (EARP)	Tinazzi 2012[160]	Ten-item questionnaires with yes or no answers asking about joint and/or tendon pain, swelling and stiffness	Patients with psoriasis but not systemic therapy. Patients with existing arthritis were excluded. The reference standard was CASPAR criteria applied by a rheumatologist	Cut-off 3/10 Sensitivity 85% Specificity 92%	N/A

(continued on next page)

Table 3
(continued)

Screening Tool	Publication(s)	Description and Caveats	Validation Population	Test Characteristics in Initial Studies	Test Characteristics in Subsequent Studies
CEPPA screening tool	Garg 2014[161]	5 questions inquiring about history of joint pain or swelling, morning stiffness, diagnosis of PsA, history of joint radiographs, and presence of nail changes	All adults presenting for psoriasis evaluation within dermatology (with or without PsA). Only patients reporting joint pain were examined. The reference standard was a rheumatologist's diagnosis	Cut-off 3/5 Sensitivity 86.9% Specificity 71.3%	N/A
CONTEST and CONTESTjt	Coates 2014[162]	Developed from combinations of questions from PASE, PEST, and TOPAS. Validated within Dublin and Utah cohorts using data from Haroon et al and Walsh et al	Patients with psoriasis. Patients reaching the previously published cut-off for either PASE, PEST, or ToPAS were invited for physical exam. The reference standard was CASPAR criteria	CONTEST: Cut-off 4/8 Sensitivity 38%–86% Specificity 35%–89% CONTESTjw: Cut-off 5/8 Sensitivity 57%–89% Specificity 37%–71%	N/A

The sensitivity and specificity used for the subsequent studies were for the cohort of patients with psoriasis but without previous diagnoses of psoriatic arthritis.

Box 2
Comorbidities associated with psoriatic arthritis

Hypertension[60,180–182]

Dyslipidemia[60,180–182]

Diabetes/insulin resistance[183,184,a]

Metabolic syndrome[185–187]

Obesity[11,185,186]

Cardiovascular disease including myocardial infarction and cerebrovascular disease[1,165,188–190,a]

Depression and anxiety[191]

Crohn disease[192,193,a]

Ulcerative colitis[192]

Keratoconjunctivitis sicca[194]

Hypothyroidism[195]

Giant cell arteritis[192]

Pulmonary fibrosis[192]

[a] Denotes an increased risk of incident comorbidity.

COMORBIDITIES IN PSORIATIC ARTHRITIS

Over the past decade, the understanding of PsA as systemic disease has significantly expanded.[163] Approximately 40% of patients with PsA had 3 or more comorbid conditions, and the presence of a comorbidity was associated with decreased quality of life.[164] Comorbidities reported to have an increased prevalence or incidence in PsA are reported in **Box 2**. The increased risk for metabolic abnormalities including cardiovascular disease and diabetes have been the most striking and of greatest importance to management of patients with PsA.[165] Although one study has suggested a risk of malignancy similar to RA, population-based studies have not suggested an increased risk of cancer, including lymphoma, compared with controls.[166–168] Osteoporosis is similarly debated; however, most studies do not suggest an increased prevalence of osteoporosis.[169–171] Increased prevalence of diffuse skeletal hyperostosis,[172] monoclonal gammopathy,[173] and iridocyclitis[174] compared with general population statistics have also been reported. Despite the increased prevalence of comorbidities, recent studies have not found an increased risk of mortality among patients with PsA.[5,175–179]

SUMMARY

PsA is a chronic inflammatory arthritis with potentially significant functional disability and poor outcomes, including cardiovascular disease. Early detection of PsA is important for improvement in long-term outcomes. Use of screening tools and improved knowledge of risk factors could improve early detection.

REFERENCES

1. Ogdie A, Yu Y, Haynes K, et al. Risk of major cardiovascular events in patients with psoriatic arthritis, psoriasis and rheumatoid arthritis: a population-based cohort study. Ann Rheum Dis 2015;74(2):326–32.

2. Finzel S, Englbrecht M, Engelke K, et al. A comparative study of periarticular bone lesions in rheumatoid arthritis and psoriatic arthritis. Ann Rheum Dis 2011;70(1):122–7.
3. Eder L, Gladman DD. Psoriatic arthritis: phenotypic variance and nosology. Curr Rheumatol Rep 2013;15:316.
4. Gelfand JM, Gladman DD, Mease PJ, et al. Epidemiology of psoriatic arthritis in the population of the United States. J Am Acad Dermatol 2005;53(4):573.
5. Shbeeb M, Uramoto KM, Gibson LE, et al. The epidemiology of psoriatic arthritis in Olmsted County, Minnesota, USA, 1982–1991. J Rheumatol 2000;27(5): 1247–50.
6. Asgari MM, Wu JJ, Gelfand JM, et al. Validity of diagnostic codes and prevalence of psoriasis and psoriatic arthritis in a managed care population, 1996–2009. Pharmacoepidemiol Drug Saf 2013;22(8):842–9.
7. Cakır N, Pamuk Ö, Derviş E, et al. The prevalences of some rheumatic diseases in western Turkey: Havsa study. Rheumatol Int 2012;32(4):895–908.
8. Hanova P, Pavelka K, Holcatova I, et al. Incidence and prevalence of psoriatic arthritis, ankylosing spondylitis, and reactive arthritis in the first descriptive population-based study in the Czech Republic. Scand J Rheumatol 2010; 39(4):310–7.
9. Löfvendahl S, Theander E, Svensson Å, et al. Validity of diagnostic codes and prevalence of physician-diagnosed psoriasis and psoriatic arthritis in southern Sweden–a population-based register study. PLoS One 2014;9(5):e98024.
10. Love T, Gudbjornsson B, Gudjonsson J, et al. Psoriatic arthritis in Reykjavik, Iceland: prevalence, demographics, and disease course. J Rheumatol 2007; 34(10):2082–8.
11. Ogdie A, Langan S, Love T, et al. Prevalence and treatment patterns of psoriatic arthritis in the UK. Rheumatology (Oxford) 2013;52(3):568–75.
12. Pedersen O, Svendsen A, Ejstrup L, et al. The occurrence of psoriatic arthritis in Denmark. Ann Rheum Dis 2008;67(10):1422–6.
13. Soriano E, Rosa J, Velozo E, et al. Incidence and prevalence of psoriatic arthritis in Buenos Aires, Argentina: a 6-year health management organization-based study. Rheumatology (Oxford) 2011;50(4):729–34.
14. Li R, Sun J, Ren LM, et al. Epidemiology of eight common rheumatic diseases in China: a large-scale cross-sectional survey in Beijing. Rheumatology 2012; 51(4):721–9.
15. Yang Q, Qu L, Tian H, et al. Prevalence and characteristics of psoriatic arthritis in Chinese patients with psoriasis. J Eur Acad Dermatol Venereol 2011;25(12): 1409–14.
16. Nossent J, Gran J. Epidemiological and clinical characteristics of psoriatic arthritis in northern Norway. Scand J Rheumatol 2009;38(4):251–5.
17. Wilson F, Icen M, Crowson C, et al. Incidence and clinical predictors of psoriatic arthritis in patients with psoriasis: a population-based study. Arthritis Rheum 2009;61(2):233–9.
18. Alamanos Y, Voulgari P, Drosos A. Incidence and prevalence of psoriatic arthritis: a systematic review. J Rheumatol 2008;35(7):1354–8.
19. Carneiro JN, Paula AP, Martins GA. Psoriatic arthritis in patients with psoriasis: evaluation of clinical and epidemiological features in 133 patients followed at the University Hospital of Brasilia. An Bras Dermatol 2012;87(4):539–44.
20. Henes JC, Ziupa E, Eisfelder M, et al. High prevalence of psoriatic arthritis in dermatological patients with psoriasis: a cross-sectional study. Rheumatol Int 2014;34(2):227–34.

21. Ibrahim G, Waxman R, Helliwell P. The prevalence of psoriatic arthritis in people with psoriasis. Arthritis Rheum 2009;61(10):1373–8.
22. Jamshidi F, Bouzari N, Seirafi H, et al. The prevalence of psoriatic arthritis in psoriatic patients in Tehran, Iran. Arch Iran Med 2008;11(2):162–5.
23. Haroon M, Kirby B, FitzGerald O. High prevalence of psoriatic arthritis in patients with severe psoriasis with suboptimal performance of screening questionnaires. Ann Rheum Dis 2013;72(5):736–40.
24. Love T, Gudjonsson J, Valdimarsson H, et al. Psoriatic arthritis and onycholysis—results from the cross-sectional Reykjavik psoriatic arthritis study. J Rheumatol 2012;39(7):1441–4.
25. Mease P, Gladman D, Papp K, et al. Prevalence of rheumatologist-diagnosed psoriatic arthritis in patients with psoriasis in European/North American dermatology clinics. J Am Acad Dermatol 2013;69(5):729–35.
26. Khraishi M, Chouela E, Bejar M, et al. High prevalence of psoriatic arthritis in a cohort of patients with psoriasis seen in a dermatology practice. J Cutan Med Surg 2012;16(2):122–7.
27. Radtke M, Reich K, Blome C, et al. Prevalence and clinical features of psoriatic arthritis and joint complaints in 2009 patients with psoriasis: results of a German national survey. J Eur Acad Dermatol Venereol 2009;23(6):683–91.
28. Reich K, Krüger K, Mössner R, et al. Epidemiology and clinical pattern of psoriatic arthritis in Germany: a prospective interdisciplinary epidemiological study of 1511 patients with plaque-type psoriasis. Br J Dermatol 2009;160(5):1040–7.
29. Eder L, Chandran V, Shen H, et al. Incidence of arthritis in a prospective cohort of psoriasis patients. Arthritis Care Res (Hoboken) 2011;63(4):619–22.
30. Merola J, Wu S, Han J, et al. Psoriasis, psoriatic arthritis and risk of gout in US men and women. Ann Rheum Dis 2014;74:1495–500.
31. Mody E, Husni ME, Schur P, et al. Multidisciplinary evaluation of patients with psoriasis presenting with musculoskeletal pain: a dermatology: rheumatology clinic experience. Br J Dermatol 2007;157(5):1050–1.
32. Marchesoni A, Atzeni F, Spadaro A, et al. Identification of the clinical features distinguishing psoriatic arthritis and fibromyalgia. J Rheumatol 2012;39(4):849–55.
33. De Marco G, Cattaneo A, Battafarano N, et al. Not simply a matter of psoriatic arthritis: epidemiology of rheumatic diseases in psoriatic patients. Arch Dermatol Res 2012;304(9):719–26.
34. Tan A, Grainger A, Tanner S, et al. A high-resolution magnetic resonance imaging study of distal interphalangeal joint arthropathy in psoriatic arthritis and osteoarthritis: are they the same? Arthritis Rheum 2006;54(4):1328–33.
35. Aggarwal R, Ringold S, Khanna D, et al. Distinctions between diagnostic and classification criteria? Arthritis Care Res (Hoboken) 2015. http://dx.doi.org/10.1002/acr.22583.
36. Moll JM, Wright V. Psoriatic arthritis. Semin Arthritis Rheum 1973;3(1):55–78.
37. Amor B, Dougados M, Mijiyawa M. Criteria of the classification of spondylarthropathies. Rev Rhum Mal Osteoartic 1990;57(2):85–9.
38. Dougados M, van der Linden S, Juhlin R, et al. The European Spondylarthropathy Study Group preliminary criteria for the classification of spondylarthropathy. Arthritis Rheum 1991;34(10):1218–27.
39. Bennett RM. Psoriatic arthritis. In: McCarty DJ, editor. Arthritis and allied conditions. 9th edition. Philadelphia: Lea & Feb; 1979. p. 645.
40. Fournie B, Crognier L, Arnaud C, et al. Proposed classification criteria of psoriatic arthritis: a preliminary study in 260 patients. Rev Rhum Engl Ed 1999;66(10):446–56.

41. Vasey F, Espinoza LR. Psoriatic arthropathy. In: Calin A, editor. Spondyloarthropathies. Orlando (FL): Grune & Stratton; 1984. p. 151–85.
42. Taylor W, Helliwell P. Classification criteria for psoriatic arthritis: development of new criteria from a large international study [PsA - CASPAR]. Arthritis Rheum 2006;54:2665–73.
43. Congi L, Roussou E. Clinical application of the CASPAR criteria for psoriatic arthritis compared to other existing criteria. Clin Exp Rheumatol 2010;28(3):304–10.
44. Gunal EK, Kamali S, Gul A, et al. Clinical evaluation and comparison of different criteria for classification in Turkish patients with psoriatic arthritis. Rheumatol Int 2008;28(10):959–64.
45. D'Angelo S, Mennillo G, Cutro M, et al. Sensitivity of the classification of psoriatic arthritis criteria in early psoriatic arthritis. J Rheumatol 2009;36(2):368–70.
46. van den Berg R, van Gaalen F, van der Helm-van Mil A, et al. Performance of classification criteria for peripheral spondyloarthritis and psoriatic arthritis in the Leiden Early Arthritis cohort. Ann Rheum Dis 2012;71(8):1366–9.
47. Chandran V, Schentag C, Gladman D. Sensitivity and specificity of the CASPAR criteria for psoriatic arthritis in a family medicine clinic setting. J Rheumatol 2008;35(10):2069–70.
48. Chandran V, Schentag C, Gladman D. Sensitivity of the classification of psoriatic arthritis criteria in early psoriatic arthritis. Arthritis Rheum 2007;57(8):1560–3.
49. Coates L, Conaghan P, Emery P, et al. Sensitivity and specificity of the classification of psoriatic arthritis criteria in early psoriatic arthritis. Arthritis Rheum 2012;64(10):3150–5.
50. Lueng YY, Tam LS, Ho KW, et al. Evaluation of the CASPAR criteria for psoriatic arthritis in the Chinese population. Rheumatology 2010;49(1):112–5.
51. Rudwaleit M, van der Heijde D, Landewé R, et al. The Assessment of SpondyloArthritis International Society classification criteria for peripheral spondyloarthritis and for spondyloarthritis in general. Ann Rheum Dis 2011;70(1):25–31.
52. Rudwaleit M, van der Heijde D, Landewé R, et al. The development of Assessment of SpondyloArthritis international Society classification criteria for axial spondyloarthritis (part II): validation and final selection. Ann Rheum Dis 2009;68(6):777–83.
53. Taylor WJ, Robinson PC. Classification criteria: peripheral spondyloarthropathy and psoriatic arthritis. Curr Rheumatol Rep 2013;15(4):317.
54. Haddad A, Chandran V. Arthritis mutilans. Curr Rheumatol Rep 2013;15(4):321.
55. Gladman DD, Shuckett R, Russell ML, et al. Psoriatic arthritis (PSA)—an analysis of 220 patients. Q J Med 1987;62(238):127–41.
56. Madland T, Apalset E, Johannessen A, et al. Prevalence, disease manifestations, and treatment of psoriatic arthritis in Western Norway. J Rheumatol 2005;32(10):1918–22.
57. Lindqvist U, Alenius G, Husmark T, et al. The Swedish early psoriatic arthritis register–2-year followup: a comparison with early rheumatoid arthritis. J Rheumatol 2008;35(4):668–73.
58. Soy M, Karaca N, Umit E, et al. Joint and nail involvement in Turkish patients with psoriatic arthritis. Rheumatol Int 2008;29(2):223–5.
59. Queiro R, Tejón P, Coto P, et al. Clinical differences between men and women with psoriatic arthritis: relevance of the analysis of genes and polymorphisms in the major histocompatibility complex region and of the age at onset of psoriasis. Clin Dev Immunol 2013;2013:482691.

60. Zisman D, Eder L, Elias M, et al. Clinical and demographic characteristics of patients with psoriatic arthritis in northern Israel. Rheumatol Int 2012;32(3):595–600.
61. Queiro R, Alperi M, Alonso-Castro S, et al. Patients with psoriatic arthritis may show differences in their clinical and genetic profiles depending on their age at psoriasis onset. Clin Exp Rheumatol 2012;30(4):476–80.
62. Tillett W, McHugh N. Treatment algorithms for early psoriatic arthritis: do they depend on disease phenotypes? Curr Rheumatol Rep 2012;14(4):334–42.
63. Queiro-Silva R, Torre-Alonso JC, Tinture-Equren T, et al. A polyarticular onset predicts erosive and deforming disease in psoriatic arthritis. Ann Rheum Dis 2003;62(1):68–70.
64. Gladman D, Ziouzina O, Thavaneswaran A, et al. Dactylitis in psoriatic arthritis: prevalence and response to therapy in the biologic era. J Rheumatol 2013; 40(8):1357–9.
65. Chandran V, Tolusso D, Cook R, et al. Risk factors for axial inflammatory arthritis in patients with psoriatic arthritis. J Rheumatol 2010;37(4):809–15.
66. Queiro R, Alperi M, Lopez A, et al. Clinical expression, but not disease outcome, may vary according to age at disease onset in psoriatic spondylitis. Joint Bone Spine 2008;75(5):544–7.
67. Thavaneswaran A, Chandran V, Gladman D. Do patients with psoriatic arthritis fall into distinct clinical subgroups—a cluster analysis? Arthritis Rheum 2012; 64(Suppl):S1106.
68. Ritchlin C, Kavanaugh A, Gladman DD, et al. Treatment recommendations for psoriatic arthritis. Ann Rheum Dis 2009;68:1387–94.
69. McGonagle D, Helliwell P, Veale D. Enthesitis in psoriatic disease. Dermatology 2012;225(2):100–9.
70. Sakkas L, Alexiou I, Simopoulou T, et al. Enthesitis in psoriatic arthritis. Semin Arthritis Rheum 2013;43(3):325–34.
71. Weiss PF, Chauvin NA, Klink AJ, et al. Detection of enthesitis in children with enthesitis-related arthritis: dolorimetry compared to ultrasonography. Arthritis Rheumatol 2014;66(1):218–27.
72. D'Agostino MA, Said-Nahal R, Hacquard-Bouder C, et al. Assessment of peripheral enthesitis in the spondylarthropathies by ultrasonography combined with power Doppler: a cross-sectional study. Arthritis Rheum 2003;48(2):523–33.
73. Weiss P, Beukelman T, Schanberg L, et al. Enthesitis-related arthritis is associated with higher pain intensity and poorer health status in comparison with other categories of juvenile idiopathic arthritis: the Childhood Arthritis and Rheumatology Research Alliance Registry. J Rheumatol 2012;39(12):2341–51.
74. Healy P, Helliwell P. Measuring clinical enthesitis in psoriatic arthritis: assessment of existing measures and development of an instrument specific to psoriatic arthritis. Arthritis Rheum 2008;59(5):686–91.
75. Kaeley G. Review of the use of ultrasound for the diagnosis and monitoring of enthesitis in psoriatic arthritis. Curr Rheumatol Rep 2011;13(4):338–45.
76. Coates L, Hodgson R, Conaghan P, et al. MRI and ultrasonography for diagnosis and monitoring of psoriatic arthritis. Best Pract Res Clin Rheumatol 2012;26(6):805–22.
77. Payet J, Gossec L, Paternotte S, et al. Prevalence and clinical characteristics of dactylitis in spondylarthritis: a descriptive analysis of 275 patients. Clin Exp Rheumatol 2012;30(2):191–6.
78. Healy P, Groves C, Chandramohan M, et al. MRI changes in psoriatic dactylitis—extent of pathology, relationship to tenderness and correlation with clinical indices. Rheumatology (Oxford) 2008;47(1):92–5.

79. Tuttle KS, Vargas SO, Callahan MJ, et al. Enthesitis as a component of dactylitis in psoriatic juvenile idiopathic arthritis: histology of an established clinical entity. Pediatr Rheumatol Online J 2015;13:7.

80. Kyriakou A, Patsatsi A, Sotiriadis D. Detailed analysis of specific nail psoriasis features and their correlations with clinical parameters: a cross-sectional study. Dermatology 2011;223(3):222–9.

81. Palmou N, Marzo-Ortega H, Ash Z, et al. Linear pitting and splinter haemorrhages are more commonly seen in the nails of patients with established psoriasis in comparison to psoriatic arthritis. Dermatology 2011;223(4):370–3.

82. Love T, Gudjonsson J, Valdimarsson H, et al. Small joint involvement in psoriatic arthritis is associated with onycholysis: the Reykjavik Psoriatic Arthritis Study. Scand J Rheumatol 2010;39(4):299–302.

83. Baran R. The burden of nail psoriasis: an introduction. Dermatology 2010; 221(Suppl 1):1–5.

84. Jiaravuthisan M, Sasseville D, Vender R, et al. Psoriasis of the nail: anatomy, pathology, clinical presentation, and a review of the literature on therapy. J Am Acad Dermatol 2007;57(1):1–27.

85. Ash Z, Tinazzi I, Gallego C, et al. Psoriasis patients with nail disease have a greater magnitude of underlying systemic subclinical enthesopathy than those with normal nails. Ann Rheum Dis 2012;71(4):553–6.

86. Augustin M, Reich K, Blome C, et al. Nail psoriasis in Germany: epidemiology and burden of disease. Br J Dermatol 2010;163(3):580–5.

87. Prasad PV, Bikku B, Kaviarasan PK, et al. A clinical study of psoriatic arthropathy. Indian J Dermatol Venereol Leprol 2007;73(3):166–70.

88. McGonagle D, Palmou Fontana N, Tan A, et al. Nailing down the genetic and immunological basis for psoriatic disease. Dermatology 2010;221(Suppl 1): 15–22.

89. Scarpa R, Cuocolo A, Peluso R, et al. Early psoriatic arthritis: the clinical spectrum. J Rheumatol 2008;35(1):137–41.

90. Dalbeth N, Pui K, Lobo M, et al. Nail disease in psoriatic arthritis: distal phalangeal bone edema detected by magnetic resonance imaging predicts development of onycholysis and hyperkeratosis. J Rheumatol 2012;39(4):841–3.

91. Aydin S, Castillo-Gallego C, Ash Z, et al. Ultrasonographic assessment of nail in psoriatic disease shows a link between onychopathy and distal interphalangeal joint extensor tendon enthesopathy. Dermatology 2012;225(3):231–5.

92. Kane D, Stafford L, Bresnihan B, et al. A prospective, clinical and radiological study of early psoriatic arthritis: an early synovitis clinic experience. Rheumatology 2003;42(12):1460–8.

93. Ichikawa N, Taniguchi A, Kobayashi S, et al. Performance of hands and feet radiographs in differentiation of psoriatic arthritis from rheumatoid arthritis. Int J Rheum Dis 2012;15(5):462–7.

94. Narváez J, Narváez JA, de Albert M, et al. Can magnetic resonance imaging of the hand and wrist differentiate between rheumatoid arthritis and psoriatic arthritis in the early stages of the disease? Semin Arthritis Rheum 2012;42(3): 234–45.

95. Tehranzadeh J, Ashikyan O, Anavim A, et al. Detailed analysis of contrast-enhanced MRI of hands and wrists in patients with psoriatic arthritis. Skeletal Radiol 2008;37(5):433–42.

96. Fournié B, Margarit-Coll N, Champetier de Ribes TL, et al. Extrasynovial ultrasound abnormalities in the psoriatic finger. Joint Bone Spine 2006;73(5): 527–31.

97. Aydin S, Ash Z, Tinazzi I, et al. The link between enthesitis and arthritis in psoriatic arthritis: a switch to a vascular phenotype at insertions may play a role in arthritis development. Ann Rheum Dis 2013;72(6):992–5.

98. Freeston J, Coates L, Nam J, et al. Is there subclinical synovitis in early psoriatic arthritis? A clinical comparison with gray-scale and power Doppler ultrasound. Arthritis Care Res (Hoboken) 2014;66(3):432–9.

99. Weckbach S, Schewe S, Michaely HJ, et al. Whole-body MR imaging in psoriatic arthritis: additional value for therapeutic decision making. Eur J Radiol 2011; 77(1):149–55.

100. Augustin M, Glaeske G, Radtke M, et al. Epidemiology and comorbidity of psoriasis in children. Br J Dermatol 2010;162(3):633–6.

101. Stoll M, Zurakowski D, Nigrovic L, et al. Patients with juvenile psoriatic arthritis comprise two distinct populations. Arthritis Rheum 2006;54(11):3564–72.

102. Berard R, Tomlinson G, Li X, et al. Description of active joint count trajectories in juvenile idiopathic arthritis. J Rheumatol 2014;41(12):2466–73.

103. Guzman J, Oen K, Tucker L, et al. The outcomes of juvenile idiopathic arthritis in children managed with contemporary treatments: results from the ReACCh-Out cohort. Ann Rheum Dis 2014. http://dx.doi.org/10.1136/annrheumdis-2014-205372.

104. Nigrovic P. Juvenile psoriatic arthritis: bathwater or baby? J Rheumatol 2009; 36(9):1861–3.

105. Stoll M, Lio P, Sundel R, et al. Comparison of Vancouver and International League of Associations for rheumatology classification criteria for juvenile psoriatic arthritis. Arthritis Rheum 2008;59(1):51–8.

106. Petty R, Southwood T, Manners P, et al. International League of Associations for Rheumatology classification of juvenile idiopathic arthritis: second revision, Edmonton, 2001. J Rheumatol 2004;31(2):390–2.

107. Demirkaya E, Ozen S, Bilginer Y, et al. The distribution of juvenile idiopathic arthritis in the eastern Mediterranean: results from the registry of the Turkish Paediatric Rheumatology Association. Clin Exp Rheumatol 2011;29(1): 111–6.

108. Flatø B, Lien G, Smerdel-Ramoya A, et al. Juvenile psoriatic arthritis: longterm outcome and differentiation from other subtypes of juvenile idiopathic arthritis. J Rheumatol 2009;36(3):642–50.

109. Stoll M, Punaro M. Psoriatic juvenile idiopathic arthritis: a tale of two subgroups. Curr Opin Rheumatol 2011;23(5):437–43.

110. Häfner R, Michels H. Psoriatic arthritis in children. Curr Opin Rheumatol 1996; 8(5):467–72.

111. Stoll M, Nigrovic P. Subpopulations within juvenile psoriatic arthritis: a review of the literature. Clin Dev Immunol 2006;13(2–4):377–80.

112. Calandra S, Gallo M, Consolaro A, et al. Female sex and oligoarthritis category are not risk factors for uveitis in Italian children with juvenile idiopathic arthritis. J Rheumatol 2014;41(7):1416–25.

113. Gladman D. Early psoriatic arthritis. Rheum Dis Clin North Am 2012;38(2): 373–86.

114. Gladman D, Thavaneswaran A, Chandran V, et al. Do patients with psoriatic arthritis who present early fare better than those presenting later in the disease? Ann Rheum Dis 2011;70(12):2152–4.

115. Tillett W, Jadon D, Shaddick G, et al. Smoking and delay to diagnosis are associated with poorer functional outcome in psoriatic arthritis. Ann Rheum Dis 2013; 72(8):1358–61.

116. Haroon M, Gallagher P, Fitzgerald O. Diagnostic delay of more than 6 months contributes to poor radiographic and functional outcome in psoriatic arthritis. Ann Rheum Dis 2015;74:1045–50.
117. Kirkham B, de Vlam K, Li W, et al. Early treatment of psoriatic arthritis is associated with improved patient-reported outcomes: findings from the etanercept PRESTA trial. Clin Exp Rheumatol 2015;33(1):11–9.
118. Theander E, Husmark T, Alenius G, et al. Early psoriatic arthritis: short symptom duration, male gender and preserved physical functioning at presentation predict favourable outcome at 5-year follow-up. Results from the Swedish Early Psoriatic Arthritis Register(SwePsA). Ann Rheum Dis 2014;73(2):407–13.
119. Sørensen J, Hetland M, all Departments of Rheumatology in Denmark. Diagnostic delay in patients with rheumatoid arthritis, psoriatic arthritis and ankylosing spondylitis: results from the Danish nationwide DANBIO registry. Ann Rheum Dis 2015;74(3):e12.
120. Palazzi C, Lubrano E, D'Angelo S, et al. Beyond early diagnosis: occult psoriatic arthritis. J Rheumatol 2010;37(8):1556–8.
121. McGonagle D, Ash Z, Dickie L, et al. The early phase of psoriatic arthritis. Ann Rheum Dis 2011;70(Suppl 1):i71–6.
122. Naredo E, Möller I, de Miguel E, et al. High prevalence of ultrasonographic synovitis and enthesopathy in patients with psoriasis without psoriatic arthritis: a prospective case-control study. Rheumatology (Oxford) 2011;50(10):1838–48.
123. Emad Y, Ragab Y, Bassyouni I, et al. Enthesitis and related changes in the knees in seronegative spondyloarthropathies and skin psoriasis: magnetic resonance imaging case-control study. J Rheumatol 2010;37(8):1709–17.
124. Erdem C, Tekin N, Sarikaya S, et al. MR imaging features of foot involvement in patients with psoriasis. Eur J Radiol 2008;67(3):521–5.
125. Gisondi P, Tinazzi I, El-Dalati G, et al. Lower limb enthesopathy in patients with psoriasis without clinical signs of arthropathy: a hospital-based case-control study. Ann Rheum Dis 2008;67(1):26–30.
126. Raza N, Hameed A, Ali M. Detection of subclinical joint involvement in psoriasis with bone scintigraphy and its response to oral methotrexate. Clin Exp Dermatol 2008;33(1):70–3.
127. Offidani A, Cellini A, Valeri G, et al. Subclinical joint involvement in psoriasis: magnetic resonance imaging and X-ray findings. Acta Derm Venereol 1998; 78(6):463–5.
128. Tinazzi I, McGonagle D, Domenico B, et al. Preliminary evidence that subclinical enthesopathy may predict psoriatic arthritis in patients with psoriasis [subclinical PsA]. J Rheumatol 2011;38:2691–2.
129. Ogdie A, Gelfand J. Identification of risk factors for psoriatic arthritis [risk factors]. Arch Dermatol 2010;146(7):785.
130. Hsieh J, Kadavath S, Efthimiou P. Can traumatic injury trigger psoriatic arthritis? A review of the literature. Clin Rheumatol 2014;33(5):601–8.
131. Olivieri I, Padula A, D'Angelo S, et al. Role of trauma in psoriatic arthritis. J Rheumatol 2008;35(11):2085–7.
132. Ozden MG, Tekin NS, Gürer MA, et al. Environmental risk factors in pediatric psoriasis: a multicenter case-control study. Pediatr Dermatol 2011;28(3): 306–12.
133. Li W, Han J, Qureshi A. Smoking and risk of incident psoriatic arthritis in US women. Ann Rheum Dis 2012;71(6):804–8.
134. Huerta C, Rivero E, Rodríguez LA. Incidence and risk factors for psoriasis in the general population. Arch Dermatol 2007;143(12):1559–65.

135. Eder L, Shanmugarajah S, Thavaneswaran A, et al. The association between smoking and the development of psoriatic arthritis among psoriasis patients. Ann Rheum Dis 2012;71(2):219–24.
136. Pattison E, Harrison B, Griffiths C, et al. Environmental risk factors for the development of psoriatic arthritis: results from a case-control study. Ann Rheum Dis 2008;67(5):672–6.
137. Eder L, Law T, Chandran V, et al. Association between environmental factors and onset of psoriatic arthritis in patients with psoriasis. Arthritis Care Res (Hoboken) 2011;63(8):1091–7.
138. Tey H, Ee H, Tan A, et al. Risk factors associated with having psoriatic arthritis in patients with cutaneous psoriasis. J Dermatol 2010;37(5):426–30.
139. Ciurtin C, Roussou E. Cross-sectional study assessing family members of psoriatic arthritis patients affected by the same disease: differences between Caucasian, South Asian and Afro-Caribbean populations living in the same geographic region. Int J Rheum Dis 2013;16(4):418–24.
140. Li W, Han J, Qureshi A. Obesity and risk of incident psoriatic arthritis in US women. Ann Rheum Dis 2012;71(8):1267–772.
141. Love T, Zhu Y, Zhang Y, et al. Obesity and the risk of psoriatic arthritis: a population-based study. Ann Rheum Dis 2012;71(8):1273–7.
142. Soltani-Arabshahi R, Wong B, Feng B, et al. Obesity in early adulthood as a risk factor for psoriatic arthritis. Arch Dermatol 2010;146(7):721–6.
143. Thumboo J, Uramoto K, Shbeeb M, et al. Risk factors for the development of psoriatic arthritis: a population based nested case control study. J Rheumatol 2002;29(4):757–62.
144. Wu S, Li WQ, Han J, et al. Hypercholesterolemia and risk of incident psoriasis and psoriatic arthritis in US women. Arthritis Rheumatol 2014;66(2):304–10.
145. Taylor SL, Petrie M, O'Rourke KS, et al. Rheumatologists' recommendations on what to do in the dermatology office to evaluate and manage psoriasis patients' joint symptoms. J Dermatolog Treat 2009;20(6):350–3.
146. Dominguez P, Gladman DD, Helliwell P, et al. Development of screening tools to identify psoriatic arthritis. Curr Rheumatol Rep 2010;12(4):295–9.
147. Haddad A, Chandran V. How can psoriatic arthritis be diagnosed early? Curr Rheumatol Rep 2012;14(4):358–63.
148. Fletcher RH, Fletcher SW. Clinical epidemiology: the essentials. 4th edition. Philadelphia: Lippincott Williams & Wilkins; 2005.
149. Coates L, Aslam T, Al Balushi F, et al. Comparison of three screening tools to detect psoriatic arthritis in patients with psoriasis (CONTEST study). Br J Dermatol 2013;168(4):802–7.
150. Walsh J, Callis Duffin K, Krueger G, et al. Limitations in screening instruments for psoriatic arthritis: a comparison of instruments in patients with psoriasis. J Rheumatol 2013;40(3):287–93.
151. Mease P, Gladman D, Helliwell P, et al. Comparative performance of psoriatic arthritis screening tools in patients with psoriasis in European/North American dermatology clinics. J Am Acad Dermatol 2014;71(4):649–55.
152. Husni M, Meyer K, Cohen D, et al. The PASE questionnaire: pilot-testing a psoriatic arthritis screening and evaluation tool. J Am Acad Dermatol 2007;57(4):581–7.
153. Dominguez P, Husni M, Holt E, et al. Validity, reliability, and sensitivity-to-change properties of the psoriatic arthritis screening and evaluation questionnaire. Arch Dermatol Res 2009;301(8):573–9.

154. Ferreyra Garrott L, Soriano E, Rosa J, et al. Validation in Spanish of a screening questionnaire for the detection of psoriatic arthritis in patients with psoriasis. Rheumatology (Oxford) 2013;52(3):510–4.
155. Husni M, Qureshi A, Koenig A, et al. Utility of the PASE questionnaire, psoriatic arthritis (PsA) prevalence and PsA improvement with anti-TNF therapy: results from the PRISTINE trial. J Dermatolog Treat 2014;25(1):90–5.
156. Merola J, Husni M, Qureshi A. Screening instruments for psoriatic arthritis. J Rheumatol 2013;40(9):1623.
157. Gladman D, Schentag C, Tom B, et al. Development and initial validation of a screening questionnaire for psoriatic arthritis: the Toronto Psoriatic Arthritis Screen (ToPAS). Ann Rheum Dis 2009;68(4):497–501.
158. Ibrahim G, Buch M, Lawson C, et al. Evaluation of an existing screening tool for psoriatic arthritis in people with psoriasis and the development of a new instrument: the Psoriasis Epidemiology Screening Tool (PEST) questionnaire. Clin Exp Rheumatol 2009;27(3):469–74.
159. Khraishi M, Mong J, Mugford G, et al. The electronic Psoriasis and Arthritis Screening Questionnaire (ePASQ): a sensitive and specific tool to diagnose psoriatic arthritis patients. J Cutan Med Surg 2011;15(3):143–9.
160. Tinazzi I, Adami S, Zanolin E, et al. The early psoriatic arthritis screening questionnaire: a simple and fast method for the identification of arthritis in patients with psoriasis. Rheumatology (Oxford) 2012;51(11):2058–63.
161. Garg N, Truong B, Ku J, et al. A novel, short, and simple screening questionnaire can suggest presence of psoriatic arthritis in psoriasis patients in a dermatology clinic. Clin Rheumatol 2014. [Epub ahead of print].
162. Coates L, Walsh J, Haroon M, et al. Development and testing of new candidate psoriatic arthritis screening questionnaires combining optimal questions from existing tools. Arthritis Care Res (Hoboken) 2014;66(9):1410–6.
163. Ogdie A, Schwartzman S, Husni M. Recognizing and managing comorbidities in psoriatic arthritis. Curr Opin Rheumatol 2015;27(2):118–26.
164. Husted J, Thavaneswaran A, Chandran V, et al. Incremental effects of comorbidity on quality of life in patients with psoriatic arthritis. J Rheumatol 2013;40(8):1349–56.
165. Jamnitski A, Symmons D, Peters MJL, et al. Cardiovascular comorbidities in patients with psoriatic arthritis: a systematic review. Ann Rheum Dis 2013;72(2):211–6.
166. Gross R, Schwartzman-Morris J, Krathen M, et al. The risk of malignancy in a large cohort of patients with psoriatic arthritis. Arthritis Rheumatol 2014;66(6):1472–81.
167. Hellgren K, Smedby K, Backlin E, et al. Ankylosing spondylitis, psoriatic arthritis, and risk of malignant lymphoma: a cohort study based on nationwide prospectively recorded data from Sweden. Arthritis Rheumatol 2014;66(5):1282–90.
168. Rohekar S, Tom B, Hassa A, et al. Prevalence of malignancy in psoriatic arthritis. Arthritis Rheum 2008;58(1):82–7.
169. Pedreira P, Pinheiro M, Szejnfeld V. Bone mineral density and body composition in postmenopausal women with psoriasis and psoriatic arthritis. Arthritis Res Ther 2011;13(1):R16.
170. Grazio S, Cvijetić S, Vlak T, et al. Osteoporosis in psoriatic arthritis: is there any? Wien Klin Wochenschr 2011;123(23–24):743–50.
171. Del Puente A, Esposito A, Parisi A, et al. Osteoporosis and psoriatic arthritis. J Rheumatol Suppl 2012;89:36–8.

172. Haddad A, Thavaneswaran A, Toloza S, et al. Diffuse idiopathic skeletal hyperostosis in psoriatic arthritis. J Rheumatol 2013;40(8):1367–773.
173. Eder L, Thavaneswaran A, Pereira D, et al. Prevalence of monoclonal gammopathy among patients with psoriatic arthritis. J Rheumatol 2012;39(3):564–7.
174. Niccoli L, Nannini C, Cassarà E, et al. Frequency of iridocyclitis in patients with early psoriatic arthritis: a prospective, follow up study. Int J Rheum Dis 2012;15(4):414–8.
175. Ogdie A, Haynes K, Troxel A, et al. Mortality in patients with psoriatic arthritis compared to patients with rheumatoid arthritis, psoriasis alone, and the general population. Ann Rheum Dis 2014;73(1):149–53.
176. Arumugam R, McHugh N. Mortality and causes of death in psoriatic arthritis. J Rheumatol Suppl 2012;89:32–5.
177. Buckley C, Cavill C, Taylor G, et al. Mortality in psoriatic arthritis—a single-center study from the UK. J Rheumatol 2010;37(10):2141–4.
178. Wong K, Gladman DD, Husted J, et al. Mortality studies in psoriatic arthritis: results from a single outpatient clinic; causes and risk of death. Arthritis Rheum 1997;40(10):1868–72.
179. Ali Y, Tom BDM, Schentag CT, et al. Improved survival in psoriatic arthritis with calendar time. Arthritis Rheum 2007;56(8):2708–14.
180. Han C, Robinson DW, Hackett MV, et al. Cardiovascular disease and risk factors in patients with rheumatoid arthritis, psoriatic arthritis, and ankylosing spondylitis. J Rheumatol 2006;33:2167–72.
181. Gladman DD, Ang M, Su L, et al. Cardiovascular morbidity in psoriatic arthritis. Ann Rheum Dis 2009;68:1131–5.
182. Tam L, Tomlinson B, Chu T, et al. Cardiovascular risk profile of patients with psoriatic arthritis compared to controls–the role of inflammation. Rheumatology (Oxford) 2008;47:718–23.
183. Dubreuil M, Hee Rho Y, Man D, et al. The independent impact of psoriatic arthritis and rheumatoid arthritis on diabetes incidence: a UK population-based cohort study. Rheumatology (Oxford) 2014;53(2):346–52.
184. Solomon D, Love T, Canning C, et al. Risk of diabetes among patients with rheumatoid arthritis, psoriatic arthritis and psoriasis. Ann Rheum Dis 2010;69(12):2114–7.
185. Haroon M, Gallagher P, Heffernan E, et al. High prevalence of metabolic syndrome and of insulin resistance in psoriatic arthritis is associated with the severity of underlying disease. J Rheumatol 2014;41(7):1357–65.
186. Labitigan M, Bahče-Altuntas A, Kremer J, et al. Higher rates and clustering of abnormal lipids, obesity and diabetes mellitus in psoriatic arthritis compared with rheumatoid arthritis. Arthritis Care Res (Hoboken) 2014;66(4):600–7.
187. Pehlevan S, Yetkin D, Bahadır C, et al. Increased prevalence of metabolic syndrome in patients with psoriatic arthritis. Metab Syndr Relat Disord 2014;12(1):43–8.
188. Li W, Han J, Manson J, et al. Psoriasis and risk of nonfatal cardiovascular disease in U.S. women: a cohort study. Br J Dermatol 2012;166(4):811–8.
189. Ahlehoff O, Gislason G, Charlot M, et al. Psoriasis is associated with clinically significant cardiovascular risk: a Danish nationwide cohort study. J Intern Med 2011;270(2):147–57.
190. Chin Y, Yu H, Li W, et al. Arthritis as an important determinant for psoriatic patients to develop severe vascular events in Taiwan: a nation-wide study. J Eur Acad Dermatol Venereol 2013;27(10):1262–8.

191. Bandinelli F, Prignano F, Bonciani D, et al. Clinical and demographic factors influence on anxiety and depression in early psoriatic arthritis (ePsA). Clin Exp Rheumatol 2013;31(2):318–9.
192. Makredes M, Robinson DJ, Bala M, et al. The burden of autoimmune disease: a comparison of prevalence ratios in patients with psoriatic arthritis and psoriasis. J Am Acad Dermatol 2009;61(3):405–10.
193. Li W, Han J, Chan A, et al. Psoriasis, psoriatic arthritis and increased risk of incident Crohn's disease in US women. Ann Rheum Dis 2013;72(7):1200–5.
194. Lima F, Abalem M, Ruiz D, et al. Prevalence of eye disease in Brazilian patients with psoriatic arthritis. Clinics (Sao Paulo) 2012;67(3):249–53.
195. Antonelli A, Delle Sedie A, Fallahi P, et al. High prevalence of thyroid autoimmunity and hypothyroidism in patients with psoriatic arthritis. J Rheumatol 2006; 33(10):2026–8.

Clinical Features and Diagnostic Considerations in Psoriatic Arthritis

 CrossMark

Dafna D. Gladman, MD, FRCPC

KEYWORDS

- Psoriatic arthritis • Dactylitis • Enthesitis • Axial disease • Clinical features
- Differential diagnosis

KEY POINTS

- Psoriatic arthritis is a unique musculoskeletal disease occurring in patients with psoriasis.
- There are specific clinical and imaging features that help identify it.
- It should be differentiated from other forms of arthritis that might coexist with psoriasis.

Psoriasis is an inflammatory immune-mediated skin disease that affects 2% to 3% of the population. Some 30% of patients with psoriasis develop an inflammatory form of arthritis, termed psoriatic arthritis. Psoriatic arthritis was initially described in detail by Wright,[1] and then Wright and Moll,[2] who considered it "an inflammatory arthritis associated with psoriasis usually seronegative for rheumatoid factor." They described 5 clinical patterns of the disease, namely distal, oligoarticular, polyarticular, primarily axial, and arthritis mutilans.[2] However, it has been demonstrated that patients change their pattern over time, such that a patient may present with oligoarthritis and then develop polyarticular involvement, or present with polyarthritis and remain oligoarticular after therapy. Alternatively, patients may have primarily peripheral disease at presentation and then develop axial disease, or vice versa. Because patients may present at different points during their disease course, these patterns are not useful in terms of identifying disease.[3] Moreover, patients with psoriatic arthritis may present with peripheral arthritis, axial disease, or enthesitis. Thus, the new definition of psoriatic arthritis is "an inflammatory musculoskeletal disease associated with psoriasis."[4] More recently, most investigators consider psoriatic arthritis to consist of 5 domains: peripheral arthritis, axial disease, enthesitis, dactylitis, and skin and nail disease.[5]

In this article, the clinical features of psoriatic arthritis are discussed, together with diagnostic considerations.

Disclosure: None.
Toronto Western Hospital, University of Toronto, University Health Network, 399 Bathurst Street, 1E-410B, Toronto, Ontario M5T 2S8, Canada
E-mail address: dafna.gladman@utoronto.ca

Rheum Dis Clin N Am 41 (2015) 569–579
http://dx.doi.org/10.1016/j.rdc.2015.07.003
0889-857X/15/$ – see front matter

CLINICAL FEATURES OF PSORIATIC ARTHRITIS
Peripheral Arthritis

Psoriatic arthritis is inflammatory in nature. Thus, patients present with joint pain that is worse with inactivity, and is associated with morning stiffness of more than 30 minutes' duration. The joint pain and stiffness improve with activity. There may be joint swelling associated with the pain. Any joint may be affected, but the most common joints are the joints of the feet and hands, followed by knees, wrists, ankles, and shoulders (**Table 1**).

On physical examination, joints may be tender and swollen; however, it should be noted that patients with psoriatic arthritis are not as tender as patients with rheumatoid arthritis.[6] Moreover, the effusions may be tight and difficult to appreciate. Patients with psoriatic arthritis may demonstrate a purplish discoloration over their affected joints.[7] When assessing disease activity in psoriatic arthritis, it is important to assess 68 joints for tenderness and 66 joints for swelling, as one may otherwise underestimate the extent of the disease.[8] Because the feet are most commonly affected, a joint count that excludes the feet is inappropriate for the assessment of psoriatic arthritis.

Most patients with psoriatic arthritis present with polyarticular disease, with 5 or more joints involved (**Fig. 1**). The distribution tends to be asymmetrical, but the more joints involved the more likely the symmetry.[9] Isolated distal joint involvement may occur in 5% to 10% of the patients (**Fig. 2**). Oligoarticular disease occurs in 37% of the patients (**Fig. 3**). Oligoarticular presentations are more likely to occur in early disease. Polyarticular disease is prognostic for progression of damage.[10,11] Patients with oligoarticular disease are more likely to achieve remission.[12]

Psoriatic arthritis may appear as a rapidly destructive arthritis described as arthritis mutilans. It was recognized by Wright and Moll[2] as a unique pattern. However,

Table 1
Active and damage joint prevalence among 355 inception patients

Joints Involved	Frequency (%)	
	Active Joint Involvement	Damage Joint Involvement
Temporomandibular	19 (5.4)	0 (0.0)
Sternoclavicular	11 (3.1)	0 (0.0)
Shoulder	71 (20.0)	4 (1.1)
Elbow	43 (12.1)	2 (0.6)
Hand		
Wrist	101 (28.5)	4 (1.1)
Metacarpophalangeal	167 (47.0)	3 (0.9)
Proximal interphalangeal	203 (57.2)	21 (5.9)
Distal interphalangeal	123 (34.7)	19 (5.4)
Hip	23 (6.5)	3 (0.9)
Knee	102 (28.7)	3 (0.9)
Ankle	81 (22.8)	3 (0.9)
Foot		
Metatarsophalangeal	186 (52.4)	11 (3.1)
Proximal/distal interphalangeal	131 (36.9)	16 (4.5)

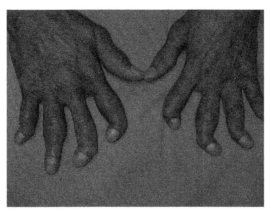

Fig. 1. Polyarticular psoriatic arthritis.

patients with other patterns may develop arthritis mutilans and therefore it is not considered a pattern but rather a specific phenotype within the disease. Clinically, one detects flail joints, although some patients demonstrate joint fusion.[13] Radiologically, there is evidence for significant osteolysis with bone resorption that may involve whole phalanges (**Fig. 4**). Fortunately, this extreme phenotype occurs in a minority of patients. In Wright and Moll's series[2] it occurred in only 5% of the patients. Two recent studies that defined arthritis mutilans as osteolysis also report low prevalence both in Nordic countries and in Bath, England.[14,15]

Patients with arthritis mutilans present at a younger age compared with other forms of psoriatic arthritis, demonstrate poorer function and more prevalent nail dystrophy, and show more radiographic axial disease/sacroiliitis. The rate of osteolysis is higher in earlier disease, and more severe in those with nail dystrophy.[15] HLA-B*27 is associated with the development of arthritis mutilans.[16]

It is important to appreciate the degree of inflammation in patients with psoriatic arthritis. Inflammation in a single joint predicts the development of damage in that joint.[17]

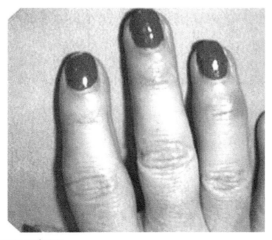

Fig. 2. Distal psoriatic arthritis.

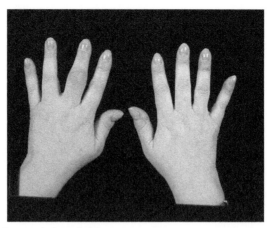

Fig. 3. Oligoarticular psoriatic arthritis.

Axial Involvement in Psoriatic Arthritis

Similar to the peripheral joints, inflammation of the back presents with inflammatory-type back pain that is worse in the morning and with inactivity, and is associated with prolonged stiffness. Both the pain and stiffness improve with activity. The pain may be felt in the sacroiliac area, or the cervical, thoracic, and lumbar spine.

On physical examination, one may find limitation of movement that may be detected using the Schober test, lateral flexion of the spine, cervical rotation, or chest expansion[18] (**Fig. 5**). Spinal mobility is correlated with radiographic progression in axial psoriatic arthritis.[19]

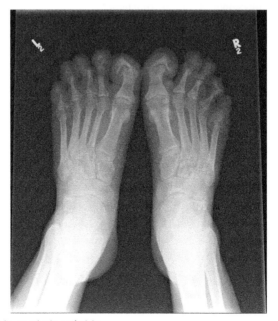

Fig. 4. Osteolysis in psoriatic arthritis.

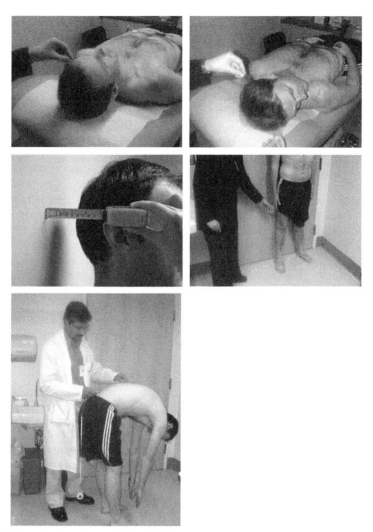

Fig. 5. Axial metrology in psoriatic arthritis.

Isolated axial disease occurs in only 2% to 4% of patients with psoriatic arthritis. Most patients with axial psoriatic arthritis present with axial as well as peripheral disease. The prevalence of axial disease among patients with psoriatic arthritis varies depending on whether radiographs are obtained.[20] Just as mentioned previously for peripheral arthritis, patients with axial psoriatic arthritis do not complain of as much pain as patients with ankylosing spondylitis.[21] Thus, many patients with axial psoriatic arthritis remain asymptomatic and their diagnosis would be missed unless radiographs were performed. On the other hand, it has been demonstrated that the assessment of patients with axial psoriatic arthritis is as reliable as the assessment of patients with ankylosing spondylitis, both in terms of clinical and radiographic assessment.[22]

Although HLA-B*27 is associated with the presence of axial disease at presentation to clinic, more severe disease, manifested by polyarticular peripheral disease and more damaged joints, is not a predictor of developing axial disease later in the course of psoriatic arthritis.[17,23]

Dactylitis

Dactylitis refers to inflammation of a whole digit. It results from inflammation in the joints, the tendon sheaths, and the soft tissues.[24] It usually presents as a painful digit with reduced mobility. The digit is often red hot and very tender. If not treated, chronic dactylitis may result with a swollen digit that is no longer painful, or red, but is often associated with reduction in range of movement (**Fig. 6**). Dactylitis commonly affects the feet, more often than the hands. The second and fifth toes are most commonly affected.[25] It is recognized as a specific feature of psoriatic arthritis, although the differential diagnosis includes trauma, sarcoidosis, gout, and reactive arthritis.

Dactylitis can be assessed by the number of "sausage digits" with or without a tenderness scale, or by the Leeds dactylitis index.[26] Tender dactylitis fingers have been demonstrated to have more severe abnormalities on MRI than those that are not tender.[27]

Dactylitis occurs in approximately 48% of the patients at some point in their disease course, and is detected in approximately 30% of the patients at presentation. It has been associated with more severe radiographic changes in the affected digits.[23]

Enthesitis

Enthesitis refers to inflammation at the insertion of tendons and ligaments into bone (**Fig. 7**). Enthesitis is a feature of all forms of spondyloarthritis, but occurs more commonly in psoriatic arthritis. It occurs in approximately 48% of patients with psoriatic arthritis. At first visit, approximately 35% of the patients present with enthesitis. Enthesitis may be the only manifestation of psoriatic arthritis and hence has been recognized as part of the stem for application of the Classification of Psoriatic Arthritis (CASPAR) criteria.[4,28,29]

Enthesitis is detected more commonly on ultrasound in patients with psoriasis without clinical evidence of psoriatic arthritis compared with healthy controls.[30] Three of 30 patients developed evidence of psoriatic arthritis after 2 years of follow-up, suggesting that enthesitis may be a clinical feature that identifies patients with psoriasis destined to develop psoriatic arthritis.[31] However, it should be noted that although ultrasound-detected enthesitis is more common and more severe in patients with psoriatic arthritis than those with psoriasis without arthritis or healthy controls, the sensitivity is only 30%, whereas the specificity is 95% compared with healthy controls and 89% when compared with patients with psoriasis without arthritis.[32] Moreover, body mass index is particularly relevant to the development of enthesitis.

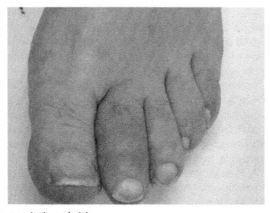

Fig. 6. Dactylitis in psoriatic arthritis.

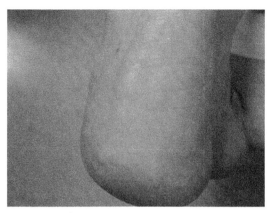

Fig. 7. Enthesitis in psoriatic arthritis.

Radiographically, enthesitis may present as spurs. It was recently demonstrated that calcaneal spurs are more common in subjects with psoriatic arthritis than controls. The presence of fluffy plantar periostitis and broad-based and longer midsegment dimensions are radiological features for inflammatory spurs.[33]

Skin and Nail Disease

Skin manifestations precede the development of psoriatic arthritis in 70% of the patients. In an additional 15% of the patients, skin and joint manifestations present simultaneously. Although the severity of skin lesions has been identified as a risk factor for developing psoriatic arthritis among patients with psoriasis,[34,35] the fact that some 15% of the patients develop psoriatic arthritis before the recognition of psoriasis suggests that it is not a very strong risk factor. Indeed, in rheumatology clinics, the severity of psoriasis tends to be lower than in dermatology clinics. Nonetheless, skin involvement is necessary for the diagnosis of psoriatic arthritis. According to the CASPAR criteria, the presence of psoriasis on current examination, a personal history of psoriasis, or a family history of psoriasis are relevant to the classification of a patient as having psoriatic arthritis.[4] Most patients with psoriatic arthritis have plaque psoriasis, with a minority having either guttate, flexural, or palmoplantar disease.

Nail lesions have also been found to be risk factors for developing psoriatic arthritis and should be sought for in patients with psoriasis. They should also be sought in patients with inflammatory arthritis who present with features of psoriatic arthritis described previously. These lesions include pits, onycholysis, hyperkeratosis, and nail bed crumbling (**Fig. 8**). A relationship between nail disease and enthesitis has been suggested, and is supported by ultrasound and MRI studies.[36]

Diagnosis of Psoriatic Arthritis

Although the CASPAR criteria are classification criteria, they have facilitated the diagnosis of psoriatic arthritis. Testing the criteria in early psoriatic arthritis, in early arthritis clinics, and in family medicine clinics demonstrated their usefulness.[37–40] However, the studies performed to date have used rheumatologists to ascertain the inflammatory musculoskeletal stem, thus making it easier to identify the patients. It is not as easy for a nonexpert to recognize the features of inflammatory musculoskeletal disease. The Group for Research and Assessment of Psoriasis and Psoriatic Arthritis (GRAPPA) is currently developing criteria to define inflammatory musculoskeletal disease that can be applied by primary care physicians and dermatologists.

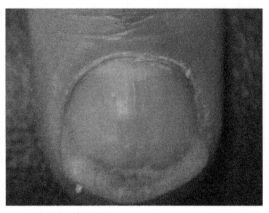

Fig. 8. Nail lesions in psoriatic arthritis.

In the meantime, there are clinical features, including the extent of psoriasis, site of psoriasis, and nail lesions, that should alert dermatologists to consider the presence of psoriatic arthritis and refer patients to a rheumatologist.[41]

Diagnostic Considerations

When a patient with psoriasis presents with peripheral inflammatory arthritis, the differential diagnosis includes not only psoriatic arthritis, but also the possible coexistence of rheumatoid arthritis and psoriasis, gout and psoriasis, or osteoarthritis and psoriasis.

Differentiating psoriatic arthritis from rheumatoid arthritis

Rheumatoid arthritis typically involves the proximal joints of the hands, whereas psoriatic arthritis affects the distal interphalangeal joints either alone or in combination with other joints in at least half the cases. Although rheumatoid arthritis usually presents with a symmetric distribution, psoriatic arthritis is most often asymmetric. Rheumatoid arthritis affects women 3 times as often as men, whereas psoriatic arthritis affects men and women equally. The presence of an erythematous change over the affected joint is more characteristic of psoriatic arthritis. In addition to the aforementioned features, the presence of inflammatory distal joint disease, dactylitis or enthesitis, axial disease, or nail lesions also helps distinguish psoriatic arthritis from rheumatoid arthritis. It has been demonstrated that the presence of 20 or more pits identifies patients with psoriatic arthritis in a rheumatology clinic.[42] On the other hand, the presence of rheumatoid nodules would favor the diagnosis of rheumatoid arthritis and psoriasis. Although it is possible for a patient to have rheumatoid arthritis and psoriatic arthritis, this co-occurrence is rare, and expected in 1:10,000 patients.

Differentiating psoriatic arthritis from gout

Gout may affect joints in a similar distribution to psoriatic arthritis. Moreover, gouty joints may have marked erythema, although it would usually extend beyond the joint and include periarticular areas. The presence of nail lesions would support a diagnosis of psoriatic arthritis, as would enthesitis and axial disease. Dactylitis may be confused with podagra, which will make the differentiation more difficult. Radiographs may be helpful, as the changes in gout are usually to a single bone, whereas in psoriatic arthritis, the erosions are marginal. The presence of tophi may support the diagnosis of gout. However, serum uric acid may be elevated in patients with psoriasis and psoriatic arthritis, making the differentiation more difficult; an increased frequency of gout has been observed among patients with psoriasis and psoriatic arthritis.

Differentiating psoriatic arthritis from osteoarthritis

Osteoarthritis is a common musculoskeletal disease and may occur concurrently with psoriasis. Because it commonly affects the distal joints in the lower extremity, it must be differentiated from psoriatic arthritis. Most of the time the differentiation is not difficult, as osteoarthritis does not usually present with inflammatory features, and the pain usually worsens with activity and improves with rest, whereas the morning stiffness, if present, tends to be short lived. Indeed, in this context, the CASPAR criteria should not be applied, as the stem requires "an inflammatory musculoskeletal disease." However, the differential diagnosis becomes particularly difficult when a patient has the inflammatory form of osteoarthritis, in which inflammatory complaints are coupled with destructive changes on radiographs. A careful evaluation, however, should allow differentiation, as the radiographs in osteoarthritis reveal focal changes that reflect cartilage loss (central joint space loss with gull wing appearance), whereas in psoriatic arthritis, the erosions are marginal and the cartilage space is less frequently affected until later in the disease. As in the case of rheumatoid arthritis or gout, the presence of nail lesions, dactylitis, and enthesitis, as well as inflammatory axial disease should help in differentiating coexisting osteoarthritis and psoriasis from psoriatic arthritis.

Differentiating psoriatic arthritis from other forms of spondyloarthritis

A difficult differential diagnosis is presented when a patient with inflammatory axial disease has psoriasis. The question that arises is whether the patient has ankylosing spondylitis and psoriasis, a situation that is recognized in approximately 10% of patients with ankylosing spondylitis, or psoriatic arthritis. According to the CASPAR criteria, if a patient has inflammatory axial disease and psoriasis with nail lesions, dactylitis, or negative rheumatoid factor, the patient would be classified as having psoriatic arthritis. As a group, patients with axial psoriatic arthritis differ from patients with ankylosing spondylitis by the severity of the pain, less severe functional limitation, less symmetric distribution of radiographic changes of sacroiliitis, and the presence of paramarginal syndesmophytes. In an individual patient, the differentiation may be more difficult. However, from a practical point of view, it probably does not matter because the management is similar, whether the patient was diagnosed with ankylosing spondylitis and psoriasis or axial psoriatic arthritis.

Reactive arthritis may be more difficult to differentiate from psoriatic arthritis, as patients have peripheral arthritis, axial disease, and skin lesions, which both clinically and pathologically may be similar to palmoplantar psoriasis. It is essential to take a careful history to determine if the patient has experienced recent enteric (*Shigella*, *Salmonella*, *Yersinia*, or *Campylobacter*) infections or symptoms suggestive of a genitourinary (*Chlamydia*) infection. Other features of reactive arthritis may be present, such as circinate balanitis or keratoderma blennorhagicum. The latter presentations also can be challenging because the appearance is psoriasiform in nature. It is important to secure a diagnosis of reactive arthritis because in many patients it does not take on a chronic course and may respond to antibiotics.

The arthritis of inflammatory bowel disease is also difficult to differentiate at times, particularly because there is an association between psoriasis and Crohn disease. The presentation can be in either the axial or peripheral skeleton and often the activity of the peripheral joint disease correlates with bowel inflammation.

SUMMARY

Psoriatic arthritis is a unique musculoskeletal disease occurring in patients with psoriasis. There are specific clinical and imaging features that help identify it. It should be differentiated from other forms of arthritis that might coexist with psoriasis.

REFERENCES

1. Wright V. Psoriatic arthritis; a comparative study of rheumatoid arthritis, psoriasis, and arthritis associated with psoriasis. AMA Arch Derm 1959;80:27–35.
2. Wright V, Moll JM. Psoriatic arthritis. Bull Rheum Dis 1971;21:627–32.
3. Khan M, Schentag C, Gladman D. Clinical and radiological changes during psoriatic arthritis disease progression: working toward classification criteria. J Rheumatol 2003;30:1022–6.
4. Taylor WJ, Gladman DD, Helliwell PS, et al. Classification criteria for psoriatic arthritis: development of new criteria from a large international study. Arthritis Rheum 2006;54:2665–73.
5. Ritchlin CT, Kavanaugh A, Gladman DD, et al. Treatment recommendations for psoriatic arthritis. Ann Rheum Dis 2009;68:1387–94.
6. Buskila D, Langevitz P, Gladman DD, et al. Patients with rheumatoid arthritis are more tender than those with psoriatic arthritis. J Rheumatol 1992;19:1115–9.
7. Jajic I. Blue coloured skin in psoriatic arthritis. Clin Exp Rheumatol 2001;19:478.
8. Coates LC, Fitzgerald O, Gladman DD, et al. Reduced joint counts misclassify psoriatic arthritis patients with oligoarthritis and miss significant active disease. Arthritis Rheum 2013;65:1504–9.
9. Helliwell PS, Hetthen J, Sokoll K, et al. Joint symmetry in early and late rheumatoid and psoriatic arthritis: comparison with a mathematical model. Arthritis Rheum 2000;43:865–71.
10. Gladman DD, Farewell VT, Nadeau C. Clinical indicators of progression in psoriatic arthritis (PSA): multivariate relative risk model. J Rheumatol 1995;22:675–9.
11. Queiro-Silva R, Torre-Alonso JC, Tinture-Eguren T, et al. A polyarticular onset predicts erosive and deforming disease in psoriatic arthritis. Ann Rheum Dis 2003;62:68–70.
12. Gladman DD, Ng Tung Hing E, Schentag CT, et al. Remission in psoriatic arthritis. J Rheumatol 2001;28:1045–8.
13. Haddad A, Chandran V. Arthritis mutilans. Curr Rheumatol Rep 2013;15:321.
14. Gudbjornsson B, Ejstrup L, Gran JT, et al. Psoriatic arthritis mutilans (PAM) in the Nordic countries: demographics and disease status. The Nordic PAM study. Scand J Rheumatol 2013;42:373–8.
15. Jadon DR, Shaddick G, Tillett W, et al. Psoriatic arthritis mutilans: characteristics and natural radiographic history. J Rheumatol Online 2015;42(7):1169–76.
16. Chandran V, Cook RJ, Thavaneswaran A, et al. Parametric survival analysis as well as multi-state analysis confirms the association between human leukocyte antigen alleles and the development of arthritis mutilans in patients with psoriatic arthritis. J Rheumatol 2012;39:1723.
17. Cresswell L, Chandran V, Farewell VT, et al. Inflammation in an individual joint predicts damage to that joint in psoriatic arthritis. Ann Rheum Dis 2011;70:305–8.
18. Gladman DD, Inman R, Cook R, et al. International spondyloarthritis interobserver reliability exercise–The INSPIRE Study: I. Assessment of spinal measures. J Rheumatol 2007;34:1733–9.
19. Chandran V, O'shea FD, Schentag CT, et al. Relationship between spinal mobility and radiographic damage in ankylosing spondylitis and psoriatic spondylitis: a comparative analysis. J Rheumatol 2007;34:2463–5.
20. Gladman DD. Axial disease in psoriatic arthritis. Curr Rheumatol Rep 2007;9:455–60.
21. Gladman DD, Brubacher B, Buskila D, et al. Differences in the expression of spondyloarthropathy: a comparison between ankylosing spondylitis and psoriatic arthritis. Genetic and gender effects. Clin Invest Med 1993;16:1–7.

22. Biagioni B, Gladman DD, Cook RJ, et al. Reliability of radiographic scoring methods in axial psoriatic arthritis. Arthritis Care Res (Hoboken) 2014;66: 1417–22.
23. Chandran V, Tolusso DC, Schentag CT, et al. Risk factors for axial inflammatory arthritis in patients with psoriatic arthritis. J Rheumatol 2010;37:809–15.
24. Olivieri I, Scarano E, Padula A, et al. Imaging of psoriatic arthritis. Reumatismo 2007;59(Suppl 1):73–6.
25. Brockbank J, Stein M, Schentag CT, et al. Dactylitis in psoriatic arthritis (PsA): a marker for disease severity? Ann Rheum Dis 2005;62:188–90.
26. Helliwell PS, Firth J, Ibrahim GH, et al. Development of an assessment tool for dactylitis in patients with psoriatic arthritis. J Rheumatol 2005;32:1745–50.
27. Healy PJ, Groves C, Chandramohan M, et al. MRI changes in psoriatic dactylitis–extent of pathology, relationship to tenderness and correlation with clinical indices. Rheumatology (Oxford) 2008;47:92–5.
28. Scarpa R, Cuocolo A, Peluso R, et al. Early psoriatic arthritis: the clinical spectrum. J Rheumatol 2008;35:137–41.
29. Bandinelli F, Prignano F, Bonciani D, et al. Ultrasound detects occult entheseal involvement in early psoriatic arthritis independently of clinical features and psoriasis severity. Clin Exp Rheumatol 2013;31:219–24.
30. Gisondi P, Tinazzi I, El-Dalati G, et al. Lower limb enthesopathy in patients with psoriasis without clinical signs of arthropathy: a hospital-based case-control study. Ann Rheum Dis 2008;67:26–30.
31. Girolomoni G, Gisondi P. Psoriasis and systemic inflammation: underdiagnosed enthesopathy. J Eur Acad Dermatol Venereol 2009;23(Suppl 1):3–8.
32. Eder L, Jayakar J, Thavaneswaran A, et al. Is the Madrid sonographic enthesitis index useful for differentiating psoriatic arthritis from psoriasis alone and healthy controls? J Rheumatol 2014;41:466–72.
33. Gladman DD, Abuffayah M, Salonen D, et al. Radiological characteristics of the calcaneal spurs in psoriatic arthritis. Clin Exp Rheumatol 2014;32:401–3.
34. Gelfand JM, Gladman DD, Mease PJ, et al. Epidemiology of psoriatic arthritis in the United States population. J Am Acad Dermatol 2005;53:573–7.
35. Wilson FC, Icen M, Crowson CS, et al. Incidence and clinical predictors of psoriatic arthritis in patients with psoriasis: a population-based study. Arthritis Rheum 2009;61:233–9.
36. Ash ZR, Tinazzi I, Gallego CC, et al. Psoriasis patients with nail disease have a greater magnitude of underlying systemic subclinical enthesopathy than those with normal nails. Ann Rheum Dis 2012;71:553–6.
37. Chandran V, Schentag CT, Gladman DD. Sensitivity of the Classification of Psoriatic Arthritis (CASPAR) criteria in early psoriatic arthritis. Arthritis Rheum 2007;57: 1560–3.
38. D'Angelo S, Mennillo GA, Cutro MS, et al. Sensitivity of the classification of psoriatic arthritis criteria in early psoriatic arthritis. J Rheumatol 2009;36:368–70.
39. Coates L, Conaghan PG, Emery P, et al. The CASPAR criteria can be used to identify early psoriatic arthritis. Arthritis Rheum 2010;62(Suppl 10):S916.
40. Chandran V, Schentag CT, Gladman DD. Sensitivity and specificity of the CASPAR criteria for psoriatic arthritis when applied to patients attending a family medicine clinic. J Rheumatol 2008;35:2069–70.
41. Gladman DD. Early psoriatic arthritis. Rheum Dis Clin North Am 2012;38:373–86.
42. Eastmond CJ, Wright V. The nail dystrophy of psoriatic arthritis. Ann Rheum Dis 1979;38:226–8.

Natural History, Prognosis, and Socioeconomic Aspects of Psoriatic Arthritis

Philip S. Helliwell, MD[a],*, Eric M. Ruderman, MD[b]

KEYWORDS

- Psoriasis • Psoriatic arthritis • Disability • Quality of life • Prognosis • Natural history
- Work • Comorbidities

KEY POINTS

- Psoriatic arthritis is a heterogeneous disease confounding generic statements about natural history and prognosis.
- A significant minority of patients manifest a relatively benign disease with little progression. The majority of cases have slowly progressive, polyarticular disease.
- An increase in cardiovascular morbidity is associated with psoriasis and psoriatic arthritis, particularly in secondary care cohorts.
- Longitudinal cohorts provide clues to adverse prognostic factors. These include the number of active and damaged joints, the presence of spinal disease, and dactylitis.
- Genetic subtypes are predictive but not practicable in the routine clinic situation. The only current biomarker with predictive value is the C reactive protein.

INTRODUCTION

Psoriatic disease, which encompasses psoriatic arthritis, has a wide variety of clinical manifestations, each of which may vary in their impact. For example, in 1 person the skin may be the most severely affected, in another the joints. Even within a single domain, such as the joints, the disease may vary from a mild nonprogressive oligoarthritis to severe, mutilating polyarticular disease. These diverse clinical manifestations undermine single statement predictions regarding outcome, although general statements may be appropriate.

Historically, psoriatic arthritis was conceived as a more benign arthropathy than rheumatoid arthritis.[1] Wright[1] acknowledged, however, that in some people the disease

Disclosures: None.
[a] Leeds Institute of Rheumatic and Musculoskeletal Medicine, Chapel Allerton Hospital, University of Leeds, 2nd Floor, Harehills Lane, Leeds LS7 4SA, UK; [b] Division of Rheumatology, Northwestern University Feinberg School of Medicine, 303 E Chicago Ave, Chicago, IL 60611, USA
* Corresponding author.
E-mail address: p.helliwell@leeds.ac.uk

Rheum Dis Clin N Am 41 (2015) 581–591
http://dx.doi.org/10.1016/j.rdc.2015.07.004   rheumatic.theclinics.com
0889-857X/15/$ – see front matter © 2015 Elsevier Inc. All rights reserved.

followed a particularly aggressive and deforming course. Subsequent clinical studies challenged the assertion that psoriatic arthritis is a more benign disease than rheumatoid arthritis.[2] It is worth noting that almost all published studies on outcome in psoriatic arthritis assessed secondary or tertiary care populations, which are composed of more severe cases, many of whom are treated more aggressively to suppress disease activity and damage.

Highly effective treatments are now available for psoriatic arthritis, and research in this field is burgeoning. Further, new drugs are effective for both skin and joints, and may also be beneficial for comorbidities and extraskeletal manifestations. Earlier referral and identification, along with more aggressive treatment, may have a significant beneficial effect on the natural course of this disease.

NATURAL HISTORY

Accurate data are limited, but clinical experience and some publications support the observation that a proportion of patients with psoriatic arthritis demonstrate mild, minimally progressive, or nonprogressive disease that may require only symptomatic treatment. This group includes those with arthralgia and low-grade inflammation, an intermittent disease that may remit for long periods of time, and, sometimes, an oligoarthritis such as a chronically swollen knee. Nevertheless, limited articular disease may still be very disabling—1 or 2 dactylitic digits on a dominant hand or a severe enthesopathy at the Achilles insertion can limit both manual tasks and mobility.

Mild, Nonprogressive Disease

Wright,[1] in his original series, identified 2 populations of patients—a group with severe disease onset followed by a complete and lasting recovery, and a more severe progressive group. Although they did not present exact figures, Wright stated that cases with mild disability outnumbered those with severe disability. In that series, 74% of the total group presented with oligoarthritis. They confirmed the observations of predominantly limited disease in a subsequent article that reported radiologic changes.[3] A later review of these patients confirmed the largely benign nature of the condition: 78% of the 178 patients were classified as mild, with only 11% of this group deteriorated over a follow-up period of more than 10 years.[4]

Later studies, particularly those from Toronto, also confirmed the presence of a milder, nonprogressive, oligoarticular population. For example, the first complete series published by Gladman and colleagues[5] included a large nonerosive group. Subsequent series reported at damage progression in a group of 33% to 36% of patients who had no evidence of damaged joints at either presentation or follow-up.[6,7] A similar proportion of patients—28%—remained without disability over a 10-year period.[8]

In unselected patients, approximately one-quarter demonstrate at least 1 erosion at presentation. Data from a study in Dublin found this proportion increased to 41% after 2 years[9]; a more recent study from an early (<2 years) cohort found that at least 27% had 1 erosion at presentation, increasing to 31% at 1 year.[10] This erosive burden will, of course, depend on treatment; psoriatic arthritis patients develop less erosive disease (at least in the hands and feet) than rheumatoid arthritis patients at all stages of disease.[11]

Prospective, community-based data are not available, but a single report identified psoriatic arthritis from health records over a 9-year period.[12] Despite the large population (population 124,277) numbers of cases were small at 66 (expected numbers in the region of 250). Only 10 people in this largely oligoarticular group received disease-modifying antirheumatic drugs (DMARDs) and only 8% developed erosions in the hands.

Progressive Deforming Arthritis

Wright reported a group of patients who developed a severely deforming arthritis, termed arthritis mutilans, with osteolysis of the digits, polyarticular involvement, and frequent spinal involvement.[13] Affected individuals often developed telescoping joints and flail digits in both hands and feet, resulting in severe disability. However, this distinctive group only represents a small proportion of affected people, less than 5% in most series. The majority of patients with psoriatic arthritis develop polyarticular arthritis with progressive deformity and damage. This mutilans group slowly accrues damaged joints and becomes progressively more disabled, as demonstrated by several cross-sectional and longitudinal surveys.[6,11,14]

Erosive disease of the peripheral joints is an indicator of progression, but other manifestations of psoriatic arthritis, particularly spinal disease, are important in the natural history. The prevalence of spinal involvement, identified by signs and symptoms, is 40%. In many patients, involvement is asymptomatic.[15] The Toronto group noted radiologic progression of spinal disease in the absence of clinical progression (as indicated by symptoms and spinal mobility) over a mean follow-up period of 57 months—clearly important to document when defining the natural history of the disease.[16]

PROGNOSIS
Cross-Sectional Studies

Cross-sectional studies provide limited data about prognostic factors owing to potential bias and confounding factors. Roberts and associates[4] identified a more severe deforming group with of psoriatic arthritis patients with an acute onset, systemic features, onset before the age of 20, and spinal involvement. Kammer and co-workers[17] found that a polyarticular group was more likely to progress and to have nail involvement. More recently, a number of studies have indicated that delay in diagnosis is associated with greater joint damage, suggesting that earlier diagnosis may improve outcomes.[18–20]

Longitudinal Studies

In longitudinal studies, significant polyarticular inflammation at onset, represented by more than 5 swollen joints and an increased erythrocyte sedimentation rate, predicts joint damage.[6] In an extension of this study, existing damage and previous steroids use were also predictive of joint damage.[21] Two other longitudinal series reported similar results. Kane and colleagues,[9] studying an inception cohort, found that patients with an oligoarticular disease onset were more likely to be in remission at 2 years. Conversely, in a separate Spanish study, polyarticular disease was the main predictor of erosions.[22]

Taken together, and recognizing that effective treatment can delay or prevent progression, these longitudinal studies suggest that earlier intervention in patients with more active disease might improve outcomes. Indeed, recent data from the Swedish early arthritis register indicates better outcomes for people with shorter symptom duration at diagnosis, confirming the data from cross-sectional studies.[20] It is likely, albeit not yet proven, that these improved outcomes with earlier referral and diagnosis are the result of earlier treatment. In addition, recent data indicate that a treat-to-target approach also improves outcomes, but additional studies are needed to examine the efficacy of this strategy in different phenotypes.[23]

Other Clinical Prognostic Factors

Dactylitis, a hallmark clinical feature of psoriatic arthritis, represents inflammation in articular, osseous, and extraarticular tissues of a digit. It is present in about 30% of cases of psoriatic arthritis at some time and may be associated with marked disability, particularly when present in the hand. Dactylitic digits are more likely to develop progressive radiologic changes compared with nondactylitic digits, thus making dactylitis an important marker of disease severity and progression in psoriatic arthritis.[24]

In cross-sectional studies, nail disease has been associated with more severe disease. In one study, describing the development of a new instrument to quantify nail involvement.[25] A Psoriatic Nail Severity Score (PNSS) score of more than 16 was associated with more hospital admissions for psoriasis and greater radiologic progression of the arthritis.

Early hip involvement is typical of ankylosing spondylitis; in psoriatic arthritis, a series from the Mayo clinic showed that patients with hip disease are significantly younger at onset (29 vs 40 years of age) and are more likely to have spondylitis.[26] Although only a few patients with established psoriatic arthritis have clinical and radiologic hip involvement, hip arthritis is often disabling and may require early arthroplasty.

HLA Studies and Serum Markers

In rheumatoid arthritis, specific HLA haplotypes are associated with disease severity and susceptibility. It seems reasonable, then, to seek such predictors in psoriatic arthritis, and genetic factors are associated with different subgroups of psoriatic arthritis.

Espinoza and associates[27] first reported an association between HLA Bw38 and peripheral polyarthritis (the subgroup most likely to progress) and this was later confirmed in a larger series from Toronto.[28] The Toronto group also found a higher prevalence of HLA DR4 in the polyarticular subgroup, providing distal interphalangeal joints were not involved. The role of HLA antigens in predicting disease progression was studied in 2 additional series from Toronto.[7,29] Progression was predicted by the following HLA antigens: combination of HLA B27 and HLA DR7 (relative risk [RR], 2.47), DQw3 (RR, 1.63), and HLA B39 (RR, 7.05). The association of DQw3 with DR7 was, however, protective (RR, 0.54). In a later Swedish study, no HLA haplotypes were predictive; the only significant variables associated with articular destruction were distal interphalangeal involvement and a polyarticular pattern.[30]

Data on cytokine polymorphisms indicate that erosive disease, and by inference the group with the worst prognosis, is associated with certain subtypes of tumor necrosis factor (TNF). Balding and colleagues[31] examined 147 patients with psoriatic arthritis and compared them to 389 healthy controls. Fifty-one psoriatic arthritis patients had sequential radiographs to assess the progression of erosive disease. TNFα -308 and TNFβ +252 were associated with erosive disease and progression of erosions. It has also been suggested that a minor allele of the interleukin (IL) 12 receptor may also be 'protective' for disease severity, as indicated by peripheral erosions (odds ratio [OR], 0.47; 95% CI, 0.18–1.20).[32]

Finally, anticitrullinated peptide antibodies, usually associated with rheumatoid arthritis, are present in low titer in less than 10% of patients with psoriatic arthritis.

These antibodies may be associated with more erosive disease, based on data from 1 cohort.[33] These data await confirmation.

MORBIDITY
Disability and Quality of Life

Psoriatic arthritis impacts significantly function and quality of life. Sokoll and Helliwell[11] compared impairment, function, and quality of life in a series of 50 patients with psoriatic arthritis and patients with rheumatoid arthritis matched for age, sex, and duration of disease. Impairment, as measured by radiologic damage score, was greater in the rheumatoid arthritis group, but both disability and quality of life were similarly impaired in both groups. Some of the impairment in psoriatic arthritis may have been attributable to the associated skin disease; patients graded for severity of skin disease showed a decline in function and quality of life with increasing severity, independent of their joint disease. A similar study from Toronto found that rheumatoid arthritis patients had markedly higher Health Assessment Questionnaire disability index scores (mean, 1.11) than psoriatic arthritis patients (mean, 0.58).[14] After adjustment for age, sex, and disease duration (the groups were not matched for these variables), only the vitality domain of the Short Form-36 separated the 2 groups. In contrast with the Leeds study, no correlation was identified between skin severity (as measured by the Psoriasis Area and Severity Index [PASI]) and quality of life.

Cardiovascular Morbidity

A number of studies have highlighted the association between cardiovascular morbidity, and associated risk factors (obesity, hypertension, type 2 diabetes mellitus, and hyperlipidemia) in psoriasis.[34] These cardiovascular risk factors were correlated with increasing extent of psoriasis.[35] The added burden of risk associated with joint disease is not completely clear, although it would be expected unresolved inflammation at a second site (joints) is significant. However, to fully understand the incremental contribution from the arthritis, it is essential to control for traditional risk factors and to acknowledge that many psoriatic arthritis patients have relatively mild psoriasis.[36] Nevertheless, the increase in cardiovascular risk in psoriatic arthritis, largely similar to that found in rheumatoid arthritis, was demonstrated in a systematic literature review.[37] This increased cardiovascular risk provides an additional domain to assess and treat in these patients. The mechanism of the association is not fully understood, but seems to be a combination of an increase in traditional risk factors and the presence of widespread systemic inflammation, a phenomenon termed the "psoriatic march."[38] Direct evidence of cardiovascular involvement comes from studies of subclinical carotid atherosclerosis that measure intimal media thickness with noninvasive methods.[39]

Most of the studies discussed were performed in a secondary care setting. Do the same considerations apply to a community setting? Some evidence suggests this may not be the case. Gelfand and colleagues[40] published widely on a UK primary care database. Allowing for the likely errors in coding in such a database, this group showed only a modest increase in major adverse cardiovascular events in psoriatic arthritis patients not taking a disease modifying drug (implying milder forms of the disease); the OR was significant at 1.24, whereas the OR of 1.17 for those on a DMARD was not significant.[40] This findings contrasts with rheumatoid arthritis, where the OR for major adverse cardiovascular events, off and on treatment, were both significant at 1.39 and 1.58.

Other Comorbidities

As indicated, an increase in traditional cardiovascular risk factors (obesity, hypertension, type 2 diabetes mellitus, and hyperlipidemia) was demonstrated in psoriasis; not surprisingly, a similar increase was shown in psoriatic arthritis.[41] As befits a condition grouped with other spondyloarthropathies, an increased prevalence of inflammatory bowel disease, either overt or covert, is observed. Finally, psychological morbidity is increased in psoriatic arthritis, particularly depression, an increase shared with psoriasis.[36,42] An increased risk of non-Hodgkin's lymphoma in rheumatoid arthritis was reported, but a population-based study in Sweden did not demonstrate a significantly increased risk in psoriatic arthritis.[43]

MORTALITY

Early studies suggested that psoriatic arthritis was a relatively mild arthropathy and, by implication, that there was little morbidity and no increase in mortality in this condition. In the original Wright series, 18 deaths were documented over a period of more than 10 years, but no age- and sex-adjusted mortality ratios were calculated, so it is hard to know how this cohort fared relative to the "general" population.[4] However, it is notable that 8 of the 18 deaths were owing to cardiovascular disease. Further studies of mortality have shown a slightly different picture. Reports from the Toronto group suggested an increase in cardiovascular mortality, but also highlighted increased mortality from respiratory diseases and injuries/poisoning, the latter particularly in men.[44] All-cause mortality was increased in this study, with a standardized mortality ratio of 1.59 for men and 1.65 for women. In a later report, the same group examined prognostic indicators for death: although recognizing that there were a small number of deaths, the poor prognostic indicators were, at presentation, prior DMARD use (RR, 1.84), radiologic damage (RR, 3.03), and an increased erythrocyte sedimentation rate (RR, 3.49).[45] The pattern of arthritis was not a prognostic indicator of mortality in this study. As this group examined mortality at later time points, it seems that recently standardized mortality ratio in psoriatic arthritis has fallen.[46] This may be owing to more aggressive treatment, as treatment may favorably influences cardiovascular morbidity, or in a decrease in the severity of cases entering the database.

The higher mortality owing to cardiovascular diseases was confirmed in a recently published literature review.[47] The authors concluded that there is an increase in cardiovascular morbidity and mortality in psoriatic arthritis, owing, in part, to an increase in conventional risk factors and also to factors, such as decreased physical activity and systemic inflammation.

However, the situation may be different in an unselected, community-based cohort. The study by Shbeeb and colleagues[12] did not find any increase in mortality in their cohort, observed over a 19-year period. However, in this small series, most (91%) had oligoarticular disease, and only a minority had ever taken DMARDs. More recently, data from a large UK general practice database provided more robust evidence; no increase in cardiovascular mortality in patients coded as having psoriatic arthritis was observed,[40] and all-cause mortality was comparable in rheumatoid arthritis and psoriasis alone (the hazard ratios for rheumatoid arthritis, psoriatic arthritis, and psoriasis were 1.59, 0.94, and 1.75, respectively, for those on DMARDs and 1.54, 1.06, and 1.08 for those not on DMARDs).[48]

Socioeconomic Factors and Work Disability

Although skin disease affects quality of life, the presence of articular involvement produces an additional impact in psoriatic arthritis. In a comparison of psoriasis and atopic dermatitis in Sweden, both were found to have significant, and comparable, impacts on quality of life, whereas patients with psoriatic arthritis reported significantly worse quality of life than either skin disease.[49] In the United States, a survey conducted by the Psoriasis Foundation found that 39% of those affected by psoriatic arthritis reported that the disease was a large problem in their everyday life, compared with just 12% of those with psoriasis.[50] More recently, the Multinational Assessment of Psoriasis and Psoriatic arthritis (MAPP) survey found significant impact of both skin and joints on quality of life.[51] Importantly, many people responding to this survey reported not seeing a health professional and/or not receiving treatment for their condition (28% of people with psoriatic arthritis were not receiving any treatment and 31% were receiving topical treatments only; equivalent figures for people with more than 10% body surface area affected by psoriasis were 37% and 52%).

A tally of the national costs of psoriatic arthritis is meaningless in this context, where treatment is incomplete or inadequate. Nevertheless, sums of great magnitude have been calculated for loss of work productivity, personal costs, and health care costs.[52] As might be expected, these costs correlate with disease severity.[53] In the last 15 years, the direct costs of this disease increased significantly, largely owing to the introduction of biologic drugs. Nevertheless, a report found that expensive therapeutics are cost effective.[54] In the UK, the National Institute of Health and Care Excellence has deemed that the cost effectiveness of TNF inhibitors is within the acceptable range.[55]

Work Disability

Data on work disability in psoriatic arthritis are beginning to appear, and it seems that the impact may be less than in rheumatoid arthritis. A prospective study of new-onset inflammatory arthritis in Finland, which included only 13 patients with psoriatic arthritis, found that 69% of them were working at 8-year follow-up, compared with 36% of those with rheumatoid arthiritis.[56] In a large recent study of employment in German patients with rheumatologic diseases, psoriatic arthritis patients were only slightly less likely to be employed than the general population (standardized employment ratio of 0.92 relative to the general population), and more likely to be employed than those with rheumatoid arthiritis.[57] As might be expected, disease duration of longer than 10 years and lower educational level were associated with a decreased likelihood of employment within diagnoses in this study. A recent systematic review found a number of factors associated with both unemployment and work disability in psoriatic arthritis, although the authors concluded that the quality of the evidence for this was not high. Duration of disease and lower educational level were also identified, along with higher joint counts, erosive disease, worse physical function, female gender, and manual work in this analysis.[58]

Examining unemployment rates hides a multitude of other occupational disability issues. More recent surveys looked at this problem in more depth using a number of different instruments. The Toronto group found reductions in work productivity, for those working both inside and outside the home; these decreases were correlated with disease severity markers, as well as demographic associations such as gender and educational status.[59] In the UK, Tillett and colleagues[60] have examined absenteeism (work time missed), presenteeism (impairment at work and reduced effectiveness), and work productivity loss in a series of 400 patients. The rates of absenteeism, presenteeism, and work productivity loss were all substantial at 14%, 39%, and 46%, respectively, and 26% were unemployed. As in the Toronto cohort, measures of disease severity were predictors of unemployment and presenteeism. In a US study, fatigue was noted to be an important correlate of work productivity loss in a cohort of 107 patients with psoriatic arthritis, independent of specific joint and skin disease activity or depression.[61] Other factors, beyond those related to the disease itself, may be at play as well; both the UK survey and the survey from Toronto confirmed that employer and work place factors were predictors of remaining in employment.

SUMMARY

Although early reports suggested that psoriatic arthritis was, with the exception of arthritis mutilans, a relatively mild arthritis, later studies have challenged this view. There is no doubt that this disease can manifest as a progressive disabling arthropathy with consequences equally severe as rheumatoid arthritis. The additional burden of skin disease adds to rates of disability and impaired quality of life. Further, patients in secondary care manifest an increased morbidity and mortality, mainly owing to cardiovascular disease. Despite these findings, the subset of patients with relatively mild disease tends not to develop significant disability and is more likely to comprise men with oligoarticular disease. The socioeconomic impact of the disease is significant both in terms of work and home. Information on the impact of early diagnosis and treatment on outcome, according to phenotype, is needed to guide future policy. Further studies are required to define the true impact of psoriatic arthritis on disability and participation, as well as to sort out the unique contributions of psoriatic plaques and inflammatory joint disease.

Research agenda

- Most data currently come from secondary care studies. More data are required on community based studies.
- We need studies to examine the impact of early identification and treatment, if possible by phenotypic variants
- Further studies are needed to define the impact of psoriatic arthritis on disability and participation across the spectrum of disease.
- More data are needed on the specific contributions of skin, musculoskeletal and extraarticular manifestations to disability and quality of life

---

REFERENCES

1. Wright V. Psoriasis and arthritis. Ann Rheum Dis 1956;15:348–56.
2. Gladman DD, Stafford-Brady F, Chang CH, et al. Longitudinal study of clinical and radiological progression in psoriatic arthritis. J Rheumatol 1990;17(6):809–12.
3. Wright V. Psoriatic arthritis: a comparative study of rheumatoid arthritis and arthritis associated with psoriasis. Ann Rheum Dis 1961;20:123.
4. Roberts ME, Wright V, Hill AG, et al. Psoriatic arthritis: follow-up study. Ann Rheum Dis 1976;35:206–12.
5. Gladman DD, Shuckett R, Russell ML, et al. Psoriatic arthritis (PSA)–an analysis of 220 patients. Q J Med 1987;62(238):127–41.
6. Gladman DD, Farewell VT, Nadeau C. Clinical indicators of progression in psoriatic arthritis: multivariate relative risk model. J Rheumatol 1995;22(4):675–9.
7. Gladman DD, Farewell VT, Kopciuk KA, et al. HLA markers and progression in psoriatic arthritis. J Rheumatol 1998;25(4):730–3.

8. Husted JA, Tom BD, Farewell VT, et al. Description and prediction of physical functional disability in psoriatic arthritis: a longitudinal analysis using a Markov model approach. Arthritis Rheum 2005;53(3):404–9.
9. Kane D, Stafford L, Bresnihan B, et al. A prospective, clinical and radiological study of early psoriatic arthritis: an early synovitis clinic experience. Rheumatology (Oxford) 2003;42:1460–8.
10. Coates L, Helliwell PS, editors. Significant erosive change is found in early psoriatic arthritis. Paris: EULAR; 2014. Ann Rheum Dis.
11. Sokoll KB, Helliwell PS. Comparison of disability and quality of life in rheumatoid and psoriatic arthritis. J Rheumatol 2001;28(8):1842–6.
12. Shbeeb M, Uramoto KM, Gibson LE, et al. The epidemiology of psoriatic arthritis in Olmsted County, Minnesota, USA 1982–1991. J Rheumatol 2000;27:1247–50.
13. Wright V. Rheumatism and psoriasis; a re-evaluation. Am J Med 1959;27:454–62.
14. Husted JA, Gladman DD, Farewell VT, et al. Health-related quality of life of patients with psoriatic arthritis: a comparison with patients with rheumatoid arthritis. Arthritis Rheum 2001;45(2):151–8.
15. Khan M, Schentag C, Gladman DD. Clinical and radiological changes during psoriatic arthritis disease progression. J Rheumatol 2003;30(5):1022–6.
16. Hanly JG, Russell ML, Gladman DD. Psoriatic spondyloarthropathy: a long term prospective study. Ann Rheum Dis 1988;47(5):386–93.
17. Kammer GM, Sotar NA, Gibson DJ. Psoriatic arthritis; a clinical, immunoligic and HLA study of 100 patients. Semin Arthritis Rheum 1979;9:513–8.
18. Haroon M, Gallagher P, Fitzgerald O. Diagnostic delay of more than 6 months contributes to poor radiographic and functional outcome in psoriatic arthritis. Ann Rheum Dis 2015;74:1045–50.
19. Gladman DD, Thavaneswaran A, Chandran V, et al. Do patients with psoriatic arthritis who present early fare better than those presenting later in the disease? Ann Rheum Dis 2011;70(12):2152–4.
20. Theander E, Husmark T, Alenius GM, et al. Early psoriatic arthritis: short symptom duration, male gender and preserved physical functioning at presentation predict favourable outcome at 5 year follow up. Results from the Swedish Early Psoriatic Arthritis Register (SwePsA). Ann Rheum Dis 2014;73:407–13.
21. Gladman DD, Farewell VT. Progression in psoriatic arthritis: role of time varying clinical indicators. J Rheumatol 1999;26(11):2409–13.
22. Queiro-Silva R, Torre-Alonso JC, Tinture-Eguren T, et al. A polyarticular onset predicts erosive and deforming disease in psoriatic arthritis. Ann Rheum Dis 2003; 62(1):68–70.
23. Coates L, Moverley A, McParland L, et al. Effect of tight control of inflammation in early psoriatic arthritis (TICOPA): a multicentre, open-label, randomised controlled trial. Lancet 2014;383(Suppl 1):S36.
24. Brockbank JE, Stein M, Schentag CT, et al. Dactylitis in psoriatic arthritis: a marker for disease severity? Ann Rheum Dis 2005;64(2):188–90.
25. Williamson L, Dalbeth N, Dockerty JL, et al. Extended report: nail disease in psoriatic arthritis–clinically important, potentially treatable and often overlooked [see comment]. Rheumatology (Oxford) 2004;43(6):790–4.
26. Michet CJ, Mason TG, Mazlumzadeh M. Hip joint disease in psoriatic arthritis: risk factors and natural history. Ann Rheum Dis 2005;64(7):1068–70.
27. Espinoza LR, Vasey FB, Oh JH, et al. Association between HLA-BW38 and peripheral psoriatic arthritis. Arthritis Rheum 1978;21:72–5.
28. Gladman DD, Anhorn KAB, Schachter RK, et al. HLA antigens in psoriatic arthritis. J Rheumatol 1986;13:586–92.

29. Gladman DD, Farewell VT. The role of HLA antigens as indicators of disease progression in psoriatic arthritis. Multivariate relative risk model. Arthritis Rheum 1995;38(6):845–50.
30. Alenius GM, Jidell E, Nordmark L, et al. Disease manifestations and HLA antigens in psoriatic arthritis in northern Sweden. Clin Rheumatol 2002;21(5):357–62.
31. Balding J, Kane D, Livingstone W, et al. Cytokine gene polymorphisms - association with psoriatic arthritis susceptibility and severity. Arthritis Rheum 2003;48: 1408–13.
32. Jadon D, Tillett W, Wallis D, et al. Exploring ankylosing spondylitis-associated ERAP1, IL23R and IL12B gene polymorphisms in subphenotypes of psoriatic arthritis. Rheumatology (Oxford) 2013;52:261–6.
33. Korendowych E, Owen P, Ravindran J, et al. The clinical and genetic associations of anti-cyclic citrullinated peptide antibodies in psoriatic arthritis. Rheumatology (Oxford) 2005;44(8):1056–60.
34. Kimball AB, Gladman D, Gelfand JM, et al. National Psoriasis Foundation clinical consensus on psoriasis comorbidities and recommendations for screening. J Am Acad Dermatol 2008;58(6):1031–42.
35. Neimann AL, Shin DB, Wang X, et al. Prevalence of cardiovascular risk factors in patients with psoriasis. J Am Acad Dermatol 2006;55(5):829–35.
36. Husted JA, Thavaneswaran A, Chandran V, et al. Cardiovascular and other comorbidities in patients with psoriatic arthritis: a comparison with patients with psoriasis. Arthritis Care Res 2011;63(12):1729–35.
37. Jamnitski A, Symmons DPM, Peters M, et al. Cardiovascular comorbidities in patients with psoriatic arthritis: a systematic review. Ann Rheum Dis 2013;72: 211–6 [systematic review].
38. Boehncke WH, Boehncke S, Schön MP. Managing comorbid disease in patients with psoriasis. BMJ 2010;340:b5666.
39. Tam LS, Shang Q, Li EK, et al. Subclinical carotid atherosclerosis in patients with psoriatic arthritis. Arthritis Rheum 2008;59:1322–31.
40. Ogdie A, Yu Y, Haynes K, et al. Risk of major cardiovascular events in patients with psoriatic arthritis, psoriasis, and rheumatoid arthritis: a population based study. Ann Rheum Dis 2015;74:326–32.
41. Khraishi M, Aslanov R, Rampakakis E, et al. Prevalence of cardiovascular risk factors in patients with psoriatic arthritis. Clin Rheumatol 2014;33:1495–500.
42. Khraishi M, MacDonald D, Rampakakis E, et al. Prevalence of patient-reported comorbidities in early and established psoriatic arthritis cohorts. Clin Rheumatol 2014;30:877–85.
43. Hellgren K, Smedby K, Backlin C, et al. Ankylosing spondylitis, psoriatic arthritis, and risk of malignant lymphoma. Arthritis Rheum 2014;66:1282–90.
44. Wong K, Gladman DD, Husted J, et al. Mortality studies in psoriatic arthritis: results from a single outpatient clinic. I. Causes and risk of death. Arthritis Rheum 1997;40(10):1868–72.
45. Gladman DD, Farewell VT, Wong K, et al. Mortality studies in psoriatic arthritis: results from a single outpatient center. II. Prognostic indicators for death. Arthritis Rheum 1998;41(6):1103–10.
46. Ali Y, Tom BD, Schentag CT, et al. Improved survival in psoriatic arthritis with calendar time. Arthritis Rheum 2007;56(8):2708–14.
47. Peters MJ, van der Horst-Bruinsma IE, Dijkmans BA, et al. Cardiovascular risk profile of patients with spondylarthropathies, particularly ankylosing spondylitis and psoriatic arthritis [Review] [76 refs]. Semin Arthritis Rheum 2004;34(3): 585–92 [systematic review].

48. Ogdie A, Haynes K, Troxel AB, et al. Risk of mortality in patients with psoriatic arthritis, rheumatoid arthritis, and psoriasis: a longitudinal cohort study. Ann Rheum Dis 2014;73:149–53.
49. Lundberg L, Johannesson M, Silverdahl M, et al. Health-related quality of life in patients with psoriasis and atopic dermatitis measured with SF-36, DLQI and a subjective measure of disease activity. Acta Derm Venereol 2000;80(6):430–4.
50. Gelfand JM, Gladman DD, Mease PJ, et al. Epidemiology of psoriatic arthritis in the population of the United States. J Am Acad Dermatol 2005;53(4):573.
51. Lebwohl MG, Bachelez H, Barker JN, et al. Patient perspectives in the management of psoriasis: results from the population-based Multinational Assessment of Psoriasis and Psoriatic Arthritis Survey. J Am Acad Dermatol 2014;70:871–81.
52. Javitz HS, Ward MM, Farber E, et al. The direct cost of care for psoriasis and psoriatic arthritis in the United States. J Am Acad Dermatol 2002;46(6):850–60.
53. Poole C, Lebmeier M, Ara R, et al. Estimation of health care costs as a function of disease severity in people with psoriatic arthritis in the UK. Rheumatology (Oxford) 2010;49:1949–56.
54. Cortesi P, Scalone L, D'Angiolella L, et al. Systematic literature review on economic implications and pharmacoeconomic issues of psoriatic arthritis. Clin Exp Rheumatol 2012;30(Suppl 73):S126–31 [systematic review].
55. National Institute of Health and Care Excellence. Etanercept, infliximab and adalimumab for the treatment of psoriatic arthritis. NICE technology appraisal guidance 199; 2010.
56. Kaarela K, Lehtinen K, Luukkainen R. Work capacity of patients with inflammatory joint diseases. An eight-year follow-up study. Scand J Rheumatol 1987;16(6): 403–6.
57. Mau W, Listing J, Huscher D, et al. Employment across chronic inflammatory rheumatic diseases and comparison with the general population. J Rheumatol 2005;32(4):721–8.
58. Tillett W, de-Vries C, McHugh N. Work disability in psoriatic arthritis: a systematic review. Rheumatology (Oxford) 2012;51:275–83 [systematic review].
59. Kennedy M, Papneja A, Thavaneswaran A, et al. Prevalence and predictors of reduced work productivity in patients with psoriatic arthritis. Clin Exp Rheumatol 2014;32(3):342–8.
60. Tillett W, Shaddick G, Askari A, et al. Factors influencing work disability in psoriatic arthritis: first results from a large UK multicentre study. Rheumatology (Oxford) 2015;54(1):157–62.
61. Walsh J, McFadden M, Morgan M, et al. Work productivity loss and fatigue in psoriatic arthritis. J Rheumatol 2014;41:1670–4.

Imaging in Psoriatic Arthritis

René Panduro Poggenborg, MD, PhD[a,b,]*, Mikkel Østergaard, MD, PhD, DMSc[a,b], Lene Terslev, MD, PhD[a,b]

KEYWORDS

- Psoriatic arthritis • Radiography • Ultrasonography • MRI

KEY POINTS

- Radiography, ultrasonography (US), and MRI are integral parts of psoriatic arthritis (PsA) management, and are increasingly used in clinical trials.
- Computed tomography is the gold standard for evaluating bone changes in arthritis, but is rarely used owing to ionizing radiation.
- Conventional radiography allows fast, feasible, and relatively inexpensive assessment of the cumulative skeletal damage in PsA.
- US can visualize the peripheral joint and entheses involved in PsA in high resolution and can guide invasive procedures.
- MRI allows detailed visualization of all structures involved in PsA, and is sensitive for peripheral and axial disease manifestations.

INTRODUCTION

Psoriatic arthritis (PsA) is a chronic inflammatory joint disease associated with the skin disease psoriasis.[1] It is characterized by arthritis, enthesitis, and/or dactylitis; cutaneous involvement may be subtle. PsA was first described as a distinct rheumatic disease in the 1950s and subsequently in the 1970s as part of the concept of spondyloarthropathy (SpA).[2–4] Until the 1950s, an inflammatory arthritis occurring in the presence of psoriasis was believed to represent rheumatoid arthritis (RA) occurring coincidentally with psoriasis. However, PsA is usually seronegative for rheumatoid factor, and today, acknowledging that diagnosing PsA can be difficult owing to its

Disclosure Statement: The authors have nothing to disclose.
[a] Copenhagen Center for Arthritis Research, Center for Rheumatology and Spine Diseases, Rigshospitalet - Glostrup, Nordre Ringvej 57, Glostrup, Copenhagen DK-2600, Denmark; [b] Department of Clinical Medicine, Faculty of Health and Medical Sciences, University of Copenhagen, Blegdamsvej 3B, Copenhagen DK-2200, Denmark
* Corresponding author. Copenhagen Center for Arthritis Research, Center for Rheumatology and Spine Diseases, Rigshospitalet - Glostrup, Nordre Ringvej 57, Glostrup, Copenhagen DK-2600, Denmark.
E-mail address: poggenborg@dadlnet.dk

varying presentation, suspicion should be raised in a patient with psoriasis and signs of arthritis, for example, RA-like arthritis, asymmetrical arthritis, involvement of the distal interphalangeal (DIP) joints or inflammatory back pain in the absence of rheumatoid factor. Occasionally, arthritis may precede the development of psoriasis. Main differential diagnoses include RA, SpA including ankylosing spondylitis (AS), osteoarthritis (OA), gout, and fibromyalgia. A range of imaging methods can be used in suspected or established PsA and provide important information on the disease process.

Different imaging procedures are used in PsA, primarily conventional radiography, ultrasonography (US) and MRI, all having different virtues and limitations.[5] Radiography is the mainstay in imaging in inflammatory joint diseases, but is not able to detect the inflammatory changes that are the earliest disease manifestations. The reference method for assessing structural damage is computed tomography (CT), but it is rarely used in arthritides owing to ionizing radiation. US and MRI allow direct visualization of both early inflammatory and destructive joint changes.[6] Other imaging modalities, such as scintigraphy, PET, single photon emission CT, and dual-emission x-ray absorptiometry, are available, but their roles in the diagnosis and management of PsA are limited, and they are not described further.[7] Research into improved techniques and novel imaging methods such as wholebody MRI, various nuclear medicine techniques, and optical imaging are exciting future options.

CONVENTIONAL RADIOGRAPHY

Conventional radiography is the most widely used imaging method in PsA, and provides a record of the cumulative joint damage.[8] It has a very high spatial resolution, and shows the skeletal structure well, whereas visualization of soft tissue is rarely of value on top of clinical examination. Radiography is a fast, feasible, reliable, and relatively inexpensive procedure allowing assessment of a large number of joints. However, radiography is a 2-dimensional visualization of a 3-dimensional anatomy, resulting in suboptimal delineation of many parts of bone, owing to projectional superimposition, particularly in anatomically complex joints. Radiography of peripheral joints requires a small dose of ionizing radiation. For evaluating the axial skeleton the dose is greater, and this concern contributes to favoring MRI, particularly in younger patients.[9] Except that radiography has been digitalized over the last decades, no major technical advances have appeared in many years.

Peripheral Psoriatic Arthritis

Although PsA shows similarities with RA there are major differences, for example, in the type and site of lesions as well as the joints involved. Although RA is characterized by mainly osteodestructive lesions, PsA involves both osteodestructive and osteoproliferative manifestations (Fig. 1).[8] In particular, juxtaarticular new bone formation, appearing as ill-defined ossification near joint margins on radiography of the hand or foot, are characteristic, and this finding is an important part of the CASPAR classification criteria for PsA.[10] The presence of joint damage on radiography has been shown to be an independent predictor of radiographic progression.[11] Structural damage can be detected and progression followed by radiography, but radiography is less sensitive to erosive damage than MRI. In PsA trials, radiographic joint damage is an established, important outcome measure of structural progression, and several radiographic scoring methods have been developed, most often as modifications of RA methods.[8] The Sharp–van der Heijde modified scoring method for PsA is the

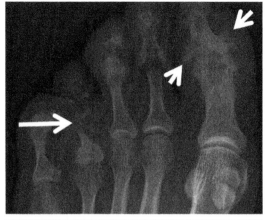

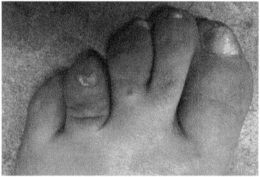

Fig. 1. Severe bone destruction (*long arrow*) and new bone proliferation (*short arrows*) in the foot as seen on radiography. Arthritis mutilans is seen in the fourth toe, and new bone formation at the interphalangeal joint of the first toe. Clinical photo shows shortening of the fourth toe, and swelling of the first and third toes. (*Courtesy of* Dr Sengül Seven; with permission.)

most frequently used method in PsA trials, and scores bone erosion and joint space narrowing (indirect measure of loss of cartilage) in hands and feet, although bone proliferation is not assessed. In contrast, the Ratingen method for PsA scores bone proliferation, in addition to scoring bone erosion.[12]

Axial Psoriatic Arthritis

For axial disease, no specific scoring systems for PsA exist, but scoring systems for AS can be applied.[13] For the sacroiliac joints (SIJ), the radiographic part of the modified New York 1984 criteria for AS may be applied to diagnose radiographic sacroiliitis, bearing in mind that MRI is more sensitive, whereas for the spine, the modified Stoke AS spine score is the generally preferred and most sensitive radiographic method for registration of structural damage progression in AS.[14,15]

A clear consensus on scoring method does not exist currently, but defining the optimal use of radiographic scores is on the research agenda of the European League Against Rheumatism (EULAR).[16] Despite its limitations, radiography of peripheral joints should generally be performed routinely when there is suspicion of PsA, because it may be of use in the differential diagnosis and provide a basis before more modern imaging, as US and/or MRI is performed. In case of suspicion of axial disease, the recent EULAR recommendations for the use of imaging in SpA recommends initial radiography of the SIJ, unless there is a short disease duration and/or young age, in which case MRI may be performed initially.[9] In the future, radiography will probably continue to play a central role in PsA, as a fast, easily accessible, and relatively inexpensive imaging method.

COMPUTED TOMOGRAPHY

CT visualizes calcified tissue with high resolution and can be considered the standard reference for assessing structural damage in inflammatory arthritides, owing to its excellent depiction of bone structures (**Fig. 2**).[17,18] By using multidetector CT, 2-dimensional images can be viewed in any given plane. However, CT is unable to detect active inflammatory lesions, and involves ionizing radiation.

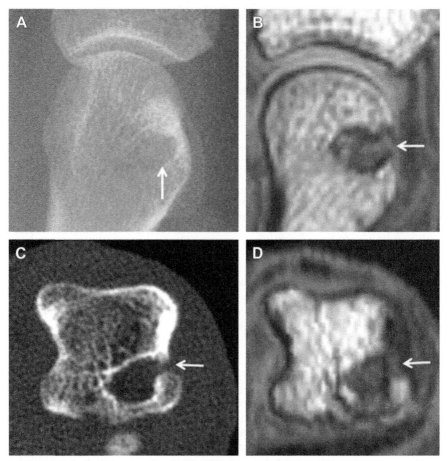

Fig. 2. Bone erosion (*arrows*) in the second metacarpal head, which was not scored on radiography (*A*), but scored on computed tomography (CT; *C*) and MRI (*B*, *D*). A bone lucency is seen on the radiograph (*A*), but because no cortical break is visible, the joint was scored as without erosions. Radiograph, posterioranterior view (*A*); CT, axial view (*C*); MRI (T1-weighted sequence, 0.6 T): coronal (*B*) and axial (*D*) views.

Peripheral Psoriatic Arthritis

Few scientific studies using CT in arthritides were available until fairly recently.[5] In peripheral joints, high-resolution CT and micro-CT have been applied in research for detailed examination of bone damages in hands with PsA.[19,20] Studies using micro-CT scans revealed Ω-shaped erosions in the metacarpophalangeal joints of PsA patients compared with RA, where the U-shaped erosions were noted.[21] Also, this technique documented new bone formation at entheses in both psoriasis patients without arthritis and PsA patients, a pattern that differed from that observed in OA.[22,23] However, in clinical practice CT has no routine role in examination of peripheral small joints in PsA.[24]

Axial Psoriatic Arthritis

In the SIJ, CT depicts bone erosion, sclerosis, and joint space alterations, including ankylosis, very well but has minimal role in clinical practice because of the ionizing radiation provided[25] and because MRI has been shown to be nearly as good in detecting SIJ bone changes.[26] In the spine, CT is not used routine, but is helpful if radiography is negative in a patient with PsA with suspected vertebral fracture.[9] Overall, CT is rarely used in PsA, but is an option for both axial and peripheral disease if radiography is inconclusive and MRI is unavailable or contraindicated.

ULTRASONOGRAPHY

US allows for high-resolution visualization of all structures involved in peripheral arthritis, and is sensitive for peripheral but not axial disease manifestations. Most attention has so far been given to the SpA group as a whole, because this patient group shows similar features in peripheral arthritis; however, in recent years studies have also been published solely on PsA patients. In the following, the US technique and findings in PsA are reviewed and the potential prognostic and diagnostic value and the use for monitoring disease activity are addressed. Finally, new potential techniques are discussed.

Ultrasound Technique and Findings

US is suitable for the evaluation of structural changes as well as changes in perfusion in joints, tendons and other soft tissues.[9,27] It can easily be performed by trained rheumatologists in relation to the clinical examination, and allows guidance of invasive procedures. US examinations are performed using B-mode US, most often in combination with color or power Doppler US. In Doppler US, color information is superimposed on the grayscale image displaying the reflection of the US by the moving erythrocytes thereby providing information about perfusion and tissue vascularization.[28] The Doppler choice depends on the most sensitive modality, which may vary from model to model.[29] In situations where the Doppler modality is less sensitive, US contrast agents in the form of microbubbles may be used to enhance the scattering reflection of erythrocytes by amplifying the Doppler signal, thereby increasing the sensitivity of the Doppler examination to low velocity flow. US has limited access in some areas and for some pathologies because it cannot penetrate bone. This limitation results in lower sensitivity than MRI and CT for diagnosing bone erosions and an inability to diagnose osteitis.[30] The main disadvantages of US versus MRI are that it is operator dependent and, for optimal information, there is a need for a trained investigator. Especially for Doppler US, there is also intermachine variability.[29]

Ultrasonography for Diagnosing Peripheral Involvement

In peripheral PsA, US is able to detect both joint involvement (synovitis and erosions) and extraarticular involvement like bursitis, tenosynovitis, and enthesitis. US seems to be more sensitive than clinical examination for the detection of synovitis, tenosynovitis, and enthesitis in patients with PsA.[31–33] In 2005, consensus definitions for US-related pathologies independent of disease were published, including definitions for synovitis, erosions, tenosynovitis, and enthesopathy,[34] enthesopathy was further elaborated in 2014, when The Outcome Measures in Rheumatology (OMERACT) US group published consensus-based definitions for US elementary lesions for enthesitis.[35]

Synovitis

The appearance of peripheral joint involvement in PsA is nonspecific and has not received as much attention as entheseal changes[36]; the diagnostic value is solely in detecting joint inflammation.[9] The occurrence of synovitis in proximal interphalangeal and metacarpophalangeal joints in PsA patients compared with RA patients are less frequent, although there is a predominance of synovitis in DIP joints in PsA.[37] This may not be the case in early PsA, where DIP involvement is found in fewer than 50% of patients investigated.[38,39] US can also detect subclinical synovitis, which is very common in early PsA, most frequently involving the wrist, knee, and/or metatarsophalangeal joints.[40] Similar findings have been found in psoriasis patients with joint symptoms, where up to 50% of clinically inactive joints had positive US findings for synovitis with or without Doppler activity.[41]

Enthesitis

Enthesitis is a very important feature in PsA, and has received most attention in US studies. The consensus-based definitions from 2014 for US enthesitis independent of SpA type was developed to ensure a greater degree of homogeneity in future clinical studies. The elementary lesions of enthesitis included presence of enthesophytes, calcifications, and erosions at the insertion site (chronic changes) and increased thickness, hypoechogenicity, and Doppler activity in the enthesis (inflammatory changes; **Fig. 3**).[35] The diagnostic value of Doppler findings at the enthesis for SpA and PsA is not elucidated fully. Enthesopathy changes such as enthesophytes and bone erosions may be found in weight-bearing entheses owing to mechanical stress.[42] Therefore, the focus for diagnosing SpA has mainly been on the inflammatory components. Doppler activity in grayscale enthesitis changes has been reported to be frequent in patients with SpA, and also specifically in PsA, as compared with patients with mechanical low back pain and healthy controls,[43,44] but Doppler findings in entheses may also be seen in RA patients, although with less severity and frequency.[45] Subclinical enthesitis is also present in PsA, and US may aid in the classification of the patients as having oligoarthritis or multiple joint involvement.[42]

Tenosynovitis and dactylitis

Some US studies have indicated that US flexor tenosynovitis is the major contributor to clinical dactylitis[46,47]; however, there is increasing evidence that other components, such as synovitis and diffuse soft tissue changes, may play a role (**Fig. 4**).[48,49] Further studies are needed to define properly the US features of dactylitis.

The Value of Ultrasound for Prediction of Development of Psoriatic Arthritis

The role of US for prognosticating PsA is not established. Entheseal involvement in patients with psoriasis, but without clinical PsA, suggests that enthesitis may be a predictor of development of PsA.[50,51] Enthesopathy seems to be associated especially with nail involvement, and this may indicate that nail disease is linked to the expression

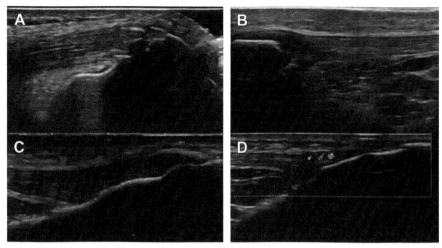

Fig. 3. Ultrasonography of the knee. (*A*) Quadriceps insertion with calcifications and erosions in the patella. (*B*) Proximal patella tendon insertion with thickened enthesis and loss of fibrillar structure. (*C*) Distal patella tendon insertion with thickened enthesis and calcification. (*D*) Distal patella tendon insertion with Doppler activity in the insertion.

of enthesitis, including subclinical disease.[52] In a cohort of patients with suspected SpA, Doppler activity in at least 1 enthesis provided good predictive value for later diagnosing the patient with SpA.[53]

Monitoring Psoriatic Arthritis by Ultrasonography

Most studies, which aim to monitor treatment response, have applied semiquantitative scoring systems for grayscale and/or Doppler changes. The scoring systems used for joint involvement are either those used in monitoring RA treatment,[54] or semiquantitative scores developed by the respective authors.[55,56] Disease-modifying antirheumatic drug–resistant knee arthritis in both RA and PsA has responded well to treatment with tumor necrosis factor-α blocker, with a significant decrease in both grayscale and Doppler semiquantitative scores after 12 months. There was no difference in treatment response between RA and PsA patients.[55] For monitoring entheseal involvement in PsA, different combinations of entheses and elementary lesions have been suggested but no consensus exists on a single scoring system. The first to propose a grayscale scoring system of lower limb enthesitis were Balint and colleagues,[57] and since then several other scoring systems have been proposed that also includes Doppler US.[43,58,59] More work is needed to develop standardized and responsive US outcome measures in PsA.

Ultrasound for Diagnosing and Monitoring Axial Involvement

The use of US for axial involvement in PsA is limited, primarily because of its inability to penetrate bone. Therefore, US cannot detect osteitis changes, but it may be used to identify the SIJ. It is, however, a deep joint and US can only visualize the superficial, posterior part of the joint. Visualization may be hampered further in obese patients. Although it has been reported that contrast-enhanced Doppler US had a high negative predictive value for sacroiliitis[60] it has no role in diagnosing SIJ involvement in PsA patients but may be used for guiding SIJ injections.[61]

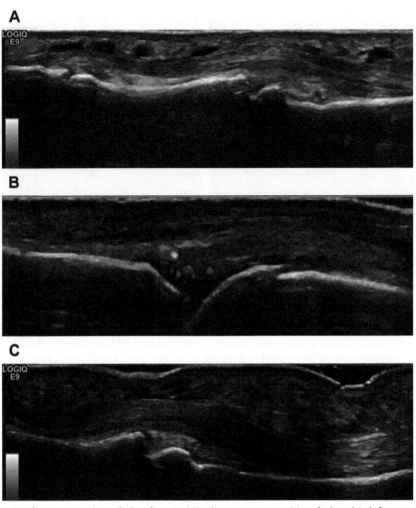

Fig. 4. Ultrasonography of the finger. (*A*) Flexor tenosynovitis of the third finger. (*B*) Minimal synovitis in third metacarpophalangeal joint. (*C*) Dactylitis with subcutaneous tissue changes, minimal flexor tenosynovitis, and minimal proximal interphalangeal joint synovial hypertrophy.

New Techniques in Ultrasonography

Recently, there has been a considerable technological development with high-frequency probes and high-frequency Doppler, which have made it possible to improve the resolution of the grayscale image and the sensitivity to low velocity flow. Some of the new probes allow elastosonography or 3-dimensional US. Elastoso-nography is a new technique for assessing tissue elasticity, and has a potential application in evaluation of tendon stiffness. Three-dimensional US is a new US modality and seems to be promising in the assessment of joint pathology in inflammatory diseases. One of the advantages may be related to the operator independence owing to image acquisition of infinite 3-dimensional datasets obtained by automated trans-ducer sweeping. Three-dimensional US has been shown to demonstrate enthesitis pathology well,[62] and seems to improve interobserver reliability in the assessment of synovitis and bone erosions.[63] Further studies are needed to validate this technique in PsA. Finally, image fusion allows simultaneous comparison and mapping of US images onto other preacquired images, for example, MRI.

MRI

Conventional MRI allows high-resolution visualization of all structures involved in arthritis, and is sensitive for peripheral and axial disease manifestations. However, MRI in PsA has received less attention than in RA and most knowledge is derived from studies of broader groups of SpA patients, including a limited number of patients with PsA.[64]

MRI Technique and Findings

For visualizing inflammation and structural damage, T1-weighted sequences (signal mainly reflecting fat content and presence of gadolinium contrast) in 1 (axial joints) or 2 (peripheral joints) planes, supplemented by a T2-weighted, fat-suppressed or short tau inversion recovery sequence (signal mainly reflecting water content) in 2 planes are generally performed.[7,65] Additional acquisition of T1-weighted sequences after intravenous injection of gadolinium-containing contrast agent can aid identification of inflamed tissue in peripheral joints, and can be done with or without fat suppression. A general agreement on which joints to examine with MRI to assess PsA activity and damage has not been established.

The main inflammatory and structural lesions visualized on MRI in peripheral PsA are synovitis, enthesitis, tenosynovitis, periarticular inflammation, bone marrow edema, bone erosion, and bone proliferation.[64,65] Consensus MRI definitions and suggestions concerning appropriate MRI sequences for use in hands with PsA were published in 2009 by the OMERACT MRI Arthritis Working Group.[65] Administration of a contrast agent is optimal for assessment of synovitis and tenosynovitis in peripheral joints, but can be omitted if the aim is to detect bone marrow edema, bone erosions, and bone proliferations.[65]

The main inflammatory and structural lesions visualized on MRI in axial PsA are bone marrow edema/osteitis, enthesitis, fat infiltration, bone erosion, bone proliferation, and ankylosis. No PsA-specific MRI definitions are published for axial disease, but findings and image sequences used in SpA, are available.[66,67] Axial enthesitis on MRI lacks a widely accepted definition in PsA and SpA; however, it may be characterized as peripheral enthesitis[65] or as a high signal on short tau inversion recovery sequences in the marrow at the entheseal insertion (or at surrounding tissue).[68,69]

MRI for Investigating Pathogenesis in Psoriatic Arthritis

Enthesitis is, in addition to the soft tissue changes also seen on US, found to be associated with perientheseal bone marrow edema.[70] Imaging studies have increased the understanding of PsA, and for example, McGonagle and colleagues[71] have proposed that synovitis is a secondary feature to enthesitis. Early MRI studies of PsA patients with dactylitic fingers have concluded that dactylitis is mainly owing to flexor tenosynovitis, but a recent systematic review conclude that it may be caused by inflammation of multiple structures in the fingers and toes, that is, also entheses, synovium, and subcutaneous tissue.[72,73] In the DIP joints, diffuse inflammation on MRI has been observed to extend to the nail bed, and an association between enthesitis, dactylitis, and nail involvement has been proposed.[74,75] An MRI study of nails in patients with skin psoriasis found characteristic nail involvement in all patients, and the authors suggested that onychopathy is preceding DIP joint damage in PsA, and that MRI of nails is of diagnostic value in undifferentiated SpA.[76] These findings have not been substantiated further. Future research using improved imaging techniques, such as microscopy high-resolution MRI coils, is needed, including studies on peripheral enthesitis, which may become a priority of the OMERACT MRI Arthritis Working Group.[77]

MRI for Diagnosing Peripheral Psoriatic Arthritis

In symptomatic PsA, synovitis, tenosynovitis, and bone marrow edema are frequent findings.[37,78,79] Inflammatory and destructive changes do not have PsA-specific features, and can involve any joint.[64] However, MRI findings may be valuable for discriminating between diagnoses. Bone marrow edema in PsA (**Fig. 5**) is often located close to the entheses, in contrast with RA, where bone marrow edema often is located close to the capsular attachments, and in OA, where bone marrow lesions are located mainly close to subchondral areas.[80] Bone erosions are seen more often adjacent to collateral ligament insertions in PsA, whereas erosions are more often located centrally in OA.[81] A comparative MRI study of the hand and wrist in PsA and RA patients found bone erosions were more frequent in RA, and periostitis more frequent in PsA.[82] Diaphyseal bone marrow edema and/or enthesitis is much more common in PsA than RA.[83] A few studies of MRI findings in psoriasis patients without arthritis have been published,[84–86] and all found higher frequency of arthritic and entheseal changes in patients than in controls. These findings suggest that MRI can detect subclinical arthritis.

MRI for Prognosticating Peripheral Psoriatic Arthritis

Based on a cross-sectional MRI study of erosive PsA patients including patients with the aggressive arthritis mutilans phenotype, a close relation between erosions and bone marrow edema was found, and this suggests that bone marrow edema is a "fore-runner" of structural joint damage in PsA.[87] In a 48-week longitudinal study of PsA patients, bone marrow edema detected by MRI was related to subsequent erosive progression as detected by CT.[18]

MRI for Monitoring Peripheral Psoriatic Arthritis

Few studies are available on the use of MRI for monitoring joint disease in PsA.[18,88–90] In a 6-month study of PsA patients receiving adalimumab, MRI of a wrist or knee showed significant improvements in both clinical measures and in bone marrow edema and effusion, but not in synovitis.[91] In another 6-month follow-up study of psoriatic dactylitis, both clinical and MRI improvements were found, but the relationship between clinical and MRI scores was weak.[92] MRI allows quantitative (contrast uptake rate), qualitative (presence/absence), and semiquantitative (scoring) evaluation of joint disease. The OMERACT MRI in Arthritis Working Group has developed an MRI scoring system for peripheral PsA in the hand, and, recently, the forefoot: the PsA MRI Scoring system (PsAMRIS), using the RA MRI Scoring system RAMRIS as template.[65,93,94] The PsAMRIS is the most validated scoring system for use in PsA, and offers good intrareader and interreader reliability, and sensitivity to change for inflammatory parameters (Glinatsi D, Bird P, Gandjbakhch F, et al: Validation of the OMERACT Psoriatic Arthritis Magnetic Resonance Imaging Score (PsAMRIS) for the hand and foot in a randomized placebo-controlled trial. J Rheumatol. Submitted for publication).[65,94] The system can be used in clinical studies. There is no consensus as to assessment methodology is most useful in clinical practice. In the future, a PsA imaging atlas could further improve the utility, because training and calibration of readers is recommended.[77,95]

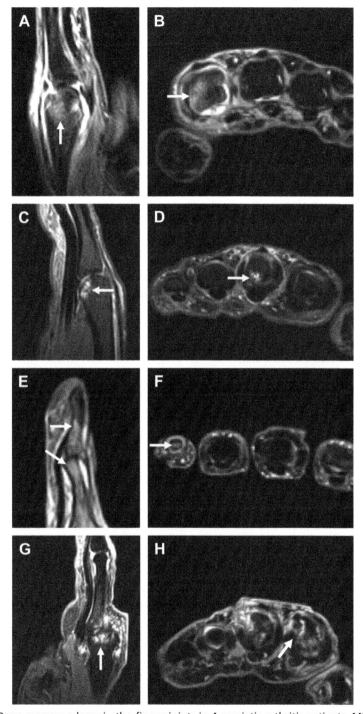

Fig. 5. Bone marrow edema in the finger joints in 4 psoriatic arthritis patients. MRI (short tau inversion recovery sequence, 0.6 T) is in sagittal (*A, C, E,* and *G*) and axial (*B, D, F,* and *H*) slice planes. Bone marrow edema (*arrows*) is visualized at the second metacarpal head (*A, B*), third metacarpal head (*C, D*), the fifth distal interphalangeal joint (*G*) and phalangeal base (*F*), and the second metacarpal head (*G, H*).

MRI in Axial Psoriatic Arthritis

Axial PsA can affect the SIJ and/or the spine.[9] In the spine, inflammatory changes, visualized as bone marrow edema or soft tissue edema/enthesitis, can characteristically be seen at the anterior and posterior corners of the vertebral bodies, and at the costovertebral, facet and costotransverse joints (**Fig. 6**). An erosive discovertebral lesion (Andersson lesion) is seen in approximately 6% of PsA and AS patients, and can be the first sign of PsA.[96] In the SIJ, inflammation is seen as bone marrow edema (see **Fig. 6**), but also soft tissue inflammation at entheses occurs frequently.[66,97] Few studies are available in axial PsA and knowledge mainly originates from SpA studies. However, findings are overall similar to findings in AS, where MRI has proven sensitive for detection of sacroiliitis and spondylitis, although more frequently asymmetric, and clinical findings in PsA is only weakly associated with sacroiliitis on MRI.[98–100] MRI signs of sacroiliac osteitis correlate with cellularity on corresponding biopsies.[101] A study from 2004 examining PsA in a rheumatology outpatient clinic found sacroiliitis

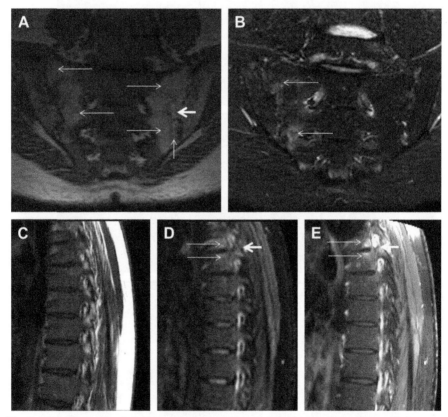

Fig. 6. MRI of sacroiliac joints (*A*, semicoronal T1-weighted image; *B*, semicoronal short tau inversion recovery [STIR]) and thoracic vertebrae 6 to 12 (*C*, sagittal T1-weighted image; *D*, sagittal STIR; *E*, sagittal postcontrast T1-weighted image with fat suppression) of patient with axial PsA. Sacroiliac joint images show bone marrow edema (*arrows in B*), massive fat infiltration (*long arrows in A*), backfill (*short arrow in A*), and ankylosis (*thick arrow in A*). Spine images show bone marrow edema (*arrows in D*) and postcontrast enhancement (*arrows in E*) in the costovertebral joint (*thin arrows in D and E*) and in facet joint (*thick arrows in D and E*) at the Th6/Th7 level.

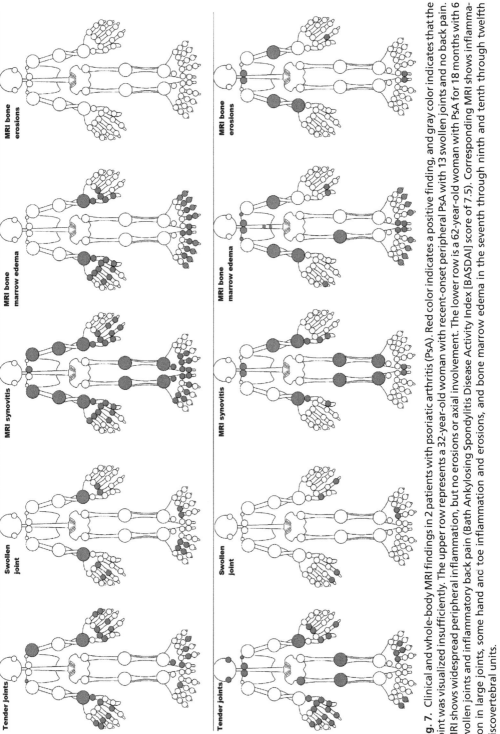

Fig. 7. Clinical and whole-body MRI findings in 2 patients with psoriatic arthritis (PsA). Red color indicates a positive finding, and gray color indicates that the joint was visualized insufficiently. The upper row represents a 32-year-old woman with recent-onset peripheral PsA with 13 swollen joints and no back pain. MRI shows widespread peripheral inflammation, but no erosions or axial involvement. The lower row is a 62-year-old woman with PsA for 18 months with 6 swollen joints and inflammatory back pain (Bath Ankylosing Spondylitis Disease Activity Index [BASDAI] score of 7.5). Corresponding MRI shows inflammation in large joints, some hand and toe inflammation and erosions, and bone marrow edema in the seventh through ninth and tenth through twelfth discovertebral units.

on MRI was common (seen in 38%).[99] A recent study reported that axial inflammation on MRI was significantly related to HLA-B27 positivity in PsA.[102] More MRI research is needed on separate PsA populations with axial disease, for example, more disease-modifying antirheumatic drug studies in MRI-positive early axial PsA, as recommended by EULAR.[16]

New MRI Methods

New MRI methods, such as dynamic contrast-enhanced (DCE)-MRI and whole-body MRI, have supplemented conventional MRI for research in arthritides. DCE-MRI allows quantification of contrast enhancement in a region of interest selected by the investigator.[103] A potential advantage of DCE-MRI is that it is possible to acquire semiautomatic recognition of the pattern of enhancement, and thereby decrease the observer dependence. Most DCE-MRI studies include RA patients, and report that DCE-MRI can measure the inflammatory activity, and correlates with histology.[88,101,104–106] Limited data from PsA patients are available, but in a small DCE-MRI study of synovitis in the wrists, no difference between matched PsA and RA patients was found. However, all PsA patients had significant higher enhancement than healthy subjects.[107]

Whole-body MRI is a novel imaging method that allows MRI of the whole body in 1 scanning session, but at the cost of lower image resolution than conventional MRI. Radiologists have applied whole-body MRI for screening for bone marrow malignancies and systemic muscle diseases.[108] In a proof-of-concept study testing whether whole-body MRI is feasible, the scans were well-tolerated by PsA patients, and the most often detected pathology was enthesitis.[109] Recently, 7 clinical enthesitis indices were examined by whole-body MRI in patients with PsA, axial SpA and healthy subjects and compared with entheseal tenderness.[110] A moderate agreement between MRI enthesitis and clinical examination was found, suggesting a role for whole-body MRI in detecting subclinical inflammation. Furthermore, a new whole-body MRI enthesitis index was proposed as a potential additional tool for assessing disease activity. An exciting possibility of whole-body MRI is the assessment of the distribution of inflammation and structural damage in the entire body (**Fig. 7**), and the possibility of providing global scores of inflammation and damage in peripheral and axial joints. Compared with healthy subjects, PsA patients have significantly higher global bone marrow edema scores as assessed by whole-body MRI, encouraging further development and longitudinal testing of this technique.[111]

SUMMARY

Various imaging modalities are useful for multiple reasons, including establishing or confirming the diagnosis, determining extent of disease, monitoring changes in inflammation and structural damage, assessing therapeutic efficacy, prognostication, and identifying complications of disease or treatment. In this article, we have provided an overview of the status, strengths, and limitations of different imaging modalities in PsA focusing on conventional radiography, US, and MRI. Although much evidence has been established in the last years, further studies are needed to fully clarify the potential and the role of modern imaging in PsA trials and clinical practice.

REFERENCES

1. Moll JM, Wright V. Psoriatic arthritis. Semin Arthritis Rheum 1973;3(1):55–78.
2. Moll JM. Psoriatic arthritis. Br J Rheumatol 1984;23(4):241–4.

3. Moll JM, Wright V. Familial occurrence of psoriatic arthritis. Ann Rheum Dis 1973;32(3):181–201.

4. Moll JM, Haslock I, Macrae IF, et al. Associations between ankylosing spondylitis, psoriatic arthritis, Reiter's disease, the intestinal arthropathies, and Behcet's syndrome. Medicine (Baltimore) 1974;53(5):343–64.

5. Ory PA, Gladman DD, Mease PJ. Psoriatic arthritis and imaging. Ann Rheum Dis 2005;64(Suppl 2):ii55–7.

6. Østergaard M, Pedersen SJ, Dohn UM. Imaging in rheumatoid arthritis–status and recent advances for magnetic resonance imaging, ultrasonography, computed tomography and conventional radiography. Best Pract Res Clin Rheumatol 2008;22(6):1019–44.

7. Tan AL, McGonagle D. Imaging of seronegative spondyloarthritis. Best Pract Res Clin Rheumatol 2008;22(6):1045–59.

8. van der Heijde D, Østergaard M. Assessment of disease activity and damage in inflammatory arthritis. In: Bijlsma JWJ, editor. The EULAR compendium on rheumatic diseases. London: BMJ publishing Group; 2009. p. 182–201.

9. Mandl P, Navarro-Compan V, Terslev L, et al. EULAR recommendations for the use of imaging in the diagnosis and management of spondyloarthritis in clinical practice. Ann Rheum Dis 2015;74(7):1327–39.

10. Taylor W, Gladman D, Helliwell P, et al. Classification criteria for psoriatic arthritis: development of new criteria from a large international study. Arthritis Rheum 2006;54(8):2665–73.

11. Gladman DD, Mease PJ, Choy EH, et al. Risk factors for radiographic progression in psoriatic arthritis: subanalysis of the randomized controlled trial ADEPT. Arthritis Res Ther 2010;12(3):R113.

12. van der Heijde D, Sharp J, Wassenberg S, et al. Psoriatic arthritis imaging: a review of scoring methods. Ann Rheum Dis 2005;64(Suppl 2):ii61–4.

13. Gladman DD. Axial disease in psoriatic arthritis. Curr Rheumatol Rep 2007;9(6):455–60.

14. van der Heijde D, Landewe R. Selection of a method for scoring radiographs for ankylosing spondylitis clinical trials, by the Assessment in Ankylosing Spondylitis Working Group and OMERACT. J Rheumatol 2005;32(10):2048–9.

15. van der Linden S, Valkenburg HA, Cats A. Evaluation of diagnostic criteria for ankylosing spondylitis. A proposal for modification of the New York criteria. Arthritis Rheum 1984;27(4):361–8.

16. Gossec L, Smolen JS, Gaujoux-Viala C, et al. European League Against Rheumatism recommendations for the management of psoriatic arthritis with pharmacological therapies. Ann Rheum Dis 2012;71(1):4–12.

17. Dohn UM, Ejbjerg BJ, Court-Payen M, et al. Are bone erosions detected by magnetic resonance imaging and ultrasonography true erosions? A comparison with computed tomography in rheumatoid arthritis metacarpophalangeal joints. Arthritis Res Ther 2006;8(4):R110.

18. Poggenborg RP, Wiell C, Boyesen P, et al. No overall damage progression despite persistent inflammation in adalimumab-treated psoriatic arthritis patients: results from an investigator-initiated 48-week comparative magnetic resonance imaging, computed tomography and radiography trial. Rheumatology (Oxford) 2014;53(4):746–56.

19. Finzel S, Kraus S, Schmidt S, et al. Bone anabolic changes progress in psoriatic arthritis patients despite treatment with methotrexate or tumour necrosis factor inhibitors. Ann Rheum Dis 2013;72(7):1176–81.

20. Poggenborg RP, Bird P, Boonen A, et al. Pattern of bone erosion and bone proliferation in psoriatic arthritis hands: a high-resolution computed tomography and radiography follow-up study during adalimumab therapy. Scand J Rheumatol 2014;43(3):202–8.

21. Finzel S, Englbrecht M, Engelke K, et al. A comparative study of periarticular bone lesions in rheumatoid arthritis and psoriatic arthritis. Ann Rheum Dis 2011;70(1):122–7.

22. Finzel S, Sahinbegovic E, Kocijan R, et al. Inflammatory bone spur formation in psoriatic arthritis is different from bone spur formation in hand osteoarthritis. Arthritis Rheum 2014;66(11):2968–75.

23. Simon D, Faustini F, Kleyer A, et al. Analysis of periarticular bone changes in patients with cutaneous psoriasis without associated psoriatic arthritis. Ann Rheum Dis 2015. [Epub ahead of print].

24. Grigoryan M, Roemer FW, Mohr A, et al. Imaging in spondyloarthropathies. Curr Rheumatol Rep 2004;6(2):102–9.

25. van der Heijde D, Østergaard M. Assessment of disease activity and damage in inflammatory arthritis. In: Bijlsma WJ, Burmester GR, Faarvang KL, editors. EULAR textbook on rheumatic diseases. London: BMJ Publishing Group Ltd; 2009. p. 35.

26. Puhakka KB, Jurik AG, Egund N, et al. Imaging of sacroiliitis in early seronegative spondylarthropathy. Assessment of abnormalities by MR in comparison with radiography and CT. Acta Radiol 2003;44(2):218–29.

27. Grassi W, Salaffi F, Filippucci E. Ultrasound in rheumatology. Best Pract Res Clin Rheumatol 2005;19(3):467–85.

28. Torp-Pedersen ST, Terslev L. Settings and artefacts relevant in colour/power Doppler ultrasound in rheumatology. Ann Rheum Dis 2008;67(2):143–9.

29. Torp-Pedersen S, Christensen R, Szkudlarek M, et al. Power and color Doppler ultrasound settings for inflammatory flow: impact on scoring of disease activity in patients with rheumatoid arthritis. Arthritis Rheum 2015;67(2):386–95.

30. Dohn UM, Terslev L, Szkudlarek M, et al. Detection, scoring and volume assessment of bone erosions by ultrasonography in rheumatoid arthritis: comparison with CT. Ann Rheum Dis 2013;72(4):530–4.

31. Delle SA, Riente L, Filippucci E, et al. Ultrasound imaging for the rheumatologist XXVI. Sonographic assessment of the knee in patients with psoriatic arthritis. Clin Exp Rheumatol 2010;28(2):147–52.

32. Galluzzo E, Lischi DM, Taglione E, et al. Sonographic analysis of the ankle in patients with psoriatic arthritis. Scand J Rheumatol 2000;29(1):52–5.

33. Milosavljevic J, Lindqvist U, Elvin A. Ultrasound and power Doppler evaluation of the hand and wrist in patients with psoriatic arthritis. Acta Radiol 2005; 46(4):374–85.

34. Wakefield RJ, Balint PV, Szkudlarek M, et al. Musculoskeletal ultrasound including definitions for ultrasonographic pathology. J Rheumatol 2005;32(12): 2485–7.

35. Terslev L, Naredo E, Iagnocco A, et al. Defining enthesitis in spondyloarthritis by ultrasound: results of a Delphi process and of a reliability reading exercise. Arthritis Care Res (Hoboken) 2014;66(5):741–8.

36. Poggenborg RP, Terslev L, Pedersen SJ, et al. Recent advances in imaging in psoriatic arthritis. Ther Adv Musculoskelet Dis 2011;3(1):43–53.

37. Wiell C, Szkudlarek M, Hasselquist M, et al. Ultrasonography, magnetic resonance imaging, radiography, and clinical assessment of inflammatory and

destructive changes in fingers and toes of patients with psoriatic arthritis. Arthritis Res Ther 2007;9(6):R119.

38. Bonifati C, Elia F, Francesconi F, et al. The diagnosis of early psoriatic arthritis in an outpatient dermatological centre for psoriasis. J Eur Acad Dermatol Venereol 2012;26(5):627–33.

39. Kane D, Stafford L, Bresnihan B, et al. A prospective, clinical and radiological study of early psoriatic arthritis: an early synovitis clinic experience. Rheumatology (Oxford) 2003;42(12):1460–8.

40. Freeston JE, Coates LC, Nam JL, et al. Is there subclinical synovitis in early psoriatic arthritis? A clinical comparison with gray-scale and power Doppler ultrasound. Arthritis Care Res (Hoboken) 2014;66(3):432–9.

41. Naredo E, Moller I, De ME, et al. High prevalence of ultrasonographic synovitis and enthesopathy in patients with psoriasis without psoriatic arthritis: a prospective case-control study. Rheumatology (Oxford) 2011;50(10):1838–48.

42. Freeston JE, Coates LC, Helliwell PS, et al. Is there subclinical enthesitis in early psoriatic arthritis? A clinical comparison with power Doppler ultrasound. Arthritis Care Res (Hoboken) 2012;64(10):1617–21.

43. D'Agostino MA, Said-Nahal R, Hacquard-Bouder C, et al. Assessment of peripheral enthesitis in the spondylarthropathies by ultrasonography combined with power Doppler: a cross-sectional study. Arthritis Rheum 2003;48(2):523–33.

44. Aydin SZ, Ash ZR, Tinazzi I, et al. The link between enthesitis and arthritis in psoriatic arthritis: a switch to a vascular phenotype at insertions may play a role in arthritis development. Ann Rheum Dis 2013;72(6):992–5.

45. Iagnocco A, Spadaro A, Marchesoni A, et al. Power Doppler ultrasonographic evaluation of enthesitis in psoriatic arthritis. A multi-center study. Joint Bone Spine 2012;79(3):324–5.

46. Kane D, Greaney T, Bresnihan B, et al. Ultrasonography in the diagnosis and management of psoriatic dactylitis. J Rheumatol 1999;26(8):1746–51.

47. Gutierrez M, Filippucci E, De Angelis R, et al. A sonographic spectrum of psoriatic arthritis: "the five targets". Clin Rheumatol 2010;29(2):133–42.

48. Fournie B, Margarit-Coll N, Champetier de Ribes TL, et al. Extrasynovial ultrasound abnormalities in the psoriatic finger. Prospective comparative power-doppler study versus rheumatoid arthritis. Joint Bone Spine 2006;73(5):527–31.

49. Olivieri I, Barozzi L, Favaro L, et al. Dactylitis in patients with seronegative spondylarthropathy. Assessment by ultrasonography and magnetic resonance imaging. Arthritis Rheum 1996;39(9):1524–8.

50. Gisondi P, Tinazzi I, El-Dalati G, et al. Lower limb enthesopathy in patients with psoriasis without clinical signs of arthropathy: a hospital-based case-control study. Ann Rheum Dis 2008;67(1):26–30.

51. Gutierrez M, Filippucci E, De AR, et al. Subclinical entheseal involvement in patients with psoriasis: an ultrasound study. Semin Arthritis Rheum 2010;40(5):407–12.

52. Ash ZR, Tinazzi I, Gallego CC, et al. Psoriasis patients with nail disease have a greater magnitude of underlying systemic subclinical enthesopathy than those with normal nails. Ann Rheum Dis 2012;71(4):553–6.

53. D'Agostino MA, Aegerter P, Bechara K, et al. How to diagnose spondyloarthritis early? Accuracy of peripheral enthesitis detection by power Doppler ultrasonography. Ann Rheum Dis 2011;70(8):1433–40.

54. Schafer VS, Fleck M, Kellner H, et al. Evaluation of the novel ultrasound score for large joints in psoriatic arthritis and ankylosing spondylitis: six month experience in daily clinical practice. BMC Musculoskelet Disord 2013;14:358.

55. Fiocco U, Ferro F, Vezzu M, et al. Rheumatoid and psoriatic knee synovitis: clinical, grey scale, and power Doppler ultrasound assessment of the response to etanercept. Ann Rheum Dis 2005;64(6):899–905.

56. Solivetti FM, Elia F, Teoli M, et al. Role of contrast-enhanced ultrasound in early diagnosis of psoriatic arthritis. Dermatology 2010;220(1):25–31.

57. Balint PV, Kane D, Wilson H, et al. Ultrasonography of entheseal insertions in the lower limb in spondyloarthropathy. Ann Rheum Dis 2002;61(10):905–10.

58. Alcalde M, Acebes J, González-Hombrado L, et al. A sonographic enthesitic index of lower limbs is a valuable tool in the assessment of ankylosing spondylitis. Ann Rheum Dis 2007;66(8):1015–9.

59. de Miguel E, Cobo T, Munoz-Fernández S, et al. Validity of enthesis ultrasound assessment in spondyloarthropathy. Ann Rheum Dis 2009;68(2):169–74.

60. Klauser A, Halpern EJ, Frauscher F, et al. Inflammatory low back pain: high negative predictive value of contrast-enhanced color Doppler ultrasound in the detection of inflamed sacroiliac joints. Arthritis Rheum 2005;53(3):440–4.

61. Klauser A, De ZT, Feuchtner G, et al. Feasibility of ultrasound-guided sacroiliac joint injection considering sonoanatomic landmarks at two different levels in cadavers and patients. Arthritis Rheum 2008;59(11):1618–24.

62. Iagnocco A, Riente L, Delle SA, et al. Ultrasound imaging for the rheumatologist. XXII. Achilles tendon involvement in spondyloarthritis. A multi-centre study using high frequency volumetric probe. Clin Exp Rheumatol 2009;27(4):547–51.

63. Naredo E, Moller I, Acebes C, et al. Three-dimensional volumetric ultrasonography. Does it improve reliability of musculoskeletal ultrasound? Clin Exp Rheumatol 2010;28(1):79–82.

64. McQueen F, Lassere M, Østergaard M. Magnetic resonance imaging in psoriatic arthritis: a review of the literature. Arthritis Res Ther 2006;8(2):207.

65. Østergaard M, McQueen F, Wiell C, et al. The OMERACT psoriatic arthritis magnetic resonance imaging scoring system (PsAMRIS): definitions of key pathologies, suggested MRI sequences, and preliminary scoring system for PsA Hands. J Rheumatol 2009;36(8):1816–24.

66. Sieper J, Rudwaleit M, Baraliakos X, et al. The Assessment of SpondyloArthritis international Society (ASAS) handbook: a guide to assess spondyloarthritis. Ann Rheum Dis 2009;68(Suppl 2):ii1–44.

67. Rudwaleit M, Jurik AG, Hermann KG, et al. Defining active sacroiliitis on magnetic resonance imaging (MRI) for classification of axial spondyloarthritis: a consensual approach by the ASAS/OMERACT MRI group. Ann Rheum Dis 2009;68(10):1520–7.

68. Eshed I, Bollow M, McGonagle DG, et al. MRI of enthesitis of the appendicular skeleton in spondyloarthritis. Ann Rheum Dis 2007;66(12):1553–9.

69. Althoff CE, Sieper J, Song IH, et al. Active inflammation and structural change in early active axial spondyloarthritis as detected by whole-body MRI. Ann Rheum Dis 2013;72(6):967–73.

70. McGonagle D. Imaging the joint and enthesis: insights into pathogenesis of psoriatic arthritis. Ann Rheum Dis 2005;64(Suppl 2):ii58–60.

71. McGonagle DG, Helliwell P, Veale D. Enthesitis in psoriatic disease. Dermatology 2012;225(2):100–9.

72. Bakewell CJ, Olivieri I, Aydin SZ, et al. Ultrasound and magnetic resonance imaging in the evaluation of psoriatic dactylitis: status and perspectives. J Rheumatol 2013;40(12):1951–7.

73. Olivieri I, Salvarani C, Cantini F, et al. Fast spin echo-T2-weighted sequences with fat saturation in dactylitis of spondylarthritis. No evidence of entheseal involvement of the flexor digitorum tendons. Arthritis Rheum 2002;46(11): 2964–7.

74. Tan AL, Fukuba E, Halliday NA, et al. High-resolution MRI assessment of dactylitis in psoriatic arthritis shows flexor tendon pulley and sheath-related enthesitis. Ann Rheum Dis 2015;74(1):185–9.

75. Tan AL, Grainger AJ, Tanner SF, et al. A high-resolution magnetic resonance imaging study of distal interphalangeal joint arthropathy in psoriatic arthritis and osteoarthritis: are they the same? Arthritis Rheum 2006;54(4):1328–33.

76. Soscia E, Scarpa R, Cimmino MA, et al. Magnetic resonance imaging of nail unit in psoriatic arthritis. J Rheumatol Suppl 2009;83:42–5.

77. Østergaard M, Bird P, Gandjbakhch F, et al. The OMERACT MRI in Arthritis Working Group - Update on Status and Future Research Priorities. J Rheumatol 2015 [pii:jrheum.141248]. [Epub ahead of print].

78. Ghanem N, Uhl M, Pache G, et al. MRI in psoriatic arthritis with hand and foot involvement. Rheumatol Int 2007;27(4):387–93.

79. Tehranzadeh J, Ashikyan O, Anavim A, et al. Detailed analysis of contrast-enhanced MRI of hands and wrists in patients with psoriatic arthritis. Skeletal Radiol 2008;37(5):433–42.

80. Totterman SM. Magnetic resonance imaging of psoriatic arthritis: insight from traditional and three-dimensional analysis. Curr Rheumatol Rep 2004;6(4):317–21.

81. Braum LS, McGonagle D, Bruns A, et al. Characterisation of hand small joints arthropathy using high-resolution MRI–limited discrimination between osteoarthritis and psoriatic arthritis. Eur Radiol 2013;23(6):1686–93.

82. Schoellnast H, Deutschmann HA, Hermann J, et al. Psoriatic arthritis and rheumatoid arthritis: findings in contrast-enhanced MRI. AJR Am J Roentgenol 2006; 187(2):351–7.

83. Narvaez J, Narvaez JA, de AM, et al. Can magnetic resonance imaging of the hand and wrist differentiate between rheumatoid arthritis and psoriatic arthritis in the early stages of the disease? Semin Arthritis Rheum 2012;42(3):234–45.

84. Offidani A, Cellini A, Valeri G, et al. Subclinical joint involvement in psoriasis: magnetic resonance imaging and X-ray findings. Acta Derm Venereol 1998; 78(6):463–5.

85. Erdem CZ, Tekin NS, Sarikaya S, et al. MR imaging features of foot involvement in patients with psoriasis. Eur J Radiol 2008;67(3):521–5.

86. Emad Y, Ragab Y, Bassyouni I, et al. Enthesitis and related changes in the knees in seronegative spondyloarthropathies and skin psoriasis: magnetic resonance imaging case-control study. J Rheumatol 2010;37(8):1709–17.

87. Tan YM, Østergaard M, Doyle A, et al. MRI bone oedema scores are higher in the arthritis mutilans form of psoriatic arthritis and correlate with high radiographic scores for joint damage. Arthritis Res Ther 2009;11(1):R2.

88. Antoni C, Dechant C, Hanns-Martin Lorenz PD, et al. Open-label study of infliximab treatment for psoriatic arthritis: clinical and magnetic resonance imaging measurements of reduction of inflammation. Arthritis Rheum 2002;47(5):506–12.

89. Marzo-Ortega H, McGonagle D, Rhodes LA, et al. Efficacy of infliximab on MRI-determined bone oedema in psoriatic arthritis. Ann Rheum Dis 2007;66(6): 778–81.

90. Yonenaga T, Saeki H, Nakagawa H, et al. Four cases of Japanese patients with psoriatic arthritis in whom effective treatments by anti-tumor necrosis factor-

alpha drugs were evaluated by magnetic resonance imaging together with improvement of skin lesions. J Dermatol 2015;42(1):49–55.

91. Anandarajah AP, Ory P, Salonen D, et al. Effect of adalimumab on joint disease: features of patients with psoriatic arthritis detected by magnetic resonance imaging. Ann Rheum Dis 2010;69(1):206–9.

92. Healy PJ, Groves C, Chandramohan M, et al. MRI changes in psoriatic dactylitis–extent of pathology, relationship to tenderness and correlation with clinical indices. Rheumatology (Oxford) 2008;47(1):92–5.

93. McQueen F, Lassere M, Bird P, et al. Developing a magnetic resonance imaging scoring system for peripheral psoriatic arthritis. J Rheumatol 2007;34(4):859–61.

94. Boyesen P, McQueen FM, Gandjbakhch F, et al. The OMERACT Psoriatic Arthritis Magnetic Resonance Imaging Score (PsAMRIS) is reliable and sensitive to change: results from an OMERACT workshop. J Rheumatol 2011;38(9):2034–8.

95. Østergaard M, Edmonds J, McQueen F, et al. An introduction to the EULAR-OMERACT rheumatoid arthritis MRI reference image atlas. Ann Rheum Dis 2005;64(Suppl 1):i3–7.

96. Queiro R, Tejon P, Alonso S, et al. Erosive discovertebral lesion (Andersson lesion) as the first sign of disease in axial psoriatic arthritis. Scand J Rheumatol 2013;42(3):220–5.

97. Poggenborg RP, Eshed I, Pedersen SJ, et al. Whole-body MRI for assessment of enthesitis in psoriatic arthritis, axial spondyloarthritis and healthy subjects - a comparison with 7 clinical enthesitis indices [abstract]. Ann Rheum Dis 2012; 71(Suppl 3):110.

98. Helliwell PS, Hickling P, Wright V. Do the radiological changes of classic ankylosing spondylitis differ from the changes found in the spondylitis associated with inflammatory bowel disease, psoriasis, and reactive arthritis? Ann Rheum Dis 1998;57(3):135–40.

99. Williamson L, Dockerty JL, Dalbeth N, et al. Clinical assessment of sacroiliitis and HLA-B27 are poor predictors of sacroiliitis diagnosed by magnetic resonance imaging in psoriatic arthritis. Rheumatology (Oxford) 2004;43(1):85–8.

100. Østergaard M, Poggenborg RP, Axelsen MB, et al. Magnetic resonance imaging in spondyloarthritis–how to quantify findings and measure response. Best Pract Res Clin Rheumatol 2010;24(5):637–57.

101. Bollow M, Fischer T, Reisshauer H, et al. Quantitative analyses of sacroiliac biopsies in spondyloarthropathies: T cells and macrophages predominate in early and active sacroiliitis- cellularity correlates with the degree of enhancement detected by magnetic resonance imaging. Ann Rheum Dis 2000;59(2): 135–40.

102. Castillo-Gallego C, Aydin SZ, Emery P, et al. Magnetic resonance imaging assessment of axial psoriatic arthritis: extent of disease relates to HLA-B27. Arthritis Rheum 2013;65(9):2274–8.

103. Kubassova O, Boesen M, Boyle RD, et al. Fast and robust analysis of dynamic contrast enhanced MRI datasets. Med Image Comput Comput Assist Interv 2007;10(Pt 2):261–9.

104. Gaffney K, Cookson J, Blake D, et al. Quantification of rheumatoid synovitis by magnetic resonance imaging. Arthritis Rheum 1995;38(11):1610–7.

105. Østergaard M, Stoltenberg M, Lovgreen-Nielsen P, et al. Quantification of synovistis by MRI: correlation between dynamic and static gadolinium-enhanced magnetic resonance imaging and microscopic and macroscopic signs of synovial inflammation. Magn Reson Imaging 1998;16(7):743–54.

106. Cimmino MA, Innocenti S, Livrone F, et al. Dynamic gadolinium-enhanced magnetic resonance imaging of the wrist in patients with rheumatoid arthritis can discriminate active from inactive disease. Arthritis Rheum 2003;48(5):1207–13.
107. Cimmino MA, Parodi M, Innocenti S, et al. Dynamic magnetic resonance of the wrist in psoriatic arthritis reveals imaging patterns similar to those of rheumatoid arthritis. Arthritis Res Ther 2005;7(4):R725–31.
108. Weckbach S. Whole-body MRI for inflammatory arthritis and other multifocal rheumatoid diseases. Semin Musculoskelet Radiol 2012;16(5):377–88.
109. Weckbach S, Schewe S, Michaely HJ, et al. Whole-body MR imaging in psoriatic arthritis: additional value for therapeutic decision making. Eur J Radiol 2011; 77(1):149–55.
110. Poggenborg RP, Eshed I, Østergaard M, et al. Enthesitis in patients with psoriatic arthritis, axial spondyloarthritis and healthy subjects assessed by 'head-to-toe' whole-body MRI and clinical examination. Ann Rheum Dis 2014; 74(5):823–9.
111. Poggenborg RP, Pedersen SJ, Eshed I, et al. Head-to-toe whole-body MRI in psoriatic arthritis, axial spondyloarthritis and healthy subjects: first steps towards global inflammation and damage scores of peripheral and axial joints. Rheumatology (Oxford) 2014;54(6):1039–49.

Early Psoriatic Arthritis

Neil John McHugh, MBChB, MD, FRCP, FRCPath

KEYWORDS

- Psoriatic arthritis • Psoriasis • Biomarkers • Genetic screening

KEY POINTS

- Early psoriatic arthritis is a heterogeneous condition that can make diagnosis difficult and can be confused with nodal osteoarthritis, fibromyalgia, and mechanical back pain.
- Screening questionnaires have highlighted that a significant number of cases are undiagnosed and delay in diagnosis may be associated with poorer long-term outcome.
- Currently, the strongest predictors for the development of psoriatic arthritis in individuals with psoriasis are nail disease, obesity, and HLA-B27.

INTRODUCTION

Psoriatic arthritis is a heterogeneous condition that may present in several different patterns; therefore, diagnosis and differentiation from other forms of arthritis can often be a challenge. Unlike conditions such as rheumatoid arthritis, systemic lupus erythematosus, or systemic vasculitis, there are no autoimmune diagnostic markers. Furthermore, once diagnosed the future course may be unpredictable and there is a relative paucity of known risk factors or biomarkers that reliably predict long-term outcome. Although there are several national and international guidelines that help to guide treatment for patients with persistently active disease, such as those who would benefit from biological therapy, there is less information to guide management of the patient with early or recently diagnosed disease. Yet the most frequently asked question from patients newly diagnosed with psoriatic arthritis relates to future outcome.

We now recognize that psoriatic arthritis is not a benign condition and, with more effective treatments available, there may never be a better opportunity for preventing its development from an early stage. Skin psoriasis precedes the development of psoriatic arthritis in the majority of cases and so represents an excellent opportunity for implementing screening strategies. Some of the evidence for the important of early detection is reviewed, as are recent epidemiologic findings, the development of screening questionnaires, and identification of high-risk groups in whom screening should be applied.

Disclosure Statement: The author has nothing to declare.
Department of Pharmacy and Pharmacology, University of Bath, Claverton Down, Bath BA2 7AY, UK
E-mail addresses: prsnjm@bath.ac.uk; N.J.McHugh@bath.ac.uk

Rheum Dis Clin N Am 41 (2015) 615–622
http://dx.doi.org/10.1016/j.rdc.2015.07.005
0889-857X/15/$ – see front matter

With the advent of more effective treatment than traditional agents, there has never been such an urgent need to focus much more attention on the natural history of early disease.

Is Psoriatic Arthritis Underdiagnosed?

There have been variable estimates of the incidence and prevalence of psoriatic arthritic, likely owing to factors such as historical differences in diagnostic criteria applied, study setting, and method of case ascertainment. Although a systematic review reported a median incidence of 6.4 in 100,000 cases per year of psoriatic arthritis in the general population,[1] a more recent population-based study from Norway found 188 incident cases over an 8-year period giving an incidence rate of 41.3 in 100,000.[2] Studies of psoriasis using information from clinical records reported a 10-year cumulative incidence of 3.1%,[3] whereas a prospective cohort study of psoriasis found an incidence of 1.8%.[4]

However, both the incidence and prevalence are likely to be higher; studies using screening questionnaires revealed that many patients are undiagnosed. For instance, 10.9% of patients from dermatology clinics in Germany were identified with undiagnosed psoriatic arthritis[5] as were 29% in a study from Dublin.[6] In a German study from 48 centers studying 1511 patients with psoriasis, 21% had psoriatic arthritis and as many as 85% of cases were newly diagnosed after assessment by rheumatology.[7] In another multinational study of 34 dermatology centers, 949 patients with plaque psoriasis were evaluated and 41% of 285 with psoriatic arthritis had not previously been diagnosed.[8] From a large, population-based, telephone survey of households in North America and Europe, 44% of patients with a diagnosis of psoriasis alone reported joint pain.[9] However, the importance of earlier detection remains uncertain because the natural history of undiagnosed psoriatic arthritis is unknown.

Observational Studies of Outcome in Psoriatic Arthritis

Long-term observational studies of psoriatic arthritis such as those from the Toronto cohort and elsewhere have provided valuable information on the natural history. For instance, health-related quality of life measures are similar to rheumatoid arthritis.[10] There are important comorbidities such as dyslipidemia and premature atherosclerosis. In 1 study of early psoriatic arthritis, joint erosions were present in 27% of patients at 10 months and in 47% of patients within 2 years of disease onset.[11] Peripheral joint disease is progressive in the majority of patients with the highest rate of progression in the first year of disease.[12]

Several more recent studies also suggest that delay in diagnosis is associated with a worse outcome. In the Toronto cohort, those patients first seen after 2 years of diagnosis compared with those seen within 2 years had a greater rate of joint damage.[13] In our own Bath cohort, delay in diagnosis as well as smoking, female gender, and older age at onset were associated with a worse physical function measured by the Health Assessment Questionnaire after 10 years.[14] Similar observations were reported in a Dublin cohort with late consulters having greater peripheral joint erosion and worse physical function.[15] Finally, results from the Swedish Early Psoriatic Arthritis Register showed that shorter duration of symptoms and lower Health Assessment Questionnaire scores independently predicted achievement of a state of minimal disease activity at 5 years.[16] Therefore, indirect evidence suggests that early intervention may be important in decreasing the burden of disease.

Some further evidence in support of early intervention comes from clinical trials. In the PRESTA, study patients receiving etanercept 50 mg once weekly with psoriatic arthritis for less than 2 years had greater improvement in efficacy measures than those with longer disease duration.[17]

Detection of Early Disease

The development of the CASPAR classification criteria helped to standardize the characteristics of patients in cohort studies and entry into clinical trials.[18] CASPAR also performs well in patients with early psoriatic arthritis.[19] However, CASPAR is mainly designed for use in rheumatology settings; therefore, other mechanisms for identifying patients with psoriatic arthritis are required.

Screening questionnaires

Several questionnaires were developed by different groups to screen for patients with psoriatic arthritis in various settings. Studies to compare the performance of the questionnaires were reported, such as 2 comparing the Psoriatic Arthritis Screening Evaluation (PASE), the Toronto Psoriatic Arthritis Screen (ToPAS), and the Psoriasis Epidemiology Screening Tool (PEST),[6,20] and another the Psoriasis and Arthritis Screening Questionnaire (PASQ) with ToPAS and PEST.[21] In general, the screening tools have not performed as well as in the setting where they were derived, although they have identified both undiagnosed psoriatic arthritis and patients who may benefit from rheumatology review. More recently, another questionnaire (CONTEST) was derived combining optimal questions from existing tools and requires further evaluation.[22] The efficacy of screening questionnaires in various health care settings, including the frequency of use and characteristics of the target population to which they are applied still, remains to be determined.

Imaging

Imaging modalities such as ultrasonography have the potential for detecting preclinical disease. Gisondi and colleagues[23] demonstrated entheseal abnormalities by ultrasonography in clinically asymptomatic patients with psoriasis. Power Doppler ultrasonography may detect vascular changes that herald the development of arthritis.[24] Also of much interest, psoriasis patients with nail changes demonstrated higher enthesitis scores at remote sites than patients with normal nails, consistent with observations that patients with psoriatic arthritis have a greater frequency of nail disease than psoriasis patients alone.[25] MRI may reveal subclinical synovitis and enthesitis inpatients with psoriasis without arthritis symptoms.[26]

Ultrasonography may also be helpful with good specificity for documenting joint and tendon involvement in early psoriatic arthritis. Furthermore, persistent change on gray scale or power Doppler ultrasonography may be a risk factor for disease progression.[27]

RISK FACTORS FOR PSORIATIC ARTHRITIS IN PSORIASIS
Clinical and Lifestyle

There may be certain types of psoriasis that put those individuals at greater risk of developing psoriatic arthritis, such as scalp and intergluteal psoriasis and nail disease (**Box 1**).[3] Certainly, nail disease has consistently been found to be a major risk factor.[28] Evidence for smoking is more conflicting, with at least 2 studies finding smoking a positive risk factor[14,29] and another reporting that smoking is protective.[30] A population-based study using The Health Improvement Network (THIN) database reported a greater incidence rate of psoriatic arthritis in a psoriasis population with increasing body mass index.[31] The severity of psoriasis seems unlikely to be a major risk factor for developing psoriatic arthritis, as most patients with psoriatic arthritis have low Psoriasis Area Severity Index (PASI) scores. However, a metaanalysis from a recent systematic literature review did show a trend between PASI score and risk of psoriatic arthritis.[32] Although it has been commonly held that psoriatic

---

Box 1
Possible risk factors for developing psoriatic arthritis in individuals with psoriasis

Lifestyle

Obesity[a]

Smoking (?)

Clinical

Severity of psoriasis

Pattern of psoriasis (scalp, intergluteal)

Nail psoriasis[a]

Imaging

Ultrasound evidence of enthesitis

Biomarkers

HLA-B27[a]

Interleukin-13

Highly sensitive C-reactive protein

Dendritic cell–specific membrane protein

Matrix metalloproteinase-3

Dickkopf-1

Macrophage colony stimulating factor

ratio of type II collagen synthesis to degradation (CPII:C2C)

[a] Denotes factors where there is strongest evidence.

---

arthritis develops most often within 10 years of onset of psoriasis, notably 1 study in European dermatology centers found the incidence rate of psoriatic arthritis remained constant with time after the diagnosis of psoriasis.[33]

Genetic Factors

There are likely to be genetic factors in psoriasis patients that confer increased susceptibility to psoriatic arthritis. This topic is thoroughly reviewed in this article. HLA-Cw6 is associated strongly with psoriasis and more so in younger onset disease, but is less common in psoriatic arthritis, suggesting that there are independent susceptibility genes for psoriatic arthritis.[34] Two such loci seem to be interleukin (IL)-13 and HLA-B27.[35] The presence of HLA-B27 is associated with a shorter interval between the onset of psoriasis and the onset of psoriatic arthritis.[34] Furthermore, it seems that there are combinations of HLA-B and C alleles/haplotypes that confer susceptibility to phenotypes and severity. In an Irish population, an HLA*B27:05:02 haplotype was associated with enthesitis, dactylitis, and symmetric sacroiliitis, whereas an HLA*08:01:01 haplotype was associated with a synovial-based pathology, including joint fusion and deformities, asymmetrical sacroiliitis, and dactylitis.[36]

Other Biomarkers

Osteoclast precursors identified with by cellular markers are upregulated in psoriatic arthritis and include dendritic cell–specific membrane protein. There are data to suggest that patients with psoriasis who develop arthritis show increased dendritic cell–specific membrane protein expression on peripheral blood mononuclear cells.[37] Measurement requires freshly isolated cells and access to flow cytometry and so is not at present a feasible strategy for screening. Other soluble biomarkers that can be more readily measured are of interest and bone turnover markers have been the subject of a recent systematic review.[38] Markers that seem to differentiate psoriatic arthritis from psoriasis include matrix metalloproteinase-3, dickkopf 1, macrophage colony stimulating factor, a ratio of type II collagen synthesis to degradation, and possibly osteoprotegerin. Increased levels of highly sensitive C-reactive protein may also be discriminatory.[39] These markers need further study in a prospective cohort of patients with psoriasis to test their predictive value.

CLINICAL PRESENTATION OF EARLY DISEASE

The distribution of the classical 5 subgroups of psoriatic arthritis as reported by Moll and Wright has varied in cohort studies, to some extent dependent on mean disease duration as subgroups may overlap and evolve.[40] Nonetheless, oligoarthritis of peripheral joints in a patient with plaque psoriasis and nail disease remains a common presenting scenario. However, the early stages of other forms of psoriatic arthritis may be difficult to distinguish, not only from other inflammatory joint disease such as rheumatoid arthritis, but even more so from osteoarthritis, fibromyalgia, and mechanical back pain. The bony proliferation that is a characteristic feature of psoriatic arthritis and contributes to the CASPAR classification criteria may yield a clinical phenotype that resembles nodal osteoarthritis when affecting the small joints of the hand. Likewise, pain and tenderness secondary to entheseal disease may be attributed to other conditions such as fibromyalgia. Enthesitis, inflammatory axial disease, and oligoarthritis contributed to 69% of undiagnosed psoriatic arthritis in a screening study of dermatology practice.[15] In a study of early psoriatic arthritis, the presence of enthesitis, inflammatory low back pain, and dactylitis were helpful diagnostic features.[41] Given the considerable heterogeneity of early psoriatic arthritis, the development of treatment algorithms can be major challenge.[42]

SUMMARY

We know that, left unchecked, the long-term outcome of psoriatic arthritis carries a high disease burden. The estimated mean health cost is high, especially in those with severe loss of physical function.[43] There are high levels of unemployment and loss of productivity that may be more readily reversible with early intervention.[44] The availability of more effective treatments with several also in the pipeline underscores the compelling case for early intervention. Individuals with psoriasis who seem to be at greatest risk are those who are obese, have nail disease, and carry the HLA-B27 allele. However, establishment of more robust bioprofiles are needed in order stratify patients into appropriate treatment pathways and to implement effective screening strategies.

REFERENCES

1. Alamanos Y, Voulgari PV, Drosos AA. Incidence and prevalence of psoriatic arthritis: a systematic review. J Rheumatol 2008;35(7):1354–8.
2. Hoff M, Gulati AM, Romundstad PR, et al. Prevalence and incidence rates of psoriatic arthritis in central Norway: data from the Nord-Trondelag Health Study (HUNT). Ann Rheum Dis 2015;74(1):60–4.

3. Wilson FC, Icen M, Crowson CS, et al. Incidence and clinical predictors of psoriatic arthritis in patients with psoriasis: a population-based study. Arthritis Rheum 2009;61(2):233–9.

4. Eder L, Chandran V, Shen H, et al. Incidence of arthritis in a prospective cohort of psoriasis patients. Arthritis Care Res 2011;63(4):619–22.

5. Henes JC, Ziupa E, Eisfelder M, et al. High prevalence of psoriatic arthritis in dermatological patients with psoriasis: a cross-sectional study. Rheumatol Int 2014;34(2):227–34.

6. Haroon M, Kirby B, FitzGerald O. High prevalence of psoriatic arthritis in patients with severe psoriasis with suboptimal performance of screening questionnaires. Ann Rheum Dis 2013;72(5):736–40.

7. Reich K, Kruger K, Mossner R, et al. Epidemiology and clinical pattern of psoriatic arthritis in Germany: a prospective interdisciplinary epidemiological study of 1511 patients with plaque-type psoriasis. Br J Dermatol 2009; 160(5):1040–7.

8. Mease PJ, Gladman DD, Papp KA, et al. Prevalence of rheumatologist-diagnosed psoriatic arthritis in patients with psoriasis in European/North American dermatology clinics. J Am Acad Dermatol 2013;69(5):729–35.

9. Lebwohl MG, Bachelez H, Barker J, et al. Patient perspectives in the management of psoriasis: results from the population-based multinational assessment of psoriasis and psoriatic arthritis survey. J Am Acad Dermatol 2014;70(5): 871–81.e30.

10. Husted JA, Gladman DD, Farewell VT, et al. Health-related quality of life of patients with psoriatic arthritis: a comparison with patients with rheumatoid arthritis. Arthritis Rheum 2001;45(2):151–8.

11. Kane D, Stafford L, Bresnihan B, et al. A prospective, clinical and radiological study of early psoriatic arthritis: an early synovitis clinic experience. Rheumatology 2003;42(12):1460–8.

12. McHugh NJ, Balachrishnan C, Jones SM. Progression of peripheral joint disease in psoriatic arthritis: a 5-yr prospective study. Rheumatology 2003;42(6):778–83.

13. Gladman DD, Thavaneswaran A, Chandran V, et al. Do patients with psoriatic arthritis who present early fare better than those presenting later in the disease? Ann Rheum Dis 2011;70(12):2152–4.

14. Tillett W, Jadon D, Shaddick G, et al. Smoking and delay to diagnosis are associated with poorer functional outcome in psoriatic arthritis. Ann Rheum Dis 2013; 72(8):1358–61.

15. Haroon M, Gallagher P, Fitzgerald O. Diagnostic delay of more than 6 months contributes to poor radiographic and functional outcome in psoriatic arthritis. Ann Rheum Dis 2015;74(6):1045–50.

16. Theander E, Husmark T, Alenius GM, et al. Early psoriatic arthritis: short symptom duration, male gender and preserved physical functioning at presentation predict favourable outcome at 5-year follow-up. Results from the Swedish Early Psoriatic Arthritis Register (SwePsA). Ann Rheum Dis 2014;73(2):407–13.

17. Kirkham B, de Vlam K, Li W, et al. Early treatment of psoriatic arthritis is associated with improved patient-reported outcomes: findings from the etanercept PRESTA trial. Clin Exp Rheumatol 2015;33(1):11–9.

18. Taylor W, Gladman D, Helliwell P, et al. Classification criteria for psoriatic arthritis: development of new criteria from a large international study. Arthritis Rheum 2006;54(8):2665–73.

19. Chandran V, Schentag CT, Gladman DD. Sensitivity of the classification of psoriatic arthritis criteria in early psoriatic arthritis. Arthritis Rheum 2007;57(8):1560–3.

20. Coates LC, Aslam T, Al Balushi F, et al. Comparison of three screening tools to detect psoriatic arthritis in patients with psoriasis (CONTEST study). Br J Dermatol 2013;168(4):802–7.
21. Mease PJ, Gladman DD, Helliwell P, et al. Comparative performance of psoriatic arthritis screening tools in patients with psoriasis in European/North American dermatology clinics. J Am Acad Dermatol 2014;71(4):649–55.
22. Coates LC, Walsh J, Haroon M, et al. Development and testing of new candidate psoriatic arthritis screening questionnaires combining optimal questions from existing tools. Arthritis Care Res 2014;66(9):1410–6.
23. Gisondi P, Tinazzi I, El-Dalati G, et al. Lower limb enthesopathy in patients with psoriasis without clinical signs of arthropathy: a hospital-based case-control study. Ann Rheum Dis 2008;67(1):26–30.
24. Aydin SZ, Ash ZR, Tinazzi I, et al. The link between enthesitis and arthritis in psoriatic arthritis: a switch to a vascular phenotype at insertions may play a role in arthritis development. Ann Rheum Dis 2013;72(6):992–5.
25. Ash ZR, Tinazzi I, Gallego CC, et al. Psoriasis patients with nail disease have a greater magnitude of underlying systemic subclinical enthesopathy than those with normal nails. Ann Rheum Dis 2012;71(4):553–6.
26. Emad Y, Ragab Y, Gheita T, et al. Knee enthesitis and synovitis on magnetic resonance imaging in patients with psoriasis without arthritic symptoms. J Rheumatol 2012;39(10):1979–86.
27. El Miedany Y, El Gaafary M, Youssef S, et al. Tailored approach to early psoriatic arthritis patients: clinical and ultrasonographic predictors for structural joint damage. Clin Rheumatol 2015;34(2):307–13.
28. Langenbruch A, Radtke MA, Krensel M, et al. Nail involvement as a predictor of concomitant psoriatic arthritis in patients with psoriasis. Br J Dermatol 2014; 171(5):1123–8.
29. Li W, Han J, Qureshi AA. Smoking and risk of incident psoriatic arthritis in US women. Ann Rheum Dis 2012;71(6):804–8.
30. Eder L, Shanmugarajah S, Thavaneswaran A, et al. The association between smoking and the development of psoriatic arthritis among psoriasis patients. Ann Rheum Dis 2012;71(2):219–24.
31. Love TJ, Zhu Y, Zhang Y, et al. Obesity and the risk of psoriatic arthritis: a population-based study. Ann Rheum Dis 2012;71(8):1273–7.
32. Rouzaud M, Sevrain M, Villani AP, et al. Is there a psoriasis skin phenotype associated with psoriatic arthritis? Systematic literature review. J Eur Acad Dermatol Venereol 2014;28(Suppl 5):17–26.
33. Christophers E, Barker JN, Griffiths CE, et al. The risk of psoriatic arthritis remains constant following initial diagnosis of psoriasis among patients seen in European dermatology clinics. J Eur Acad Dermatol Venereol 2010;24(5):548–54.
34. Winchester R, Minevich G, Steshenko V, et al. HLA associations reveal genetic heterogeneity in psoriatic arthritis and in the psoriasis phenotype. Arthritis Rheum 2012;64(4):1134–44.
35. Bowes J, Eyre S, Flynn E, et al. Evidence to support IL-13 as a risk locus for psoriatic arthritis but not psoriasis vulgaris. Ann Rheum Dis 2011;70(6):1016–9.
36. Haroon M, Winchester R, Giles JT, et al. Certain class I HLA alleles and haplotypes implicated in susceptibility play a role in determining specific features of the psoriatic arthritis phenotype. Ann Rheum Dis 2014. [Epub ahead of print].
37. Ritchlin C. Biomarker development in psoriatic arthritis. J Rheumatol Suppl 2012; 89:57–60.

38. Jadon DR, Nightingale AL, McHugh NJ, et al. Serum soluble bone turnover biomarkers in psoriatic arthritis and psoriatic spondyloarthropathy. J Rheumatol 2015;42(1):21–30.

39. Chandran V. Soluble biomarkers may differentiate psoriasis from psoriatic arthritis. J Rheumatol Suppl 2012;89:65–6.

40. Jones SM, Armas JB, Cohen MG, et al. Psoriatic arthritis: outcome of disease subsets and relationship of joint disease to nail and skin disease. Br J Rheumatol 1994;33(9):834–9.

41. Caso F, Costa L, Atteno M, et al. Simple clinical indicators for early psoriatic arthritis detection. Springerplus 2014;3:759.

42. Tillett W, McHugh N. Treatment algorithms for early psoriatic arthritis: do they depend on disease phenotype? Curr Rheumatol Rep 2012;14(4):334–42.

43. Poole CD, Lebmeier M, Ara R, et al. Estimation of health care costs as a function of disease severity in people with psoriatic arthritis in the UK. Rheumatology 2010;49(10):1949–56.

44. Tillett W, Shaddick G, Askari A, et al. Factors influencing work disability in psoriatic arthritis: first results from a large UK multicentre study. Rheumatology 2015;54(1):157–62.

Genetic, Epigenetic and Pharmacogenetic Aspects of Psoriasis and Psoriatic Arthritis

Darren D. O'Rielly, PhD, FCCMG[a], Proton Rahman, MD, MSc, FRCPC[b],*

KEYWORDS

- Genetics • Candidate genes • GWAS • Psoriasis • Psoriatic arthritis
- Pharmacogenetics • Epigenetics

KEY POINTS

- Despite the large number of genes identified in psoriatic disease, the genetic contribution identified by genome-wide association studies (GWAS) accounts for less than 25% of heritability.
- This "missing heritability" is attributed to inherent limitations of this technology and limits searches to common variants, neglecting rare variants.
- No clinically actionable information can be gleaned by a single variant from GWAS studies owing to the very low odds ratio for the individual variants.
- A genetic risk score combining multiple loci associated with psoriasis/psoriatic arthritis may hold more clinical promise.

GENETICS OF PSORIATIC DISEASE

Clinicians have long recognized a strong familial component to psoriatic disease, and this observation has been substantiated in population and cohort-based studies. Epidemiologic studies suggest that psoriatic arthritis (PsA) has a higher heritability than psoriasis vulgaris (PsV).[1] However, many of the genes identified to date are related to psoriasis, whereas genes specific to PsA remain elusive.

Initial genetic studies in psoriatic disease involved interrogation of *HLA* alleles, which was subsequently followed by candidate gene studies within and outside the major histocompatibility complex (MHC) region. With the emergence of genome-wide microarrays, multiple genome-wide linkage studies were performed using either

Competing Interests: None declared.
[a] Faculty of Medicine, Health Sciences Centre, Memorial University of Newfoundland, 300 Prince Philip Drive, Room 1J440, St. John's, Newfoundland and Labrador A1B 3V6, Canada;
[b] St. Clare's Mercy Hospital, Memorial University of Newfoundland, 154 Le Marchant Road, St. John's, Newfoundland and Labrador A1C 5B8, Canada
* Corresponding author.
E-mail address: prahman@mun.ca

Rheum Dis Clin N Am 41 (2015) 623–642
http://dx.doi.org/10.1016/j.rdc.2015.07.002
0889-857X/15/$ – see front matter © 2015 Elsevier Inc. All rights reserved.

rheumatic.theclinics.com

large multiplex families or sibling pairs. These strategies were followed by genome-wide association studies (GWAS), which also included metaanalyses. These large, international, single nucleotide polymorphism–based studies have identified numerous additional genes reaching genome-wide significance, which can be broadly classified into those involved in maintaining skin barrier functions, innate immunity, and acquired immunity. New technologies are being used to investigate the genetic basis of psoriatic disease using next-generation sequencing, copy number variation (CNV) analysis, and epigenetics.

Major Histocompatibility Complex Associations in Psoriatic Disease

The MHC region located on the short arm of chromosome 6 continues to be the dominant susceptibility region in psoriatic disease. Recent estimates suggest that at least one-third of the entire genetic contribution of psoriasis and PsA resides within this region. The major genetic determinant of psoriasis was initially localized to ~300 kb segment in the MHC I region, known as *PSORS1*; subsequent resequencing studies concluded that *HLA-Cw6* is the *PSORS1* risk variant that confers susceptibility to PsV.[2] There is also consistent association between *HLA-Cw0602* and PsA; however, the magnitude of the association with PsA is lower compared with PsV.[3] The *HLA-C*0602* allele seems to be associated with subphenotypes of PsV and PsA. In patients with PsV, *HLA-C*0602* is associated with type 1 psoriasis, guttate psoriasis, Koebner phenomenon, and amelioration of psoriasis during pregnancy.[4] Among patients with PsA, the *HLA-C*0602* allele is associated with delayed onset of arthritis and there is an inverse correlation with psoriatic nail disease, as summarized elswhere.[5]

The *HLA-B*27* allele seems to be a specific genetic marker for PsA; however, its magnitude is not as strong as in ankylosing spondylitis.[6] The prevalence of *HLA-B*27* is only about 20% compared with 70% to 90% in ankylosing spondylitis. The *HLA-B*27* allele is also associated with selected subphenotypes of PsA, including axial involvement, dactylitis, and greater burden of articular damage.[7] Thus, the presence of the *HLA-B*27* allele in PsA may lead to a more severe form of disease.

The 3 most consistently reported *HLA-B* alleles that are specific to PsA are *HLA-B*38*, *HLA-B*08*, and *HLA-B*39*.[6,8] A recent large fine-mapping study of psoriatic disease within the MHC region using an HLA-variant imputation approach, has shed new light regarding HLA associations within this region for PsV and PsA.[9] In this elegant study, Okada and colleagues[9] defined the 4-digit *HLA* allele and amino acid resolutions. This study included 9247 affected individuals (3038 PsA subjects, 3098 cutaneous psoriasis (PsC) subjects, and 3111 subjects of unknown PsA or PsC status) and 13,589 control individuals of European ancestry. They found that the *HLA-B*27* allele was the most discriminative allele separating PsA from PsC. A more refined analysis revealed that the presence of glutamine in position 45 of the *HLA-B* antigen conferred the strongest risk for PsA. This polymorphic site is located in the binding groove of HLA-B and can influence the binding of a peptide to the HLA molecule. The PsA-specific alleles noted (*HLA-B*27*, *B*39*, and *B*38*) all encode proteins that contain Glu at position 45.

Non–Major Histocompatibility Complex Candidate Genes Studies in Psoriatic Arthritis

Multiple association studies of non-MHC genes have been conducted in PsA. Most association studies reporting an initial association have not been replicated and the majority have failed to demonstrate independence from association with known *HLA* alleles. *MICA* represents the non-*HLA* gene within the MHC region that has received the most interest. This gene is in close proximity to the *HLA-B* locus and, in a Spanish cohort, the trinucleotide repeat polymorphism, *MICA-A9* (which corresponds with *MICA*002*), was associated with PsA independent of *HLA-Cw6*, *MICB*, or *TNF*.[10] However, the large fine-mapping study failed to demonstrate an association between *MIC* alleles and PsA.[9]

The killer-cell immunoglobulin-like receptors (KIR) do not reside in the MHC region, but interact with class I HLA antigens, and therefore are covered in this article. KIRs are encoded by a highly polygenic and polymorphic locus on chromosome 19q13.4 and located on natural killer cells.[11] The frequency of *KIR2DS2* is increased in PsA compared with unaffected controls and this association is amplified when *KIR2DS2* is coupled with various HLA-C ligands. The *KIR2DS2* may be specific to PsA because the association is maintained when PsA and PsV were compared (odds ratio, 1.34; 95% CI, 1.04, 1.73; $P = .024$).[12]

Genome-wide Linkage Scans in Psoriasis Vulgaris and Psoriatic Arthritis

Genome-wide linkage studies are only of historical significance because no convincing susceptibility variants can be attributed reliably to the linkage peaks in psoriasis. Nine genome-wide linkage studies were completed in PsV and these efforts identified 10 loci (*PSORS1* to *PSORS10*) with the strongest and most consistent association being *PSORS1* at chromosome 6p21.3, as summarized by O'Rielly and Rahman.[13] Only 1 genome-wide linkage study was completed in PsA and this study revealed evidence for significant linkage on chromosome 16q only when conditioned on paternal transmission.[14]

Meanwhile, GWAS have resulted in multiple new candidate genes in psoriasis and PsA. The candidate genes achieving genome-wide significance are grouped into skin barrier function genes, innate immune response genes involving nuclear factor-kappa B (NF-κB) and interferon (IFN) signaling, and adaptive immune response genes involving CD8 T-lymphocytes and T helper (Th)-17 lymphocyte signaling.

Skin Barrier Function

Psoriasis is characterized by keratinocyte hyperplasia, which may develop as a result of the effects of cytokines produced by immune cells. The potential role for epidermal keratinocytes as triggers for the initiation of psoriasis has also been proposed. CNV GWAS and functional studies have identified significant associations with *DEFB* genes and late cornified envelope (*LCE*) genes and an Asian GWAS study identified Connexin, all reaching genome-wide significance. β-Defensins are responsible for maintaining a chemical barrier by generating small antimicrobial peptides that possess a broad spectrum of antimicrobial activity.[15] Each additional copy above 2 copies of *DEFB4* increases the relative risk of psoriasis.[16] The *DEFB4* gene, which encodes for the hBD-2 protein, is induced dramatically in skin as a part of the inflammatory response in psoriasis and psoriatic keratinocytes are programmed to secrete large amounts of β-defensins in response to 'Th1' or 'Th17' cytokines.[17]

LCE gene cluster encodes cornified envelope proteins that are important for epidermal cell differentiation. A genome-wide investigation targeting CNVs identified a significant association within the *PSORS4* locus that encompassed both *LCE3B* and *LCE3C* genes with increased susceptibility to PsV in multiple populations.[18] GWAS followed by targeted candidate gene studies been confirmed associations with *LCE3* gene in multiple populations.[19,20] A gene–gene interaction (epistasis) between *LCE3C_LCE3B-del* and *HLA-Cw6* has also been noted.[21]

Connexin 26 is expressed at the cell periphery of keratinocytes in psoriatic plaques and is not present in normal, unaffected skin.[22] When keratinocytes release connexin-mediated adenosine triphosphate, this indirectly results in epidermal proliferation and differentiation resembling a characteristic response in psoriasis.[23] Connexin 26 is encoded by *GJB2* and a variant residing in this gene was identified in an Asian GWAS as a PsV susceptibility locus.[24]

Innate Immune Response

The innate immune response, which is present from birth and not adapted or persistently amplified as a result of exposure to microorganisms, is composed of physical epithelial barriers, phagocytic leukocytes, dendritic cells, natural killer cells, and circulating plasma proteins. An important cellular regulator of the innate response is the immediate–early response transcription factor NF-κB. NF-κB accumulation triggers transcription of numerous target genes, which contributes to the pathogenesis of inflammatory disease in PsV and PsA. Genes reaching genome-wide significance in psoriasis that encode proteins crucial for NF-κB signaling and subsequent transcription include *REL, TNIP1, TNFAIP3, NFKBIA, FBXL19, NOS2, CARD14, CARM1, TYK2,* and *UBE2L3* (**Table 1**).[24–33] *REL* genes encode 1 of the 4 subunits comprising the

Table 1
Genetic associations identified in psoriasis and PsA with respect pathways involved in skin barrier function and the innate immune response

Gene/Locus	Chr.	Ethnic Ancestry	Psoriatic Disease	
			Psoriasis	PsA
Skin barrier function				
LCE3B/LCE3C	1q21.3	European	X	—
DEFB4	8p23.1	European	X	—
KLF4	9q31	European	X	—
GJB2	13q11-q12	Asian	X	—
Innate immune response				
Interferon signaling				
IFNLR1/IL-28RA	1p36.11	European	X	—
IFIH1	2q24	European	X	—
ELMO1	7p14.1	European	X	—
DDX58	9p12	European	X	—
SOCS1	16p13.13	European	X	—
TYK2	19p13.2	European	X	X
RNF114	20q13.13	European	X	—
NF-κB signaling				
REL	2p13-p12	European	X	X
TNIP1	5q32-q33.1	European	X	X
TNFAIP3	6q23	European	X	—
NFKBIA	14q13	European	X	—
FBXL19	16p11.2	European	X	X
NOS2	17q11.2-q12	European	X	—
CARD14	17q25	European	X	—
CARM1	19p13.2	European	X	—
TYK2	19p13.2	European	X	X
UBE2L3	22q11.21	European	X	—

Abbreviations: NF-κB, nuclear factor-κB; PSA, psoriatic arthritis.

NF-κB complex and belong to the family of the NF-κB (REL) transcription factor, which is essential for proper signaling.[25] Tumor necrosis factor (TNF) α–induced protein 3-interacting protein 1 (*TNIP1*) encodes ABIN-1, which interacts with the zinc finger protein, A20, to inhibit TNF-α–induced, NF-κB–dependent gene expression.[34] It inhibits both transduction by transmembrane receptors, such as TNF-α–receptor, epidermal growth factor receptor, and Toll-like receptor, and nuclear receptors peroxisome proliferator activated receptor and retinoic acid receptor activity.[35] Multiple autoimmune diseases implicated *TNIP1* through GWAS, including PsV and rheumatoid arthritis.[36] TNF-α–inducible protein 3 (*TNFAIP3*) encodes the inducible zinc finger protein A20, a critical protein in the inhibition of NF-κB signaling. Activation of NF-κB signaling triggers ubiquitination of A20, which prevents subsequent NF-κB activation.[37] *TNFAIP3* polymorphisms are associated with susceptibility to multiple autoimmune diseases, including psoriasis, systemic lupus erythematosus, rheumatoid arthritis, systemic sclerosis, and celiac disease.[13] A large metaanalysis of the *TNFAIP3* region revealed multiple associations, with the top variant being rs582757 ($P = 6.07 \times 10^{-12}$). Further analysis of *TNFAIP3* haplotypes revealed that the psoriasis risk haplotype is distinct from other autoimmune diseases, highlighting the complex genetic architecture of this locus.[38] *NFKBIA* encodes an inhibitory protein that interferes with nuclear localization, which inactivates NF-κB dimers in the absence of inflammatory stimuli.[39] *FBXL19* is a member of the F-box family and the encoded protein is reported to bind to the transmembrane receptor interleukin (IL) 1 receptor-like 1 and regulate its ubiquitination and degradation. FBXL19 is also known to reversibly inhibit NF-kB signaling.[40] *FBXL19* expression is increased significantly in psoriatic skin, suggesting a role in its pathogenesis. *NOS2* encodes an inducible form of nitric oxide synthase, which is a known effector of the innate immune system, and whose transcription may be induced by NF-κB.[41] *CARD14* encodes a member of the family of caspase recruitment domain-containing scaffold proteins and mediates recruitment and activation of the NF-κB pathway,[42] whereas *CARM1* encodes a transcriptional coactivator of NF-κB and functions as a promoter-specific regulator of NF-κB recruitment to chromatin. *TYK2* encodes a tyrosine kinase involved in the initiation of IFN-α signaling and NF-κB activation.[43] *UBE2L3* encodes an ubiquitin-conjugating enzyme, UBCH7, which is involved in the ubiquitination of the NF-κB precursor p105 which prevents NF-κB activation.[44]

Genes reaching genome-wide significance in psoriasis that encode proteins important for IFN signaling include *IFNLR1/IL-28RA*, *IFIH1*, *ELMO1*, *DDX58*, *SOCS1*, *TYK2*, and *RNF114* (see **Table 1**).[24–33] IL-28 receptor, alpha subunit (IL-28RA) gene, which encodes a protein that forms a receptor complex with IL-10 receptor β (IL-10RB), can influence IFN type III signaling.[45] *IFIH1* initiates a transduction cascade that induces several cytokines, including interferons, whereas *ELMO1* encodes a member of the engulfment and cell motility protein family, which is essential for Toll-like receptor-mediated IFN-α induction by plasmacytoid dendritic cells.[46] *DDX58*, which encodes the RIG-I receptor, is induced by IFN-γ and regulates the production of IFN-α and INF-γ.[47] *SOCS1* is a member of the suppressor of cytokine signaling family of proteins and inhibits signaling events downstream of INF-γ and interacts with TYK2 in cytokine signaling.[48] *RNF114* encodes an ubiquitin binding protein that enhances production of IFN-α through dysregulation of RIG-I/MDA5 signaling.[49]

With respect to PsA, *TNIP1*, *REL*, *TYK2*, and *FBXL19* have reached genome-wide significance in PsA as summarized by O'Rielly and Rahman.[13] Collectively, these data strongly support an important role of NF-κB and IFN signaling in psoriasis and PsA pathology.

Acquired Immune Response

The conventional model underling psoriasis and PsA pathogenesis was that these conditions were autoimmune based and driven by activated T cells reacting to skin or synovial antigens presented by macrophages or dendritic cells.[50] Indeed, an inflammatory milieu characterized by a perivascular lymphocytic infiltrate of activated T cells with signs of organ-specific migration have been documented in both the skin and joints.[51] Traditionally, psoriasis and PsA have been considered 'Th-1' diseases involving differentiation of naive T cells into Th-1 cells. More recently, IL-17–producing Th-17 cells maintained via IL-23 signaling by activated dendritic cells[52] have emerged as a critical signaling pathway contributing to psoriasis and PsA pathogenesis.

Antigen presentation

Disruption of antigen presentation by genetic variation can result in inappropriate targeting and destruction of cells, thereby contributing to psoriasis and PsA pathogenesis. Variations located within *RUNX3*, *TNFRSF9*, *MBD2*, *ETS1*, *IRF4*, *TAGAP*, *B3GNT2*, *ERAP1*, and *HLA-B/C*, which encode proteins crucial for antigen presentation, have been identified in GWAS investigating susceptibility to psoriasis (**Table 2**).[24–33] We do not discuss the genetic contribution of HLA-B/C loci to psoriasis pathogenesis because this has been covered in a previous section. *RUNX3*, *TNFRSF9*, and *MBD2* encode proteins involved in the generation of CD8 T cells.[53–55] Similarly, *ETS1*, *IRF4*, *TAGAP*, and *B3GNT2* encode proteins involved in the activation and differentiation of CD8 T cells.[53,56,57] That *ERAP1* codes for a protein that trims peptides in the endoplasmic reticulum before their MHC class I presentation,[58] and that it interacts with HLA-C indicates that this gene is important for antigen presentation. Collectively, these genes encode proteins that are important in proper antigen presentation and may underlie psoriasis pathogenesis. With respect to PsA, only variations within *HLA-B/C* have been identified in GWAS (see **Table 2**).

T helper-1 signaling pathway

The Th-1 signaling pathway was originally considered to play a prominent role in the pathogenesis of psoriasis and PsA. TNF-α, IFN-λ, IFN-α, IL-6, and IL-1β induce the secretion of IL-12 by myeloid dendritic cells resulting in differentiation of Th-1 cells.[59] Disruption of this signaling pathway by genetic variation can result in a shift toward a Th-1 phenotype contributing to the pathogenesis of psoriasis and PsA. Variations within numerous genes that encode proteins crucial for Th-1 signaling have been identified in GWAS investigating susceptibility to psoriasis, including *ZC3H12C*, *IL-12β*, *TYK2*, *STAT5A*, *STAT5B*, and *ILF3* (see **Table 2**). *ZC3H12C* encodes a zinc-finger protein regulating macrophage activation.[60] *IL-12β* is involved in IL-12 receptor activation, and *TYK2*, which encodes Tyk2, binds directly to IL-12Rβ1, and is involved in IL-12–mediated signaling.[61] *STAT5A* and *STAT5B* encode members of the STAT family of transcriptional activators and participate in signaling downstream of the IL-2 family of cytokines, including IL-2, IL-7, IL-15, and IL-21.[62] *ILF3* encodes a double-stranded RNA-binding protein and is a subunit of the nuclear factor of activated T cells, a transcription factor required for the expression in T cells of IL-2.[63] Collectively, these genes encode proteins that play an important role in Th-1 signaling. To date, only a single genetic locus (*IL-12β*) involved in Th-1 signaling has also reached genome-wide level of significance in PsA.

T helper-17 signaling pathway

The discovery of the Th-17 signaling pathway, also known as the IL-23/IL-17 axis, has enhanced dramatically our understanding of the pathogenesis of psoriasis and PsA

Table 2
Genetic associations identified in PsV and PsA with respect pathways involved in the acquired immune response

| Gene/Locus | Chr. | Ethnic Ancestry | Psoriatic Disease | |
			Psoriasis	PsA
Antigen presentation				
RUNX3	1p36	European	X	—
TNFRSF9	1p36	European	X	—
B3GNT2	2p15	European	X	—
ERAP1	5q15	European	X	—
TAGAP	6p25.3	European	X	—
IRF4	6p25-p23	European	X	—
HLA-B/C	6p21.3	European	X	X
ETS1	11q23.3	European	X	—
MBD2	18q21	European	X	—
Th-1 signaling pathway				
IL-12β	5q31.1-q33.1	European	X	X
ZC3H12C	11q22.3	European	X	—
STAT5A/B	17q21.31	European	X	—
TYK2	19p13.2	European	X	X
ILF3	19p13.2	European	X	—
Th-17 signaling pathway				
IL-23R	1p31.3	European	X	X
IL-1RN	2q14.2	European	X	—
IL-17RD	3p14.3	European	X	—
IL-2/IL-21	4q27	European	X	—
IL-12β	5q31.1-q33.1	European	X	X
TRAF3IP2	6q21	European	X	X
IRF4	6p25-p23	European	X	—
IL-6	7p21	European	X	—
KLF4	9q31	European	X	—
ETS1	11q23.3	European	X	—
IL-23A	12q13.3	European	X	X
IL-22	12q15	Asian	X	—
SOCS1	16p13.13	European	X	—
STAT3	17q21.31	European	X	—
TYK2	19p13.2	European	X	X

Abbreviations: PSA, psoriatic arthritis; PsV, psoriasis vulgaris; Th, T helper.

disease. Specifically, Th-17 cells produce IL-17, which induces proinflammatory cytokines and angiogenic factors[60] and commits naive T cells to the Th-17 lineage representing a positive feedback mechanism.[52] Moreover, through its intermediaries, the Th-17 pathway forms a complex interplay with TNF-α and NF-κB[64–67] and, consequently, also plays an important role in the innate immune response. That IL-17 displays synergistic effects with TNF-α, and that both IL-23 and IL-17 activate the NF-κB pathway in multiple ways,[68] is consistent with suppression of IL-17 signaling with a TNF-α inhibitor in psoriasis.[69] Genetically driven dysfunction of IL-23 signaling may enhance Th-17 cell expansion, with consequent IL-17–mediated upregulation of cytokines, chemokines, and tissue-degrading matrix metalloproteases, culminating in an inflammatory environment.[70] Indeed, GWAS have identified genetic variants associated with susceptibility to psoriasis and PsA (see **Table 2**), which are involved in Th-17 differentiation effector signaling.

IL-17–promoting cytokines (eg, transforming growth factor (TGF)-β, IL-6, IL-1β, and IL-23) and their signaling pathways induce Th-17 cell differentiation culminating in a psoriatic phenotype. With the exception of IL-23, all other cytokines are covered briefly in this review. Although *TGF-β1* is increased in the epidermis and the serum of psoriatic patients[71] and TGF-β1 serum level correlates closely with disease severity,[72,73] presently *TGF-β1* polymorphisms have not been reported to be associated with susceptibility to psoriasis or PsA. IL-6 is involved in the differentiation of Th-17 cells and in the IL-23–induced skin inflammation.[74] IL-6 signaling through STAT3 is required for both IL-23 receptor expression and for IL-17A and IL-17F induction.[75] Unfortunately, there have been no studies in PsA; however, the *IL-6* single nucleotide polymorphism rs1800795 was associated with a lower risk of PsV.[76] Sustained differentiation of Th-17 cells requires IL-1β and IL-23.[77,78] A role for IL-1 in PsV pathogenesis is supported by IL-1 family members being enhanced in psoriatic skin.[79] Although GWAS studies in psoriasis failed to detect an association with *IL-1β*,[22–33] *IL-1RN* was associated significantly with cutaneous disease severity and nail involvement in purely cutaneous psoriasis.[80] Although the *IL-1* locus was initially considered a PsA susceptibility locus,[81,82] this finding was not confirmed in follow-up studies.[27–29,83]

IL-23 is a heterodimeric cytokine that binds IL-23R and IL-12Rβ1, promotes the expansion and survival of Th-17 cells,[83,84] and acts as a proinflammatory mediator.[85] That IL-23 plays a prominent role in psoriasis and PsA is supported by increased serum levels and skin expression of *IL-23* in patients compared with healthy controls[86,87] and monocytes producing higher levels of IL-23 in patients with psoriasis or PsA.[88] GWAS analysis has revealed that variations located within *IL-12β*, *IL-23A*, *IL-23R*, *TYK2*, *STAT3*, *SOCS1*, and *ETS1* are associated with psoriasis susceptibility (see **Table 2**).[24–33] Whereas *IL-12β*, *IL-23A*, and *IL-23R* are involved in IL-23 receptor activation, *TYK2*, *STAT3*, *SOCS1*, and *ETS1* are involved with downstream signaling.[84,89] *TYK2* encodes Tyk2, which binds directly to IL-12Rβ1 and is essential for IL-23–mediated signaling and Th-17 cell differentiation.[61] *STAT3* and *SOCS1* encode for Stat3 and Socs1, respectively, and are required for the differentiation of Th-17 cells.[90,91] *ETS1* encodes Ets1, which is a negative regulator of Th-17 differentiation.[92]

Th-17 effector signaling (eg, IL-17, IL-21, and IL-22) produces autoimmunity, setting the stage for the development of psoriatic disease, and candidate gene studies, GWAS, and gene expression profiling evidence a genetic component in Th-17–mediated signaling. With the exception of IL-17, other cytokines are covered briefly in this review. IL-17 binds to IL-17RA and IL-17RC receptors[93,94] and activates macrophages, dendritic cells, endothelial cells, fibroblasts, chondrocytes, and osteoblasts culminating in a proinflammatory, destructive environment.[95,96] The relevance of the IL-17 in psoriatic disease is supported by the elevation of *IL-17/IL-17R* in psoriatic skin and synovial fluid from PsA patients.[97–100] GWAS have revealed that variations located within *TRAF3IP2*, *KLF4*, and *IRF2* are associated with psoriasis susceptibility (see **Table 2**).[24–33] TRAF3 interacting protein 2 (TRAF3IP2) is required for Th-17–mediated inflammatory responses,[66] and the *TRAF3IP2* variant associated with PsA (rs33980500) nearly abolished the interaction with TRAF6.[25] *KLF4* binds to the IL-17A promoter and positively regulates its expression.[101] Similarly, *IRF4* encodes a transcription factor that regulates IL-17A promoter activity.[102] Although GWAS have not identified an association of *IL-17* with either psoriasis or PsA,[24–33] a family-based association study in Tunisian familial PsV revealed an association between *IL-17RD* (rs12495640), which is a member of the IL-17 receptor (IL-17R) family.[103] However, in PsA patients of northern Italian origin, *IL-17A* and *IL17-RA* allelic variants were not associated with disease susceptibility.[104]

IL-22, a newly discovered Th-17 cytokine, contributes to proliferation and differentiation of keratinocytes,[105] which is supported by enhanced *IL-22* receptor (*IL-22R*) expression in the epidermis of psoriatic compared with normal skin.[106] Although an association was not detected in Caucasian GWAS, an *IL-22* association with psoriasis was identified in a Japanese population.[107] *IL-22* gene copy number correlated with clinical manifestations of psoriasis with high copy numbers being more prone to the appearance of nail manifestations.[105] IL-21 binds to IL-21R, which activates the JAK-STAT signaling pathway[108] and increases IL-17 production and IL-23R expression.[109,110] *IL-21* gene and protein expression is increased in lesional skin of psoriatic patients compared with nonlesional samples,[111] and serum IL-21 levels in patients with psoriasis are increased and positively correlate with Psoriasis Area and Severity Index scores.[112] Although there was a trend toward an association of within the IL-2/IL-21 region in psoriasis GWAS,[28] strong evidence of association with 2 variants in the *IL-2/IL-21* (rs6822844 and rs2069778) region was reported in a subsequent study.[113]

In PsA, only 2 genetic loci (ie, *IL-12B*, *TRAF3IP2*) involved in Th-17 signaling have reached a genome-wide level of significance.[25,31] However, results from candidate gene studies have revealed an association of *IL-23A*, *IL-23R*, and *STAT3*.[114–116] A prominent role of Th-17 signaling in the pathogenesis of PsA is supported by increased Th-17 cells in peripheral blood of PsA patients, which correlated with disease activity,[117] and IL-17 and IL-23 being involved in osteoclastogenesis and bone erosion in PsA joints.[118] Moreover, anti–IL-17 and anti–TNF-α agents suppress IL-23–induced osteoclastogenesis,[119] and treatment with human IL-12/23 p40 monoclonal antibody is able to reduce the signs and symptoms of joint inflammation in PsA.[120] The lack of identified genetic susceptibility loci involved in the adaptive immune response is attributed largely to the much smaller number of PsA patients interrogated with genome-wide scans and the greater degree of clinical heterogeneity observed with PsA compared with psoriasis.

EPIGENETICS OF PSORIASIS AND PSORIATIC ARTHRITIS SUSCEPTIBILITY

That the discordance of psoriasis between monozygotic twins,[121] and that abnormal keratinocyte differentiation is tightly linked with the epigenetic state of the basal keratinocytes,[122] strongly suggests that, in addition to genetic predisposition factors, the envlronment and other epigenetic factors play a role in the onset and progression of psoriasis and PsA. Environmental factors contributing to pathogenesis or progression of psoriasis and PsA include infections, psychological stress, cigarette smoking, and obesity. In particular, gene–environment interactions have been noted for smoking with smoking delaying the onset of inflammatory arthritis in psoriasis patients, particularly for those patients with selected IL-13 polymorphisms.[123,124]

DNA methylation is an epigenetic silencing mechanism that occurs at the 5'-carbon of cytosine residue within the CpG dinucleotides by DNA methyltransferases (DNMTs).[125] That DNA methylation is relevant to psoriasis and PsA pathogenesis is evidenced by higher DNMT1 expression in psoriatic peripheral blood mononuclear cells compared with normal controls.[126] Currently, there have been 8 genome-wide DNA methylation studies performed in psoriasis, including 6 and 2 beadchip and methylated DNA immunoprecipitation followed by next-generation sequencing (MeDIP-Seq), respectively. A genome-wide methylation study involving CD4$^+$ and CD8$^+$ T cells of monozygotic twins discordant for psoriasis identified differentially methylated CpG regions,[121] and hypomethylated regions in CD4$^+$ T cells have been detected in psoriasis patients compared with healthy controls,[127] suggesting that methylation changes in naïve CD4$^+$ T cells may affect CD4$^+$ T-cell polarization, especially in the pathogenesis of psoriasis. A third genome-wide methylation study identified 1108 differentially methylated CpG sites in the psoriatic involved skin compared with normal skin, including 12 CpG sites mapped to genes associated with epidermal differentiation and function.[128] Similarly, genome-wide DNA methylation profiling of epidermal cells revealed a distinct DNA methylation pattern in psoriasis compared with controls, including 3665 differentially methylated sites with an overall hypomethylation.[129] Importantly, both studies reported that the methylation pattern reversed after 1 month of TNF-α inhibitor treatment or at the end of phototherapy.[128,129] Furthermore, aberrant promoter methylation of several genes in dermal mesenchymal stem cells from psoriatic patients compared with the normal controls,[126] and increased global DNA methylation in psoriatic peripheral blood mononuclear cells compared with the normal controls have been reported.[130]

MeDIP-Seq has revealed a much greater number of hypermethylated DMRs in the affected skin of psoriatic patients, including in genes enriched for the immune system, cell cycle regulation, and apoptotic mechanisms.[131] The MeDIP-Seq results for methylation status of PDCD5 and TIMP2 were confirmed and the messenger RNA expression levels of these 2 genes were consistent with their DNA methylation profiles.[131] Likewise, MeDIP-Seq of CD4$^+$ T cells from psoriatic patients revealed global DNA hypermethylation compared with healthy controls, and hypermethylated regions were enriched in gene promoters.[132] Unfortunately, studies of genome-wide DNA methylation in PsA patients are lacking.

PHARMACOGENETICS OF PSORIATIC DISEASE

That disease severity varies from patient to patient, that comorbidities are frequent and that patient response to therapy (ie, efficacy and adverse events) is quite variable and unpredictable underscores the importance of personalization with respect to therapy. Biologic agents such as etancerpt (Enbrel), adalumimab (Humira), infliximab (Remicade), and ustekinumab (Stelara) are used increasingly to treat moderate-to-severe PsA in patients refractory to traditional therapy, and are the focus of this section. Because these biologics are newer medications for the treatment of psoriasis and PsA compared with systemic agents, studies investigating their pharmacogenetic profile are limited. Consequently, adequately powered pharmacogenetic studies in psoriasis and PsA are currently lacking.

Tumor Necrosis Factor-α Inhibitors

The potential importance of TNF-α in the pathogenesis of psoriasis is underscored by (1) the report of increased levels of TNF-α in both the affected skin and serum of patients with psoriasis; (2) the increased levels correlate with psoriasis severity as measured by the Psoriasis Area and Severity Index score; and (3) the decrease in TNF-α levels, returning to normal after successful treatment of psoriasis.[133] TNF-α blockade represents a major advancement in the treatment of psoriasis and PsA.[134] Controlled trials with etanercept, infliximab, and adalimumab have demonstrated impressive improvement in most response measures.[135–140] However, response to treatment is still variable with 20% to 40% of patients experiencing an inadequate response.

It has been proposed that genetic factors contribute substantially to clinical responses to TNF-α inhibitors. PsA patients with the *TNFα* -308 GG genotype responded better to TNF-α inhibitors than those with the AA or AG genotypes,[141] and the *TNF-α* +489A allele showed a trend of association with the response to PsA treatment with etanercept, although there is as yet no evidence for a causal relationship.[142] The *TNFRSF10A* CC genotype (rs20575) was associated with European League Against Rheumatism (EULAR) response to infliximab at 6 months, whereas the *TNFR1A* AA genotype (rs767455) was associated with a better EULAR response at 3 months in PsA patients.[143] This finding is consistent with evidence that *TNFRSF10A* is expressed in PsA patients, where it can induce cell cycle arrest of proinflammatory cells and apoptosis in arthritic synovium.[144,145] An interaction between the *HLA-Cw6* and *LCE* genotypes on disease improvement among psoriatic patients treated with TNF-α inhibitors,[146] and a highly significant association between *PDE3A-SLCO1C1* and clinical response to TNF-α inhibitors in psoriasis have been recently reported.[146] Furthermore, PsA patients with high-affinity *FCGR2A* (p.H131R) genotypes (homozygous wild-type or heterozygous combinations) achieved a EULAR response at 6 months compared with patients with the low-affinity genotype (homozygous mutant).[147] Although these results require confirmation in larger prospective cohorts, they do suggest that variants affecting genes involved in general immunity and the TNF-α signaling pathway might functionally affect the response to TNF-α inhibitors.

Expression profiling studies investigating response to TNF-α inhibitors in psoriasis is also limited. Psoriasis disease improvement at 1 month after treatment with etanercept was highly correlated with IL-1, matrix metalloproteinase-12, and several type 1 pathway products, including STAT-1, IL-23, MIG, IL-8, and inducible nitrous oxide synthase.[148] Comparisons of responders and nonresponders to TNF-α inhibitors revealed rapid downregulation of innate IL-1β, IL-8, and IL-17 pathway genes with administration of etanercept.[69] Thus, the effective treatment of psoriasis with etanercept is linked to IL-17 signaling. Large, prospective psoriasis cohorts are needed to identify pharmacogenetic markers influencing TNF-α inhibitors.

Interleukin-12/23 Inhibitors

Ustekinumab is a targeted monoclonal antibody directed against the common p40 subunit of IL-12 and IL-23. Ustekinumab has demonstrated superior efficacy and safety in the treatment of plaque psoriasis by its unique mechanism of inhibiting IL-12/23 inflammatory pathways.[149,150] There is growing evidence that genes participating in IL-12/23 signaling play a prominent role in the pathogenesis of chronic epithelial inflammation, as observed in psoriasis.[151] Pharmacogenetic studies of ustekinumab are lacking in psoriasis patients, with only a single study being published. In that study, a faster and increased response to ustekinumab has been reported in HLA-Cw6–positive psoriasis patients.[152]

There have been 3 studies, which have performed gene expression profiling after ustekinumab treatment. The expression of numerous genes was significantly reduced in responders 2 weeks after anti–IL-12p40 administration in psoriasis patients.[122] Four weeks after a single ustekinumab injection, *NGF* showed a significant decrease, whereas *GATA3* and *IL-22RA1* expression increased, indicative of reduced responsiveness to epidermal triggering.[153] *IL-20, IL-21*, and *p40* messenger RNA expression in lesional psoriatic skin at baseline were upregulated significantly among nonresponders compared with responders.[154] These findings suggest that the development of a "genetic signature" could identify responders versus nonresponders to ustekinumab therapy and identify candidate genes, which can be investigated further in larger psoriasis cohorts.

SUMMARY

Despite the large number of genes identified in psoriatic disease, in particular psoriasis, the genetic contribution identified by GWAS accounts for less than 25% of psoriasis heritability. This "missing heritability" is attributed, at least in part, to inherent limitations of this technology as GWAS primarily assesses 1 type of genetic variation (ie, single nucleotide polymorphisms) and limits searches to common variants and neglects rare variants, which may also contribute to disease susceptibility. No clinically actionable information can be gleaned by a single variant from GWAS studies owing to the very low odds ratio for the individual variants. A genetic risk score combining multiple loci associated with psoriasis/PsA might hold more clinical promise.

Additional complexities that need to be assessed include gene–gene and gene–environment interactions, with gene–gene interaction being reported in psoriasis with respect to defective processing of antigens indicated by the epistatic association of the *ERAP1* and *HLA-Cw6* in PsV.[32] With respect to study design, family-based designs focusing on highly penetrant, rare variants, segregating in multiplex families should be encouraged. With respect to technologies, discovery of rare variants with extensive resequencing studies may prove fruitful. Moreover, searching for different types of genetic variants, such as small CNVs and insertions/deletions using multiple platforms, is recommended.

Additional pharmacogenetic studies in psoriasis or PsA are required, because those conducted to date are often too small (ie, underpowered), have modest effect sizes, and have produced inconsistent results. A priori knowledge of pharmacogenetic mechanisms associated with psoriasis and PsA pharmacotherapy has the potential to identify and therefore stratify patients into clinically important treatment categories (ie, responders vs nonresponders; tolerant vs intolerant).

REFERENCES

1. Chandran V, Schentag CT, Brockbank JE, et al. Familial aggregation of psoriatic arthritis. Ann Rheum Dis 2009;68:664–7.
2. Nair RP, Stuart PE, Nistor I, et al. Sequence and haplotype analysis supports HLA-C as the psoriasis susceptibility 1 gene. Am J Hum Genet 2006;78:827–51.
3. Eder L, Chandran V, Pellett F, et al. Differential human leucocyte allele association between psoriasis and psoriatic arthritis: a family-based association study. Ann Rheum Dis 2012;71:1361–5.
4. Gudjonsson JE, Karason A, Runarsdottir EH, et al. Distinct clinical differences between HLA-Cw*0602 positive and negative psoriasis patients–an analysis of 1019 HLA-C- and HLA-B-typed patients. J Invest Dermatol 2006;126:740–5.
5. Eder L, Chandran V, Gladman DD. What have we learned about genetic susceptibility in psoriasis and psoriatic arthritis? Curr Opin Rheumatol 2015;27:91–8.
6. Winchester R, Minevich G, Steshenko V, et al. HLA associations reveal genetic heterogeneity in psoriatic arthritis and in the psoriasis phenotype. Arthritis Rheum 2012;64:1134–44.
7. Haroon M, Winchester R, Giles JT, et al. Certain class I HLA alleles and haplotypes implicated in susceptibility play a role in determining specific features of the psoriatic arthritis phenotype. Ann Rheum Dis 2014. [Epub ahead of print].

8. Eder L, Chandran V, Pellet F, et al. Human leucocyte antigen risk alleles for psoriatic arthritis among patients with psoriasis. Ann Rheum Dis 2012;71: 50–5.

9. Okada Y, Han B, Tsoi LC, et al. Fine mapping major histocompatibility complex associations in psoriasis and its clinical subtypes. Am J Hum Genet 2014;95: 162–72.

10. Gonzalez S, Martinez-Borra J, Torre-Alonso JC, et al. The MICA-A9 triplet repeat polymorphism in the transmembrane region confers additional susceptibility to the development of psoriatic arthritis and is independent of the association of Cw*0602 in psoriasis. Arthritis Rheum 1999;42:1010–6.

11. Lanier LL. NK cell recognition. Annu Rev Immunol 2005;23:225–74.

12. Chandran V, Bull SB, Pellett FJ, et al. Killer-cell immunoglobulin-like receptor gene polymorphisms and susceptibility to psoriatic arthritis. Rheumatology 2014;53:233–9.

13. O'Rielly DD, Rahman P. Genetics of susceptibility and treatment response in psoriatic arthritis. Nat Rev Rheumatol 2011;7:718–32.

14. Karason A, Gudjonsson JE, Upmanyu R, et al. A susceptibility gene for psoriatic arthritis maps to chromosome 16q: evidence for imprinting. Am J Hum Genet 2003;72:125–31.

15. Schroder JM, Harder J. Human beta-defensin-2. Int J Biochem Cell Biol 1999; 31:645–51.

16. Hollox EJ, Huffmeier U, Zeeuwen PL, et al. Psoriasis is associated with increased β defensin genomic copy number. Nat Genet 2008;40:23–5.

17. Niyonsaba F, Ogawa H, Nagaoka I. Human β defensin 2 functions as a chemotactic agent for tumour necrosis factor α-treated human neutrophils. Immunology 2004;111:273–81.

18. Filer C, Ho P, Smith RL, et al. Investigation of association of the IL12B and IL23R genes with psoriatic arthritis. Arthritis Rheum 2008;58:3705–9.

19. Li M, Wu Y, Chen G, et al. Deletion of the late cornified envelope genes LCE3C and LCE3B is associated with psoriasis in a Chinese population. J Invest Dermatol 2011;131:1639–43.

20. Coto E, Santos-Juanes J, Coto-Segura P, et al. Mutation analysis of the LCE3B/LCE3C genes in Psoriasis. BMC Med Genet 2010;11:45.

21. Riveira-Munoz E, He SM, Escaramís G, et al. Meta-analysis confirms the LCE3C_LCE3B deletion as a risk factor for psoriasis in several ethnic groups and finds interaction with HLA-Cw6. J Invest Dermatol 2011;131:1105–9.

22. Labarthe MP, Bosco D, Saurat JH, et al. Upregulation of connexin 26 between keratinocytes of psoriatic lesions. J Invest Dermatol 1998;111:72–6.

23. Djalilian AR, McGaughey D, Patel S, et al. Connexin 26 regulates epidermal barrier and wound remodeling and promotes psoriasiform response. J Clin Invest 2006;116:1243–53.

24. Sun LD, Cheng H, Wang ZX, et al. Association analyses identify six new psoriasis susceptibility loci in the Chinese population. Nat Genet 2010;42:1005–9.

25. Hüffmeier U, Uebe S, Ekici AB, et al. Common variants at TRAF3IP2 are associated with susceptibility to psoriatic arthritis and psoriasis. Nat Genet 2010;42: 996–9.

26. Tsoi LC, Spain SL, Knight J, et al. Identification of 15 new psoriasis susceptibility loci highlights the role of innate immunity. Nat Genet 2012;44(12):1341–8.

27. Ellinghaus D, Ellinghaus E, Nair RP, et al. Combined analysis of genome-wide association studies for Crohn disease and psoriasis identifies seven shared susceptibility loci. Am J Hum Genet 2012;90:636–47.

28. Liu Y, Helms C, Liao W, et al. A genome-wide association study of psoriasis and psoriatic arthritis identifies new disease loci. PLoS Genet 2008;4:e1000041.
29. Stuart PE, Nair RP, Ellinghaus E, et al. Genome-wide association analysis identifies three psoriasis susceptibility loci. Nat Genet 2010;42:1000–4.
30. Nair RP, Duffin KC, Helms C, et al. Genome-wide scan reveals association of psoriasis with IL-23 and NF-kappaB pathways. Nat Genet 2009;41:199–204.
31. Ellinghaus E, Ellinghaus D, Stuart PE, et al. Genome-wide association study identifies a psoriasis susceptibility locus at TRAF3IP2. Nat Genet 2010;42: 991–5.
32. Strange A, Capon F, Spencer CC, et al. A genome-wide association study identifies new psoriasis susceptibility loci and an interaction between HLA-C and ERAP1. Nat Genet 2010;42:985–90.
33. Zhang XJ, Huang W, Yang S, et al. Psoriasis genome-wide association study identifies susceptibility variants within LCE gene cluster at 1q21. Nat Genet 2009;41:205–10.
34. Verstrepen L, Carpentier I, Verhelst K, et al. ABINs: A20 binding inhibitors of NF-kappa B and apoptosis signaling. Biochem Pharmacol 2009;78:105–14.
35. Hayden MS, Ghosh S. NF κB in immunobiology. Cell Res 2011;21:223–44.
36. Orozco G, Eyre S, Hinks A, et al. Study of the common genetic background for rheumatoid arthritis and systemic lupus erythematosus. Ann Rheum Dis 2011; 70:463–8.
37. Vereecke L, Beyaert R, van Loo G. Genetic relationships between A20/TNFAIP3, chronic inflammation and autoimmune disease. Biochem Soc Trans 2011;39: 1086–91.
38. Nititham J, Taylor KE, Gupta R, et al. Meta-analysis of the TNFAIP3 region in psoriasis reveals a risk haplotype that is distinct from other autoimmune diseases. Genes Immun 2015;16:120–6.
39. De Molfetta GA, Lucíola Zanette D, Alexandre Panepucci R, et al. Role of NFKB2 on the early myeloid differentiation of CD34+ hematopoietic stem/progenitor cells. Differentiation 2010;80:195–203.
40. Lowenstein CJ, Padalko E. iNOS (NOS2) at a glance. J Cell Sci 2004;117: 2865–7.
41. Strobl B, Stoiber D, Sexl V, et al. Tyrosine kinase 2 (TYK2) in cytokine signaling and host immunity. Front Biosci 2011;16:3214–32.
42. Blonska M, Lin X. NF-κB signaling pathways regulated by CARMA family of scaffold proteins. Cell Res 2011;21(1):55–70.
43. Lu T, Jackson MW, Wang B, et al. Regulation of NF-kappaB by NSD1/FBXL11-dependent reversible lysine methylation of p65. Proc Natl Acad Sci U S A 2010; 107:46–51.
44. Orian A, Whiteside S, Israël A, et al. Ubiquitin-mediated processing of NF-kappa B transcriptional activator precursor p105. Reconstitution of a cell-free system and identification of the ubiquitin-carrier protein, E2, and a novel ubiquitin-protein ligase, E3, involved in conjugation. J Biol Chem 1995; 270(37):21707–14.
45. Zhou Z, Hamming OJ, Ank N, et al. Type III interferon (IFN) induces a type I IFN-like response in a restricted subset of cells through signaling pathways involving both the Jak-STAT pathway and the mitogen-activated protein kinases. J Virol 2007;81(14):7749–58.
46. Gotoh K, Tanaka Y, Nishikimi A, et al. Selective control of type I IFN induction by the Rac activator DOCK2 during TLR-mediated plasmacytoid dendritic cell activation. J Exp Med 2010;207(4):721–30.

47. Negishi H, Osawa T, Ogami K, et al. A critical link between Toll-like receptor 3 and type II interferon signaling pathways in antiviral innate immunity. Proc Natl Acad Sci U S A 2008;105(51):20446–51.

48. Piganis RA, De Weerd NA, Gould JA, et al. Suppressor of cytokine signaling (SOCS) 1 inhibits type I interferon (IFN) signaling via the interferon alpha receptor (IFNAR1)-associated tyrosine kinase Tyk2. J Biol Chem 2011;286(39): 33811–8.

49. Bijlmakers MJ, Kanneganti SK, Barker JN, et al. Functional analysis of the RNF114 psoriasis susceptibility gene implicates innate immune responses to double-stranded RNA in disease pathogenesis. Hum Mol Genet 2011;20(16): 3129–37.

50. Veale DJ, Barnes L, Rogers S, et al. Immunohistochemical markers for arthritis in psoriasis. Ann Rheum Dis 1994;53(7):450–4.

51. Pitzalis C, Cauli A, Pipitone N, et al. Cutaneous lymphocyte antigen-positive T lymphocytes preferentially migrate to the skin but not to the joint in psoriatic arthritis. Arthritis Rheum 1996;39(1):137–45.

52. Miossec P. IL-17 and Th17 cells in human inflammatory diseases. Microbes Infect 2009;11(5):625–30.

53. Bowcock AM, Shannon W, Du F, et al. Insights into psoriasis and other inflammatory diseases from large-scale gene expression studies. Hum Mol Genet 2001; 10(17):1793–805.

54. Kersh EN. Impaired memory CD8 T cell development in the absence of methyl-CpG-binding domain protein 2. J Immunol 2006;177(6):3821–6.

55. Zamisch M, Tian L, Grenningloh R, et al. The transcription factor Ets1 is important for CD4 repression and Runx3 up-regulation during CD8 T cell differentiation in the thymus. J Exp Med 2009;206(12):2685–99.

56. Chang IF, Hsiao HY. Induction of RhoGAP and pathological changes characteristic of Alzheimer's disease by UAHFEMF discharge in rat brain. Curr Alzheimer Res 2005;2(5):559–69.

57. Togayachi A, Kozono Y, Kuno A, et al. Beta3GnT2 (B3GNT2), a major polylactosamine synthase: analysis of B3GNT2-deficient mice. Methods Enzymol 2010; 479:185–204.

58. Yan J, Parekh VV, Mendez-Fernandez Y, et al. In vivo role of ER associated peptidase activity in tailoring peptides for presentation by MHC class Ia and class Ib molecules. J Exp Med 2006;203(3):647–59.

59. Ryan C, Abramson A, Patel M, et al. Current investigational drugs in psoriasis. Expert Opin Investig Drugs 2012;21(4):473–87.

60. Liang J, Wang J, Azfer A, et al. A novel CCCH-zinc finger protein family regulates proinflammatory activation of macrophages. J Biol Chem 2008;283(10): 6337–46.

61. Robinson RT. IL12Rβ1: the cytokine receptor that we used to know. Cytokine 2015;71(2):348–59.

62. Wei L, Laurence A, O'Shea JJ. New insights into the roles of Stat5a/b and Stat3 in T cell development and differentiation. Semin Cell Dev Biol 2008;19(4): 394–400.

63. Marcoulatos P, Avgerinos E, Tsantzalos DV, et al. Mapping interleukin enhancer binding factor 3 gene (ILF3) to human chromosome 19 (19q11-qter and 19p11-p13.1) by polymerase chain reaction amplification of human-rodent somatic cell hybrid DNA templates. J Interferon Cytokine Res 1998;18(5):351–5.

64. Cheung PF, Wong CK, Lam CW. Molecular mechanisms of cytokine and chemokine release from eosinophils activated by IL-17A, IL-17F, and IL-23: implication

for Th17 lymphocytes-mediated allergic inflammation. J Immunol 2008;180: 5625–35.

65. Bulek K, Liu C, Swaidani S, et al. The inducible kinase IKKi is required for IL-17-dependent signaling associated with neutrophilia and pulmonary inflammation. Nat Immunol 2011;12:844–52.

66. Sønder SU, Saret S, Tang W, et al. IL-17-induced NF-kappaB activation via CIKS/Act1: physiologic significance and signaling mechanisms. J Biol Chem 2011;286:12881–90.

67. Fujioka S, Niu J, Schmidt C, et al. NF-kappaB and AP-1 connection: mechanism of NF-kappaB-dependent regulation of AP-1 activity. Mol Cell Biol 2004;24: 7806–19.

68. Chiricozzi A, Guttman-Yassky E, Suárez-Faripas M, et al. Integrative responses to IL-17 and TNF-α in human keratinocytes account for key inflammatory pathogenic circuits in psoriasis. J Invest Dermatol 2011;131:677–87.

69. Zaba LC, Suárez-Fariñas M, Fuentes-Duculan J, et al. Effective treatment of psoriasis with etanercept is linked to suppression of IL-17 signaling, not immediate response TNF genes. J Allergy Clin Immunol 2009;124:1022–30.

70. Tesmer LA, Lundy SK, Sarkar S, et al. Th17 cells in human disease. Immunol Rev 2008;223:87–113.

71. Flisiak I, Chodynicka B, Porebski P, et al. Association between psoriasis severity and transforming growth factor beta(1) and beta (2) in plasma and scales from psoriatic lesions. Cytokine 2002;19:121–5.

72. Flisiak I, Zaniewski P, Chodynicka B. Plasma TGF-beta1, TIMP-1, MMP-1 and IL-18 as a combined biomarker of psoriasis activity. Biomarkers 2008;13: 549–56.

73. Nockowski P, Szepietowski JC, Ziarkiewicz M, et al. Serum concentrations of transforming growth factor beta 1 in patients with psoriasis vulgaris. Acta Dermatovenerol Croat 2004;12:2–6.

74. Lindroos J, Svensson L, Norsgaard H, et al. IL-23-mediated epidermal hyperplasia is dependent on IL-6. J Invest Dermatol 2011;131:1110–8.

75. Yang XP, Ghoreschi K, Steward-Tharp SM, et al. Opposing regulation of the locus encoding IL-17 through direct, reciprocal actions of STAT3 and STAT5. Nat Immunol 2011;12:247–54.

76. Boca AN, Talamonti M, Galluzzo M, et al. Genetic variations in IL6 and IL12B decreasing the risk for psoriasis. Immunol Lett 2013;156:127–31.

77. Di Cesare A, Di Meglio P, Nestle FO. The IL-23/Th17 axis in the immunopathogenesis of psoriasis. J Invest Dermatol 2009;129:1339–50.

78. Korn T, Bettelli E, Oukka M, et al. IL-17 and Th17 Cells. Annu Rev Immunol 2009; 27:485–517.

79. Blumberg H, Dinh H, Dean C Jr, et al. IL-1RL2 and its ligands contribute to the cytokine network in psoriasis. J Immunol 2010;185:4354–62.

80. Julià A, Tortosa R, Hernanz JM, et al. Risk variants for psoriasis vulgaris in a large case-control collection and association with clinical subphenotypes. Hum Mol Genet 2012;21:4549–57.

81. Rahman P, Sun S, Peddle L, et al. Association between the interleukin-1 family gene cluster and psoriatic arthritis. Arthritis Rheum 2006;54:2321–5.

82. Ravindran JS, Owen P, Lagan A, et al. Interleukin 1alpha, interleukin 1beta and interleukin 1 receptor gene polymorphisms in psoriatic arthritis. Rheumatology (Oxford) 2004;43:22–6.

83. Bowes J, Ho P, Flynn E, et al. Investigation of IL1, VEGF, PPARG and MEFV genes in psoriatic arthritis susceptibility. Ann Rheum Dis 2012;71:313–4.

84. Oppmann B, Lesley R, Blom B, et al. Novel p19 protein engages IL-12p40 to form a cytokine, IL-23, with biological activities similar as well as distinct from IL-12. Immunity 2000;13:715–25.
85. Pappu R, Ramirez-Carrozzi V, Sambandam A. The interleukin-17 cytokine family: critical players in host defence and inflammatory diseases. Immunology 2011; 134:8–16.
86. Szodoray P, Alex P, Chappell-Woodward CM, et al. Circulating cytokines in Norwegian patients with psoriatic arthritis determined by a multiplex cytokine array system. Rheumatology (Oxford) 2007;46:417–25.
87. Lee E, Trepicchio WL, Oestreicher JL, et al. Increased expression of interleukin 23 p19 and p40 in lesional skin of patients with psoriasis vulgaris. J Exp Med 2004;199:125–30.
88. Tang C, Chen S, Qian H, et al. Interleukin-23: as a drug target for autoimmune inflammatory diseases. Immunology 2012;135:112–24.
89. Langrish CL, Chen Y, Blumenschein WM, et al. IL-23 drives a pathogenic T cell population that induces autoimmune inflammation. J Exp Med 2005;201: 233–40.
90. Harris TJ, Grosso JF, Yen HR, et al. Cutting edge: an in vivo requirement for STAT3 signaling in TH17 development and TH17-dependent autoimmunity. J Immunol 2007;179:4313–7.
91. Tanaka K, Ichiyama K, Hashimoto M, et al. Loss of suppressor of cytokine signaling 1 in helper T cells leads to defective Th17 differentiation by enhancing antagonistic effects of IFN-gamma on STAT3 and Smads. J Immunol 2008;180: 3746–56.
92. Moisan J, Grenningloh R, Bettelli E, et al. Ets-1 is a negative regulator of Th17 differentiation. J Exp Med 2007;204:2825–35.
93. Novatchkova M, Leibbrandt A, Werzowa J, et al. The STIR-domain superfamily in signal transduction, development and immunity. Trends Biochem Sci 2003;28: 226–9.
94. Toy D, Kugler D, Wolfson M, et al. Cutting edge: interleukin 17 signals through a heteromeric receptor complex. J Immunol 2006;177:36–9.
95. Lubberts E. IL-17/Th17 targeting: on the road to prevent chronic destructive arthritis? Cytokine 2008;41:84–91.
96. Chabaud M, Lubberts E, Joosten L, et al. IL-17 derived from juxta-articular bone and synovium contributes to joint degradation in rheumatoid arthritis. Arthritis Res 2001;3:168–77.
97. Raychaudhuri SP, Raychaudhuri SK, Genovese MC. IL-17 receptor and its functional significance in psoriatic arthritis. Mol Cell Biochem 2012;359:419–29.
98. Mrabet D, Laadhar L, Sahli H, et al. Synovial fluid and serum levels of IL-17, IL-23, and CCL-20 in rheumatoid arthritis and psoriatic arthritis: a Tunisian cross-sectional study. Rheumatol Int 2013;33:265–6.
99. Tonel G, Conrad C, Laggner U, et al. Cutting edge: a critical functional role for IL-23 in psoriasis. J Immunol 2010;185:5688–91.
100. Wilson NJ, Boniface K, Chan JR, et al. Development, cytokine profile and function of human interleukin 17-producing helper T cells. Nat Immunol 2007;8: 950–7.
101. Feinberg MW, Cao Z, Wara AK, et al. Kruppel-like factor 4 is a mediator of proinflammatory signaling in macrophages. J Biol Chem 2005;280(46):38247–58.
102. Huber M, Brüstle A, Reinhard K, et al. IRF4 is essential for IL-21-mediated induction, amplification, and stabilization of the Th17 phenotype. Proc Natl Acad Sci U S A 2008;105(52):20846–51.

103. Ammar M, Bouchlaka-Souissi C, Zaraa I, et al. Family-based association study in Tunisian familial psoriasis. Int J Dermatol 2012;51:1329–34.
104. Catanoso MG, Boiardi L, Macchioni P, et al. IL-23A, IL-23R, IL-17A and IL-17R polymorphisms in different psoriatic arthritis clinical manifestations in the northern Italian population. Rheumatol Int 2013;33:1165–76.
105. Prans E, Kingo K, Traks T, et al. Copy number variations in IL22 gene are associated with Psoriasis vulgaris. Hum Immunol 2013;74:792–5.
106. Tohyama M, Hanakawa Y, Shirakata Y, et al. IL-17 and IL-22 mediate IL-20 subfamily cytokine production in cultured keratinocytes via increased IL-22 receptor expression. Eur J Immunol 2009;39:2779–88.
107. Saeki H, Hirota T, Nakagawa H, et al. Genetic polymorphisms in the IL22 gene are associated with psoriasis vulgaris in a Japanese population. J Dermatol Sci 2013;71:148–50.
108. Yang XO, Pappu BP, Nurieva R, et al. T helper 17 lineage differentiation is programmed by orphan nuclear receptors ROR alpha and ROR gamma. Immunity 2008;28:29–39.
109. Korn T, Bettelli E, Gao W, et al. IL-21 initiates an alternative pathway to induce proinflammatory T(H)17 cells. Nature 2007;448:484–7.
110. Nurieva R, Yang XO, Martinez G, et al. Essential autocrine regulation by IL-21 in the generation of inflammatory T cells. Nature 2007;448:480–3.
111. Caruso R, Botti E, Sarra M, et al. Involvement of interleukin-21 in the epidermal hyperplasia of psoriasis. Nat Med 2009;15:1013–5.
112. He Z, Jin L, Liu ZF, et al. Elevated serum levels of interleukin 21 are associated with disease severity in patients with psoriasis. Br J Dermatol 2012;167:191–3.
113. Warren RB, Smith RL, Flynn E, et al. A systematic investigation of confirmed autoimmune loci in early-onset psoriasis reveals an association with IL2/IL21. Br J Dermatol 2011;164:660–4.
114. Bowes J, Orozco G, Flynn E, et al. Confirmation of TNIP1 and IL23A as susceptibility loci for psoriatic arthritis. Ann Rheum Dis 2011;70:1641–4.
115. Zhu KJ, Zhu CY, Shi G, et al. Association of IL23R polymorphisms with psoriasis and psoriatic arthritis: a meta-analysis. Inflamm Res 2012;61:1149–54.
116. Cénit MC, Ortego-Centeno N, Raya E, et al. Influence of the STAT3 genetic variants in the susceptibility to psoriatic arthritis and Behcet's disease. Hum Immunol 2013;74:230–3.
117. Leipe J, Grunke M, Dechant C, et al. Role of Th17 cells in human autoimmune arthritis. Arthritis Rheum 2010;62(10):2876–85.
118. van Kuijk AW, Reinders-Blankert P, Smeets TJ, et al. Detailed analysis of the cell infiltrate and the expression of mediators of synovial inflammation and joint destruction in the synovium of patients with psoriatic arthritis: implications for treatment. Ann Rheum Dis 2006;65(12):1551–7.
119. Yago T, Nanke Y, Kawamoto M, et al. IL-23 induces human osteoclastogenesis via IL-17 in vitro, and anti-IL-23 antibody attenuates collagen-induced arthritis in rats. Arthritis Res Ther 2007;9(5):R96.
120. Gottlieb A, Menter A, Mendelsohn A, et al. Ustekinumab, a human interleukin 12/23 monoclonal antibody, for psoriatic arthritis: randomised, double-blind, placebo-controlled, crossover trial. Lancet 2009;373(9664):633–40.
121. Gervin K, Vigeland MD, Mattingsdal M, et al. DNA methylation and gene expression changes in monozygotic twins discordant for psoriasis: identification of epigenetically dysregulated genes. PLoS Genet 2012;8(1):e1002454.

122. Gudjonsson JE, Krueger G. A role for epigenetics in psoriasis: methylated Cytosine-Guanine sites differentiate lesional from nonlesional skin and from normal skin. J Invest Dermatol 2012;132(3 Pt 1):506–8.
123. Duffin KC, Freeny IC, Schrodi SJ, et al. Association between IL13 polymorphisms and psoriatic arthritis is modified by smoking. J Invest Dermatol 2009; 129(12):2777–83.
124. Eder L, Chandran V, Pellett F, et al. IL13 gene polymorphism is a marker for psoriatic arthritis among psoriasis patients. Ann Rheum Dis 2011;70(9):1594–8.
125. Chatterjee R, Vinson C. CpG methylation recruits sequence specific transcription factors essential for tissue specific gene expression. Biochim Biophys Acta 2012;1819(7):763–70.
126. Zhang P, Su Y, Chen H, et al. Abnormal DNA methylation in skin lesions and PBMCs of patients with psoriasis vulgaris. J Dermatol Sci 2010;60(1):40–2.
127. Han J, Park SG, Bae JB, et al. The characteristics of genome-wide DNA methylation in naïve CD4+ T cells of patients with psoriasis or atopic dermatitis. Biochem Biophys Res Commun 2012;422(1):157–63.
128. Roberson ED, Liu Y, Ryan C, et al. A subset of methylated CpG sites differentiate psoriatic from normal skin. J Invest Dermatol 2012;132(3 Pt 1):583–92.
129. Gu X, Nylander E, Coates PJ, et al. Correlation between reversal of DNA methylation and clinical symptoms in psoriatic epidermis following narrow-band UVB phototherapy. J Invest Dermatol 2015;135(8):2077–83.
130. Hou R, Yin G, An P, et al. DNA methylation of dermal MSCs in psoriasis: identification of epigenetically dysregulated genes. J Dermatol Sci 2013;72(2):103–9.
131. Zhang P, Zhao M, Liang G, et al. Whole-genome DNA methylation in skin lesions from patients with psoriasis vulgaris. J Autoimmun 2013;41:17–24.
132. Park GT, Han J, Park SG, et al. DNA methylation analysis of CD4+ T cells in patients with psoriasis. Arch Dermatol Res 2014;306(3):259–68.
133. Mizutani H, Ohmoto Y, Mizutani T, et al. Role of increased production of monocytes TNF-alpha, IL-1beta and IL-6 in psoriasis: relation to focal infection, disease activity and responses to treatments. J Dermatol Sci 1997; 14(2):145–53.
134. Anandarajah A, Ritchlin CT. Treatment update on spondyloarthropathy. Curr Opin Rheumatol 2005;17(3):247–56.
135. Gottlieb AB, Leonardi CL, Goffe BS, et al. Etanercept monotherapy in patients with psoriasis: a summary of safety, based on an integrated multistudy database. J Am Acad Dermatol 2006;54(Suppl):S92–100.
136. Krueger GG, Langley RG, Finlay AY, et al. Patient-reported outcomes of psoriasis improvement with etanercept therapy: results of a randomized phase III trial. Br J Dermatol 2005;153:1192–9.
137. Moore A, Gordon KB, Kang S, et al. A randomized, open-label trial of continuous versus interrupted etanercept therapy in the treatment of psoriasis. J Am Acad Dermatol 2007;56:598–603.
138. Gottlieb AB, Masud S, Ramamurthi R, et al. Pharmacodynamic and pharmacokinetic response to anti-tumor necrosis factor-alpha monoclonal antibody (infliximab) treatment of moderate to severe psoriasis vulgaris. J Am Acad Dermatol 2003;48:68–75.
139. Menter A, Gottlieb A, Feldman SR, et al. Guidelines of care for the management of psoriasis and psoriatic arthritis: section 1. Overview of psoriasis and guidelines of care for the treatment of psoriasis with biologics. J Am Acad Dermatol 2008;58(5):826–50.

140. Menter A, Tyring SK, Gordon K, et al. Adalimumab therapy for moderate to severe psoriasis: a randomized, controlled phase III trial. J Am Acad Dermatol 2007;58:106–15.

141. Seitz M, Wirthmüller U, Möller B, et al. The -308 tumour necrosis factor-alpha gene polymorphism predicts therapeutic response to TNFalpha-blockers in rheumatoid arthritis and spondyloarthritis patients. Rheumatology (Oxford) 2007;46:93–6.

142. Murdaca G, Gulli R, Spanò F, et al. TNF-α gene polymorphisms: association with disease susceptibility and response to anti-TNF-α treatment in psoriatic arthritis. J Invest Dermatol 2014;134:2503–9.

143. Morales-Lara MJ, Cañete JD, Torres-Moreno D, et al. Effects of polymorphisms in TRAILR1 and TNFR1A on the response to anti-TNF therapies in patients with rheumatoid and psoriatic arthritis. Joint Bone Spine 2012;79:591–6.

144. Pundt N, Peters MA, Wunrau C, et al. Susceptibility of rheumatoid arthritis synovial fibroblasts to FasL- and TRAIL-induced apoptosis is cell cycle-dependent. Arthritis Res Ther 2009;11:R16.

145. Hofbauer LC, Schoppet M, Christ M, et al. Tumour necrosis factor-related apoptosis-inducing ligand and osteoprotegerin serum levels in psoriatic arthritis. Rheumatology (Oxford) 2006;45:1218–22.

146. Batalla A, Coto E, González-Fernández D, et al. The Cw6 and late-cornified envelope genotype plays a significant role in anti-tumor necrosis factor response among psoriatic patients. Pharmacogenet Genomics 2015;25(6):313–6.

147. Ramírez J, Fernández-Sueiro JL, López-Mejías R, et al. FCGR2A/CD32A and FCGR3A/CD16A variants and EULAR response to tumor necrosis factor-α blockers in psoriatic arthritis: a longitudinal study with 6 months of followup. J Rheumatol 2012;39:1035–41.

148. Gottlieb AB, Chamian F, Masud S, et al. TNF inhibition rapidly down-regulates multiple proinflammatory pathways in psoriasis plaques. J Immunol 2005;175:2721–9.

149. Krueger GG, Langley RG, Leonardi C, et al. A human interleukin-12/23 monoclonal antibody for the treatment of psoriasis. N Engl J Med 2007;356(6):580–92.

150. Chien AL, Elder JT, Ellis CN. Ustekinumab: a new option in psoriasis therapy. Drugs 2009;69(9):1141–52.

151. Chen X, Tan Z, Yue Q, et al. The expression of interleukin-23 (p19/p40) and inteleukin-12 (p35/p40) in psoriasis skin. J Huazhong Univ Sci Technolog Med Sci 2006;26(6):750–2.

152. Talamonti M, Botti E, Galluzzo M, et al. Pharmacogenetics of psoriasis: HLA-Cw6 but not LCE3B/3C deletion nor TNFAIP3 polymorphism predisposes to clinical response to interleukin 12/23 blocker ustekinumab. Br J Dermatol 2013;169(2):458–63.

153. Baerveldt EM, Onderdijk AJ, Kurek D, et al. Ustekinumab improves psoriasis-related gene expression in noninvolved psoriatic skin without inhibition of the antimicrobial response. Br J Dermatol 2013;168(5):990–8.

154. Gedebjerg A, Johansen C, Kragballe K, et al. IL-20, IL-21 and p40: potential biomarkers of treatment response for ustekinumab. Acta Derm Venereol 2013;93(2):150–5.

Etiology and Pathogenesis of Psoriatic Arthritis

Jennifer L. Barnas, MD, PhD, Christopher T. Ritchlin, MD, MPH*

KEYWORDS

- Psoriatic arthritis • IL-23 • IL-17 • Psoriasis • Spondyloarthropathy • Enthesitis
- Inflammatory arthritis • Dactylitis

KEY POINTS

- Psoriatic arthritis appears to be triggered by autoinflammatory cytokine networks responding to microbiome and mechanical stress signals.
- Interleukin (IL)-23, IL-17, and tumor necrosis factor-α are instrumental in pathogenesis and have served as clinically effective therapeutic targets.
- Alterations in bone resorption and formation are due to interplay of several signaling networks, including RANK-L, Wnt, and BMP.

Arthritis associated with psoriasis was first described in 1956 by Wright.[1] It was not until 1973, however, that Moll and Wright[2] defined the various clinical phenotypes, including asymmetric arthritis, enthesitis, dactylitis, and nail disease. The following year, these authors introduced the concept of spondyloarthritis, a cluster of diseases with shared clinical and immunogenetic features.[3] Despite these advances, the immunopathogenesis of psoriatic arthritis (PsA) remained poorly understood, awaiting a more detailed understanding of immune networks and the inflammatory response. In particular, discovery of the interleukin (IL-23)/T helper 17 (Th17) axis transformed the understanding of mechanisms that underlie not only PsA but also the spondyloarthritis family in general. Data derived from animal models, human tissues, and clinical trials underscore the concept that PsA is fundamentally different from rheumatoid arthritis (RA) (**Table 1**). Although RA is considered an autoimmune disorder given the strong association with shared epitopes in the DRβ region of the major histocompatibility complex (MHC) and antibodies against citrullinated peptides, a parallel autoimmune response has not been identified in PsA. Indeed, the data point to an immune response that is largely innate in composition, promoting differentiation of both type 1 and 17 T lymphocytes. Moreover, the link between infections and spondyloarthritis raises the possibility that the composition of the microbiome, in the skin, the gut, or

Disclosures: Consultant for Abbvie, Amgen, Novartis, Sanolfi, Regeneron Research support from Janssen, Amgen, Abbvie (C.T. Ritchlin); None (J.L. Barnas).
Allergy, Immunology and Rheumatology, University of Rochester Medical Center, 601 Elmwood Avenue, Box 695, Rochester, NY 14642, USA
* Corresponding author.
E-mail address: Christopher_Ritchlin@urmc.rochester.edu

Table 1
Psoriatic arthritis versus rheumatoid arthritis

	Psoriatic Arthritis	Rheumatoid Arthritis
Inflammatory arthritis	Yes	Yes
Autoantibodies	No	Anti-cyclic citrullinated peptides
Erosive disease	Yes	Yes
Genetic associations	MHC I	MHC II
Peripheral involvement	Yes	Yes
Axial involvement	Sacroiliac joint, spine	Rarely cervical spine
DIP involvement	Yes	No
Enthesitis	Yes	No
Dactylitis	Yes	No
Skin disease	Yes	No
New bone formation	Yes	No
Symmetry	Often asymmetric	Symmetric
Origin of joint inflammation	Enthesis	Synovium
Responds to rituximab	No	Yes
Responds to abatacept	Arthritis but not psoriasis	Yes
Responds to TNF blockade	Yes	Yes
Responds to IL-17 blockade	Yes	No
Responds to apremilast	Yes	No

both sites, may be important in the cause and persistence of skin and joint inflammation in PsA.

GENETIC FACTORS

PsA is a highly heritable, polygenic disease. The recurrence risk (λ) ratio, defined as the ratio of a disease manifestation in family members to the affected individual compared with the prevalence in the general population, is significantly higher in PsA than RA and psoriasis.[4–6] This high ratio underscores the strong familial component of this disease; the genetic risk factors are discussed in the article in this issue. In contrast to RA, which shows an association with specific MHC class II alleles, psoriasis and PsA are associated with MHC class I alleles. In particular, HLA-C*06 (previously called HLA-Cω06) is the genetic risk factor most strongly linked to psoriasis.[7] Interestingly, this MHC I allele does not track with joint and nail disease.[8] HLA-B*08, B*27, B*38 are found in increased frequency in PsA, and a recent study showed that the presence of glutamine in the HLA-B27 gene at amino acid position 45 significantly increased the risk for PsA, but not psoriasis.[9] Immunochip genotype array case-controlled analysis also identified HLA-C*0602, amino acid position 67 of HLA-B, and HLA-A*0201 as independently associated with PsA in a study that included nearly 2000 PsA patients and 9000 controls.[10] The presence of HLA-B*27 correlates with the severity of axial involvement on MRI studies[11] as well as a shortened interval between the development of skin and joint disease.[12]

ENVIRONMENTAL FACTORS

The concept that psoriatic plaques develop in response to bacterial antigens originated from clinical observations of a close temporal relationship between streptococcal tonsillitis and guttate psoriasis in young individuals.[13] Streptococci produce a virulence factor (M protein) with sequence homology to keratin 16 and 17. Peripheral blood CD8+ cells from psoriasis patients react to keratin peptides so molecular mimicry was initially proposed to explain plaque development.[14] Subsequent studies found identical T-cell clones in both the skin and the tonsils of patients who developed psoriasis following streptococcal infections.[15] Moreover, psoriatic patients undergoing tonsillectomy for recurrent tonsillitis demonstrated improvement in skin disease not observed in psoriasis patients who did not undergo the procedure.[16] In preclinical studies, immunization of rabbits with *Streptococcus pyogenes* yielded antibodies reactive against several keratinocyte proteins,[17] and interestingly, sera taken from psoriasis patients also reacted against these keratinocyte proteins. Homology was found between keratinocyte proteins and *Streptococcus* proteins FcR, RecF, and RopA along with M protein.[17] Individually, these studies support a molecular mimicry hypothesis of autoimmunity driven by CD8+ T cells, yet taken together show different sets of keratinocyte proteins and *Streptococcus* proteins with molecular homology, suggesting that multiple antigens are important for the development of psoriasis.

The immune response in psoriasis may be dominated by an autoinflammatory rather than an autoimmune response. Danger signals, released from dying cells, bind pattern recognition receptors on innate immune cells and activate the NFκB signaling cascade, resulting in sterile inflammation. Pattern recognition receptors include the Toll-like (TLR) and NOD receptors. A specific antigen is not required, and any event that generates a danger signal may ignite psoriasis in the proper genetic context, including infection and trauma. In 1877, Koebner (a German dermatologist) observed the widely recognized phenomena that psoriatic plaques can arise at sites of prior trauma. Similar reports have been published on PsA (reviewed in Ref.[18]), and these findings increase the possibility that mechanical stress at the enthesis or joint may precipitate PsA.

MICROBIOME

Humans can be viewed as a superorganism living in harmony with more than 10,000 microbial species of viral, fungal, and bacterial origin.[19] Symbiosis refers to the mutually beneficial relationship between different organisms living in close proximity. Recent studies suggest that colonization with different commensal skin organisms may induce specific T-cell responses that serve as a rheostat for dynamic barrier immunity and a means of educating the adaptive immune system.[20] A fungal microbiota with increased numbers of *Firmicutes* and *Actinobacterium* species was identified in psoriasis skin compared with healthy controls.[21,22] Dysbiosis implies a change within normal microbiome or misrecognition of or aberrant response to normal microbiota within another body environment. Dysbiosis has been proposed as a mechanism for the development of an altered immune response in diseases like psoriasis and inflammatory bowel disease. Thus, multiple organisms might incite disease as opposed to typical infections, where one specific microbe is causal. The innate immune system is capable of recognizing evolutionarily conserved pathogens-associated molecular patterns expressed on a wide variety of microbes through pattern recognition receptors. Examples of pattern recognition receptors include the TLRs, NOD-like receptors, RIG-I-like receptors, and C-type-lectin-like receptors.[23] Links between the gut and psoriasis have been proposed.

Subclinical gut inflammation was found in PsA patients undergoing colonoscopy (without gastrointestinal complaint) compared with control patients undergoing colonoscopy due to a history of benign colon polyps.[24] Patients with psoriasis and particularly those with PsA are at increased risk of developing Crohn disease, as shown in the Nurses' Health Study.[25] The gut microbiota profile in PsA is reported to be similar to that of inflammatory bowel disease. Psoriasis and PsA patients have a narrower spectrum of gut flora in comparison to healthy controls.[26] Therefore, dysbiosis has been suggested as a mechanism to generate an autoinflammatory response that may precipitate psoriasis and PsA.

ROLE OF OBESITY

A range of other inflammatory conditions are linked to the development of PsA. Obesity, or overabundance of adipose tissue, is an inflammatory state characterized by a type 1 immune response.[27] Adipocytes produce adipokines, which include classical cytokines such as IL-6 and tumor necrosis factor (TNF)-α, but also soluble molecules such as resistin and leptin (reviewed in Ref.[28]). Leptin regulates body weight by causing satiety and stimulating expenditure of energy. Leptin has a diverse array of effects on the immune system, and leptin-deficient mice are prone to death by infection. Leptin inhibits T-regulatory cells, promotes naïve T-cell and natural killer (NK) cell proliferation, induces monocyte proliferation, increases macrophage production of TNF-α, IL-6, and IL-12, and increases neutrophil chemotaxis (reviewed in Ref.[28]). These adipokines are elevated in the sera of PsA and psoriasis patients and fluctuate with disease activity.[29–32] Epidemiologic studies indicate that obesity is a risk factor for incident psoriasis.[33] Moreover, a meta-analysis of 2.1 million people, which included 200,000 psoriasis patients, found a dose-response relationship between obesity and psoriasis; the odds ratio of obesity was 1.46 for mild psoriasis and 2.23 for severe psoriasis compared with the general population.[34] Obesity was also shown to be a risk factor for PsA, and increasing body mass index was associated with increased psoriasis risk.[35] A causal link between obesity and psoriasis awaits additional research, but one plausible explanation is that unresolved inflammation associated with obesity fosters development of skin and, in some cases, joint inflammation in the genetically predisposed patient. An increased prevalence of type II diabetes mellitus has also been found in patients with psoriasis and PsA.[36] Weight loss intervention through calorie reduction,[37] exercise,[38] or gastric bypass[39,40] reduces psoriasis severity and improves response to anti-TNF agents in PsA.[41] These studies indicate that obesity may be an essential cofactor in the development of psoriatic disease and may present an opportunity for therapeutic intervention.

IMMUNOPATHOLOGY: HISTORICAL CONTEXT

Cytokines generated by innate immune cells promote the differentiation of T lymphocytes, key effectors of adaptive immunity. Mosmann and Coffman[42] described 2 types of T-helper lymphocytes in 1986 and proposed a Th1-Th2 paradigm. In this paradigm, interferon (IFN)-γ, released by Th1 cells, inhibit differentiation of IL-4-producing Th2 cells and vice versa. This reciprocal interaction results in a polarized immune response dependent on the type of invading pathogen (virus, bacteria, fungus, or parasite) and, subsequently, the cytokine milieu. In this model, IL-12 triggers a Th1 response and IL-4, a Th2 response. This paradigm proved inadequate though when a new cytokine, IL-23, was described in 2000, which shared a subunit with IL-12. IL-12, comprising p35 and p40 subunits, is released by dendritic cells and leads to differentiation of naïve T CD4+ cells to IFN-γ-producing Th1 cells. The finding that the p40 subunit was shared between IL-12 and IL-23 required the scientific community to reassess years of literature in which anti-p40 antibodies were thought to block or identify IL-12, given that IL-23 also possessed this subunit. Despite the shared p40 subunit, it was apparent that IL-12 remained the key cytokine for Th1 differentiation. In 2005, IL-17-producing CD4+ T-helper cells were described independently by 2 groups, and this finding required a revision of theTh1-Th2 paradigm.[43,44] Interestingly, IL-17A (then called CTL8) was initially discovered in 1993 as a transcript from a rat CD8+ T-cell hybridoma.[45] Nevertheless, IL-17 research predominately centered on CD4+ helper T cells for years. Subsequent studies revealed several cytokines are required for the differentiation of naïve T lymphocytes to IL-17-producing Th17 cells. In humans, these include IL-1β and transforming growth factor-β along with IL-6, IL-21, or IL-23 to induce the STAT3 transcription factor.[46] The characterization of Th17 as a distinct subset from Th1 became increasingly blurred with the description of IFN-γ and IL-17 double-producer T-helper cells.[47,48] With these discoveries, it became apparent that helper T-cell subsets showed a great deal of plasticity in the immune response.[49] The discovery of the IL-23-Th-17 axis would have great therapeutic implication for autoimmune diseases, particularly spondyloarthritis and PsA.

ESTABLISHING A ROLE FOR INTERLEUKIN-17 IN PSORIATIC ARTHRITIS

Researchers sought to define the role of Th17 cells in inflammatory arthritis. In RA and PsA, serum levels of IL-17 were not elevated compared with healthy controls.[50] However, an increased percentage of IL-17-producing cells was identified in both RA and PsA compared with controls when peripheral blood T cells are stimulated ex vivo.[50] Moreover, the CD4+ IL-17+ subset was present at higher levels in RA and PsA synovial fluid, whereas CD8+ IL-17− T cells were elevated only in PsA synovial fluid.[51] Furthermore, the number of CD8+ IL-17-producing cells in the PsA patients correlated with disease activity and musculoskeletal ultrasound signals.[51] These findings suggest that CD4+ IL-17+ cells contribute to inflammation in rheumatoid and psoriatic joints, while the IL-17 response in psoriatic synovial tissues involves CD4− cells, specifically, CD8+ cells and innate lymphocytes.

Enthesitis, dactylitis, spondylitis, synovitis, nail disease, and skin plaques are features of PsA. The pathogenetic pathways that underlie this diverse array of phenotypic features remained enigmatic until the discovery of the IL-23/Th17 axis. It is now apparent that cellular events triggered by cytokines in this pathway provide key insights into the disease mechanisms associated with the heterogeneous clinical features associated with both PsA and spondyloarthritis.

SKIN

Psoriasis is characterized by hallmark raised, erythematous plaques with silver scale. New psoriatic plaques may form in response to danger signals from infection or injury (Koebner phenomena). In research models, these lesions develop following intradermal injection of IFN-α. Psoriatic skin plaques are thought to develop because DNA released by stressed keratinocytes binds to the antibacterial peptide, cathelicidin LL-37 (**Fig. 1**). The DNA-LL37 complex binds TLR-9 in plasmacytoid dendritic cells (pDC). In response to TLR-9 activation, the pDC cells release IFN-α activating dermal dendritic cells, which migrate to draining lymph nodes. In the lymph node, the DCs stimulate differentiation of naïve T lymphocytes to Th1 and Th17 cells, which migrate back to the skin through blood vessels. Th1 cells release IFN-γ and TNF-α, while the Th17 cells produce TNF-α, IL-1, IL-17, and IL-22. In the dermis, populations of CD8+ T cells also produce IL-17. When referring to T cells, the α-β T cell receptor is often assumed; however, a greater frequency of γ-δ T cells, also capable of producing IL-17, reside in psoriatic plaques than in peripheral blood.[52] Many T-cell subsets

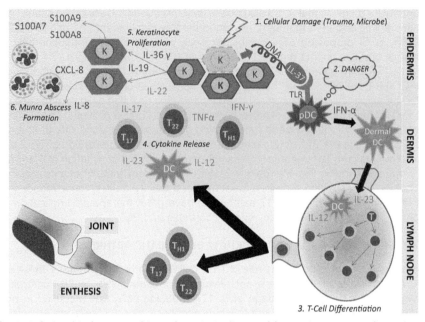

Fig. 1. Relationship between skin and psoriatic disease. (1) Keratinocytes may be activated by mechanical trauma or pathogens. (2) DNA and RNA released by damaged keratinocytes are recognized by pattern recognition receptors on pDC, which induce IFN-α release. (3) Interferon-α activates dermal dendritic cells, which traffic to draining lymph nodes where they release cytokines that influence T-cell differentiation. IL-23 triggers the development of IL-17-producing T cells, while IL-12 promotes development of IFN-γ-producing T lymphocytes. (4) T cells migrate from the draining lymph node back to the skin and to distant sites, which include the enthesis and joints, where they release cytokines such as IL-17 and IL-22. (5) IL-22 stimulates keratinocyte proliferation. Proliferating keratinocytes produce IL-19, IL-36γ, and antibacterial proteins S100 proteins. (6) IL-17 triggers release of neutrophil chemotactic factors from keratinocytes. Neutrophils accumulate, leading to the formation of Munro's abscesses. The abscesses and keratinocyte proliferation lead to the development of a psoriatic plaque.

release IL-22, a cytokine responsible for keratinocyte proliferation, including Th17 cells, Th22 cells, and minor populations of CD8+ cells as well as NK cells.[49] Keratinocytes release large amounts of IL-1, IL-6, and TNF-α as well as chemokines. Dermal dendritic cells synthesize IL-23, which leads to further proliferation and survival of Th17 cells. A combination of IL-17A, IL-22, and TNF-α leads to the greatest amount of IL-19 production in skin and in human tissues. IL-19 is strongly upregulated in psoriatic plaques compared with normal skin.[53] Moreover, IL-19 induces production of antibacterial proteins in keratinocytes, including S100A7, S100A8, and S100A9, along with IL-1β, IL-20, CXCL-8, and matrix metalloproteinase-1, and IL-19 levels decrease following phototherapy or anti-TNF therapy.[53] IL-36γ, upregulated by LL-37, is also found in abundance in psoriatic plaques and stimulates release of neutrophil-attracting IL-8 and CXCL1.[54] Neutrophil collections, termed Munro's abscesses, are formed that develop into psoriatic plaques.

Recent clinical trials document impressive clinical responses in psoriasis patients treated with agents directed toward molecules in the IL-23/Th17 pathway. Specifically, antibodies blocking the common p40 subunit of IL-23 and IL-12 (ustekinumab)[55] and more recently anti-p19 antibodies markedly reduce psoriasis.[56]

Antibodies against IL-17A (secukinumab, ixekizumab) and its receptor (brodalumab) show high efficacy in the treatment of skin and nail disease.[55,57] The clinical efficacy of blocking the IL-17 pathway underscores its central importance in human psoriatic disease.

NAILS

Nail disease is associated with joint disease, particularly distal interphalangeal (DIP) joint involvement, in PsA. The mechanisms responsible for the inflammatory changes in these adjacent structures are not well understood. McGonagle and colleagues,[58] using cadaver specimens, noted the extensor tendon enthesis fuses directly with the nail root, providing a potential link to explain contiguous arthritis and onycho-dystrophy in the DIP joint and the nail, respectively. They proposed that the nail is part of the enthesis complex.[58]

The nail is composed of 4 epithelial layers (nail matrix, proximal nail fold, nail bed, and hyponychium) and the nail plate (**Fig. 2**).[59] The nail plate arises from below the proximal nail fold. It comprises dead epithelial cells pushed forward by the dividing cells of the lunula. Psoriasis may affect any part of the nail.[60] If the matrix is involved, pitting, leukonychia, red patches in the lunula, or onchodystrophy may develop. Desquamation of poorly adherent keratinocytes in areas of parakeratosis lead to the nail pits. If the nail bed becomes involved, oncholysis, "oil spots," splinter hemorrhage, subungual parakeratosis, and hyperkeratosis may be observed.[60]

ENTHESIS

Enthesitis is considered a key feature of PsA and spondyloarthritis. The enthesis is the attachment site of the joint capsule, tendon, or ligament to bone. MRI studies revealed that inflammation at the enthesis is more widespread than originally thought, involving

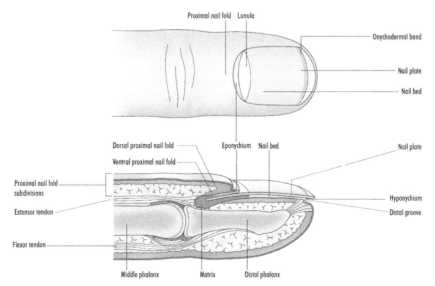

Fig. 2. Nail anatomy. Longitudinal cross-section demonstrating the close proximity of the extensor tendon attachment site, nail, and DIP joint. (*From* Carney CK, Cantrell W, Elewski BE. Nail psoriasis: a review of current topical and systemic therapies. Adv Psor Inflamm Skin Dis 2010;1(3):90; with permission.)

the bone, synovium, and several contiguous structures.[61] An organ is a collection of interactive tissues that carry out the same function. Therefore, the "enthesis organ" comprises tissues that may include sesamoid, periosteal cartilage, or fibrocartilage adjacent to a synovial cavity.[62] The tissues of the enthesis organ cooperate to dissipate mechanical stress at the attachment site to the skeleton. Under normal conditions, the enthesis lacks vasculature or cells. The adjacent enthesis and synovial tissues form a functionally integrated anatomic unit labeled the synovial-enthesial complex.[58] During times of mechanical stress or enthesial damage, danger signals released by stressed tendons or ligaments lead to cytokine and growth factor production by cells of the synovium, including lymphocytes and monocytes. Thus, in PsA, it is hypothesized that the enthesis is the site of origin for the inflammatory response, which is in contrast to RA, where inflammation originates in the synovium (reviewed in Ref.[63]). This view is controversial, however, and several studies have questioned the primacy of the enthesis in PsA pathogenesis.[61,64] Mechanical trauma may be an inciting factor for the development of enthesitis as demonstrated in preclinical models. In the TNF (Δ ARE) mouse model, unloading of the hind limbs results in decreased inflammation of the Achilles tendon, supporting a role for biomechanical stress as an early event.[65] Although these findings are of great interest, the relevance to PsA or spondyloarthritis remains to be established.

The enthesial interface of tendon and bones in both murine axial and peripheral joints contains cells that express IL-23 receptor. These IL-23R-expressing cells were further characterized in mice as double-negative T lymphocytes (CD3+ CD4− CD8− Rorγt+).[66] This population was found only at the interface of the tendon and bone and not in the belly of the tendon. In response to IL-23, the enthesis produces IL-17A, IL-22, and Bmp7. Using IL-23 minicircle technology in B10.R111 mice, overexpression of IL-23 resulted in paw swelling, sacroiliitis, axial enthesitis, and arthritis with evidence of erosion and new bone formation and psoriasiform lesions, findings reminiscent of PsA. This model also had aortic wall, aortic valve inflammation, and uveitis,[66] also clinical features of PsA and spondyloarthritis. Furthermore, enthesitis persisted after CD4+ cell depletion, demonstrating that inflammation was not dependent on T-helper cells. Cartilage, osteoid, and new bone were evident at the periosteum. CXCL1 recruited neutrophils to the bone. CCL20 recruited additional IL-23 receptor + cells to the site. Furthermore, transcriptome analyses on murine tissues exposed to IL-22 and IL-23 minicircles demonstrated that IL-17 triggered inflammatory and osteoclast pathways, whereas IL-22 was associated with inflammation and osteogenic signatures. Subsequent studies in several different murine models also provided strong support for the importance of IL-22 and IL-23 in the development of enthesitis (**Table 2**).

DACTYLITIS

Dactylitis, derived from the Greek "daktylos," meaning "finger," is the diffuse swelling of a finger or toe producing a "sausage digit." Dactylitis may be acute (usually tender, frequently erythematous, and warm) or chronic (painless swelling).[67] Dactylitis is not unique to PsA and may be seen in any of the spondyloarthropathies, sickle cell disease, sarcoid, crystalline arthritis, and infections such as tuberculosis and syphilis. Trauma was proposed as the inciting factor for dactylitis. For instance, if immunologically intact DBA/1 male mice housed together under conditions to increase territorial behavior, spontaneous ankyloses and arthritis in the hind limbs with dactylitis develop similar to ankylosing spondylitis.[68,69] Also, dactylitis often accompanies enthesitis in murine models (discussed later). TNF inhibition, ustekinumab (anti-p40), and IL-17

Table 2
Animal models

Species	Manipulation	Skin or Nail	Joint	Enthesitis	Dactylitis	Author
Baboon	Spontaneous	—	+	—	—	Rothschild,[116] 2005
Mouse	Act1-D10N transgenic	+	—	—	—	Wang et al,[117] 2013
Mouse	Amphiregulin expression under control of INF-AR	+	+	—	—	Cook et al,[114] 2004
Mouse	Collagen-induced arthritis	—	+	—	—	Courtenay et al,[118] 1980
Mouse	IL-23 minicircle	—	+	+	—	Adamopoulos et al,[119] 2011; Sherlock et al,[66] 2012
Mouse	Inducible epidermal deletion of JunB and c-Jun	+	+	—	+	Zenz et al,[109] 2005
Mouse	Lacks endogenous MHC class II molecules	+	—	—	—	Bardos et al,[110] 2002
Mouse	Spontaneous in DBA/1 (male)	—	—	+	+	Lories et al,[69] 2004
Mouse	TNF transgenic	—	+	—	—	Keffer et al,[120] 1991
Mouse	β2-microglobulin knockout	+	—	—	+	Khare et al,[111] 1995
Mouse	β-Glucan-Zap70	—	+	+	+	Ruutu et al,[113] 2012
Rat	HLA-B27/B2 transgene	+	+	—	—	Hammer et al,[121] 1995; Yanagisawa et al,[112] 1995

inhibition (anti-IL-17/brodalumab and anti-IL-17R/secukinumab) have shown efficacy for the treatment of dactylitis (reviewed in Ref.[63]), suggesting a role for the IL-23-Th17 pathway in the pathogenesis of both dactylitis and enthesitis. Methotrexate and sulfasalazine are not effective in the treatment of dactylitis.[63]

SYNOVIUM

Histologic studies of PsA and RA demonstrate lining-layer hyperplasia and a subsynovial infiltrate with T lymphocytes, B lymphocytes, and monocytes. In comparison to RA, PsA synovial tissue samples demonstrated increased tortuous vascularity, fewer T lymphocytes, and more neutrophils.[70] Interestingly, the histopathologic findings in PsA have more in common with synovial tissues from spondyloarthritis than RA patients despite the observation that expression of TNF-α, IL-1β, IL-6, IL-18, matrix metalloproteinases, vascular makers, and adhesion markers are comparable between these two entities.[71,72] In addition, lymphoid neogenesis has been identified in both RA and PsA.[73] IL-17-expressing cells were identified in psoriatic synovium.[74] Studies by Baeten[70] reported mast cells expressing IL-17 in synovial tissue from spondyloarthritis patients, but subsequent work showed that these cells take up IL-17 from the microenvironment but do not synthesize this cytokine. Low IL-17 expression in RA synovium has been cited as the reason for lack of response to anti-IL-17 therapy in this patient population.[75] Other studies, however, reported similar heterogeneous expression of IL-17 in the synovium of RA, PsA, and osteoarthritis patients,[76] suggesting the patient heterogeneity may have been the reason for the lack of clinical response seen in RA anti-IL-17 clinical trials. It is also important to note, however, that RA patients did not respond to ustekinumab either, which suggests divergent disease mechanisms compared with PsA.

ALTERED BONE REMODELING IN PSORIATIC ARTHRITIS

One of the remarkable clinical features of PsA is the marked heterogeneity of bone phenotypes. These marked heterogeneities range from extensive bone damage characterized by arthritis mutilans and large eccentric erosions to spinal ankyloses, bony fusion of digits, and enthesophytes (bone formation in and around enthesis). Thus, unlike RA, a disease characterized by extensive erosion and inadequate bone repair, in PsA both extensive resorption and exuberant new bone formation may be present, and widely disparate PsA bone phenotypes can be viewed on plain radiographs (reviewed in Ref.[2]). Both bone erosions and new bone formation may co-occur in one extremity or even in the joints of a single digit. Isolated small joints may demonstrate severe destruction, whereas other MTP and metacarpophalangeal (MCP) joints remain relatively spared. The radiographic features are frequently asymmetric in appearance and include acro-osteolysis (erosion) of the terminal phalangeal tufts and whittling, "pencil-in-cup" deformities, ankyloses of phalanges, metacarpals, and metatarsals (reviewed in the article in this issue). The striking appearance of varied bone phenotypes (ankylosis, marked erosion) in different digits of the same hand suggests that local factors may be important, but these remain enigmatic. In the axial skeleton, sacroiliitis (often asymmetric), vertebral osteitis, and syndesmophytes bridging vertebrae are present in up to 40% of patients. MRI evaluation of bone in PsA patients is associated with bone marrow edema, an imaging correlate of osteitis, and microcomputed tomographic scans of psoriatic MCP joints show omega-shaped erosions that differ from the U-shaped erosions in RA.[77] In addition, the location and appearance of new bone formation in the MCPs differ from that observed in osteoarthritis and RA.[77] Recognition of the IL-23/Th17 axis has allowed for a better understanding of how these changes might occur in PsA through the enhanced activity of normal bone remodeling pathways (**Fig. 3**).

Osteoclasts and osteoblasts, through highly coordinated interactions, maintain bone homeostasis in the human skeleton. Osteoclasts resorb bone, whereas osteoblasts lay down new osteoid. Osteoclasts are multinucleated cells that differentiate from the macrophage/monocyte lineage. They possess a ruffled border that seals off a section of bone and releases enzymes that degrade the inorganic matrix. During inflammation, the frequency of circulating CD14+ monocytes increases in the blood. A subset of these monocytes differentiates into circulating and tissue resident osteoclast precursors in response to M-CSF and RANKL, expressed by Th17 cells, bone marrow stromal cells, and type B synoviocytes in inflamed joints and form osteoblasts in bone. TNF-α induces increased expression of the osteoclast-associated receptor (OSCAR) on monocytes[78] and potentiates osteoclastogenesis.[79] Activation of this receptor acts as a second signal, following RANK engagement by RANKL to trigger osteoclastogenesis. A variety of cytokines, including TNF-α, IL-1, IL-6, IL-17, and vascular endothelial growth factor, induce expression of RANKL. RANKL in combination with M-CSF, a growth factor that initiates initiation and survival of osteoclast precursors, promotes osteoclast differentiation. The binding of RANKL to RANK on osteoclasts leads to NFκB and AP-1 signaling, activating these cells. Several lines

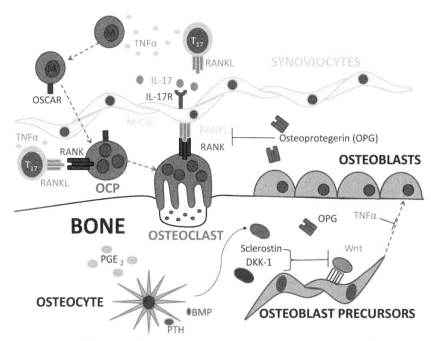

Fig. 3. Bone metabolism pathways. Monocytes express OSCAR receptor in the presence of TNF-α, which enhances their differentiation to osteoclasts. RANKL is found on Th17 cells, bone marrow stromal cells, and type B synoviocytes in inflamed synovium. Th17 cells produce IL-17 leading to upregulation of RANKL on synoviocytes. Osteoclast differentiation and activation are induced through binding of RANK and RANKL as well as through synoviocyte production of M-CSF. Activated osteoclasts resorb bone, and osteoclastogenesis is inhibited by OPG. Osteoblasts differentiate from mesenchymal precursors through the Wnt pathway. The Wnt pathway and osteoblast differentiation can be inhibited by sclerostin and DKK-1 produced by osteocytes as well as by TNF-α. PTH, prostaglandin E2, and BMP also modify bone metabolism.

of evidence from in vitro studies and animal models indicate that both IL-23 and Th17 cells promote bone destruction.[80] Th17 cells express RANKL, which facilitates the transition of an osteoclast from a nonresorptive to resorptive phenotype.[81] Th17 cells also induce expression of RANKL on mesenchymal cells via IL-17.[80] Both IL-23 and IL-17 knockout mice exhibit significantly less inflammatory bone destruction than wild-type mice in the lipopolysaccharide-induced mouse models of arthritis underscoring the central Importance of the IL-23/Th17 axis in erosive arthritis.

Bone remodeling is a finely balanced process that depends on interaction of several factors. For instance, osteoprotegerin (OPG), a soluble decoy receptor, binds to RANKL and prevents engagement with the RANK receptor. Thus, the ratio of RANKL to OPG in the bone marrow or target tissues modulates resorption and ultimately bone mass. Osteocytes, osteoblasts, and osteogenic stromal stem cells secrete OPG, protecting the body from excessive bone resorption. In PsA synovial tissue, synoviocytes express high levels of RANKL, whereas OPG surface expression was low. These findings indicate the presence of a pro-osteoclastogenic environment in the psoriatic joint.[82] In addition, a markedly elevated frequency of circulating CD14+ osteoclast precursor cells (OCP) was observed in PsA patients compared with controls. The OCP frequency correlated with extent of radiographic damage and dropped rapidly following treatment with anti-TNF agents.[83] Erosions in PsA are explained by increased number and activity of osteoclasts. However, the mechanisms responsible for new bone formation in PsA are not well understood. Musculoskeletal ultrasound studies indicate that bone erosions and new bone formation in the region of the Achilles tendon in psoriatic joint take place at different locations, supporting uncoupling of the homeostatic bone response.[84] Both endochondral and membranous bone formation are operative in the pathologic bone response.[85,86] Several signaling pathways may be key, including the Wnt, bone morphogenetic protein (BMP), and Hedgehog signaling pathways.[85,86]

The canonical Wnt/β-catenin signaling pathway is required for osteoblast differentiation from mesenchymal progenitor or bone marrow stromal cells (**Fig. 4**). Wnt ligands bind the frizzled and Lrp5/6 receptor, which allows β-catenin to accumulate in the cell cytoplasm, translocate to the nucleus, and regulate gene expression. Osteocytes, which represent mature osteoblasts entombed in the mineralized bone matrix, may produce inhibitors of Wnt signaling: sclerostin and Dickkopf-related protein 1 (DKK-1).[87] Both DKK-1 and sclerostin serve as negative regulators of bone mass (reviewed in Ref.[88]). Release of sclerostin is regulated by mechanical shear stress on osteocytes and TNF-α. Sclerostin promotes bone resorption through increased osteoclastogenesis,[89] while inhibiting osteoblastogenesis.[90] Sclerostin expression is suppressed in patients administered parathyroid hormone. Thus, parathyroid hormone indirectly modulates Wnt-signaling leading to increased bone formation; however, cross-talk between bone metabolism pathways is complex, and ultimately, parathyroid hormone may exert both anabolic and catabolic effects on bone metabolism. DKK-1, like sclerostin, is a soluble factor with inhibitory actions

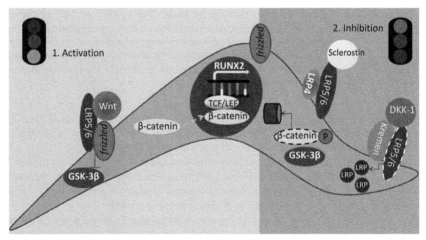

Fig. 4. Canonical Wnt signaling activation and inhibition in osteoblast precursor. 1. Activation. β-Catenin resides in the cytoplasm, where it undergoes ubiquitination and degradation. Wnt binding to frizzled and LPR5/6 coreceptors on the surface of osteoblast precursors leads to disruption of the β-catenin degradation complex. β-Catenin accumulates in the cytoplasm and translocates to the nucleus. β-Catenin interacts with TCF/LEF to allow for transcription and expression of osteoblast differentiation genes, such as RUNX2 (also called Cbfa1). 2. Inhibition. Sclerostin and DKK-1 have sequence homology to Wnt. 2a. Sclerostin binds to LPR5/6 and LPR4, preventing signaling from Wnt leading to the phosphorylation and then ubiquitination of β-catenin and subsequent destruction by the proteasome. 2b. Binding of DKK-1 to Kremen and LPR5/6 leads to the internalization and destruction of LRP5/6.

on the canonical Wnt/β-catenin pathway.[91] It is also induced by TNF-α.[92] Of note, antibody blockade of DKK-1 protects TNF transgenic (hTNFtg) mice from inflammatory bone destruction mediated by TNF-α.[93] In studies comparing ankylosing spondylitis to RA patients, anti-TNF therapy reduced DKK-1 levels in the RA patients but demonstrated the opposite effect in AS patients; yet, the biological activity was diminished, suggesting the molecule is dysfunctional in spondyloarthritis.[94] The BMP and WNT signaling pathway interactions are complex and may be of central importance in PsA and spondyloarthritis. For example, BMP-2 and BMP-7 were upregulated in areas of new bone formation in the DBA/1 mouse model of oncychoperiostitis and ankylosis, whereas downstream signaling molecules Smad1 and Smad5 were phosphorylated in a bone biopsy from an ankylosing spondylitis patient.[85] A role for BMP was hypothesized for new bone formation in PsA as well.[91–93] In ankylosing spondylitis patients with elevated serum C-reactive protein levels, nonsteroidal anti-inflammatory drugs inhibit new bone formation by blocking prostaglandin E2, suggesting this pathway is also involved in pathologic bone formation.[95] IL-1 and IL-22 may also drive osteoproliferation in axial disease (reviewed in Ref.[96]).

As mentioned earlier, Th17 cells congregate in peripheral joints in RA and PsA, but this trend is reversed following anti-TNF treatment. In the collagen-induced arthritis mouse model, anti-TNF therapy was associated with a decreased number of Th17 cells in joints, but associated with increased numbers in the draining lymph nodes.[97] Translational studies of human cells and tissues in patients treated with biologics provide additional insights into disease mechanisms in PsA. Anti-TNF therapy reduced the frequency of circulating OCP in PsA peripheral blood.[83] Blockade of TNF also directly affects bone metabolism and alters trafficking of T lymphocytes. These observations[97] are consistent with induced transit of Th17 cells from the synovium to adjacent nodes and circulation following TNF therapy.[98] Also, return of Th17 cells to peripheral blood was observed earlier in RA compared with PsA patients following anti-TNF therapy.[99] Although anti-TNF therapy has effects on bone erosion, TNF blockade does not influence the formation of osteophytes or syndesmophytes with well-established disease.[100] The ability of anti-TNF agents to block new bone formation in patients with early PsA and spondyloarthritis is currently under study. TNF is expressed in two forms: transmembrane and soluble. Of potential relevance is the report that transmembrane TNF overexpression is associated with a spondyloarthropathy phenotype, while soluble TNF is associated with an RA-like phenotype in transgenic mouse models, although the relevance of this finding to human disease is unknown (reviewed in Ref.[96]).

The surge in effective therapeutic options for treatment of PsA illustrates the key role of the phosphodiesterase (PDE4) and IL-23/Th17 pathways in disease pathogenesis. Apremilast, a small molecule inhibitor of PDE4, is effective in both psoriasis and PsA.[101] PDE4 is the predominate phosphodiesterase In immune cells. In mouse models, apremilast inhibited production of CXCL9, CXCL10, IFN-γ, TNF-α, IL-2, IL-12, and IL-23.[102] Secukinumab (anti-IL-17A), brodalumab (anti-IL-17R), and ustekinumab (anti-p40 of Il-12 and IL-23) significantly improved both psoriasis and PsA.[103–105] Intravenous secukinumab has shown efficacy in the treatment of uveitis, an eye disorder associated with PsA and spondyloarthropathy.[106] It is interesting to note that for each of the agents that target the IL-23/Th17 pathway outlined earlier, efficacy is significantly higher in psoriasis than in PsA, suggesting that joint inflammation arises as a result of complex interactions between cells and cytokines of the innate and acquired inflammatory immune response or the presence of other factors that remain to be identified.

Approximately 30% of psoriasis patients develop arthritis, but the events that underlie this transition are poorly understood. In a proteomic study that compared skin biopsies from psoriasis patients with and without PsA, PSME3, C1QC, RENBP, GRHPR, POLE, POSTN, and IGLV3-21 were identified as potential biomarkers for PsA.[107] Of these, POSTN and ITGB5 could be measured in the serum. POSTN (or periostin) interacts with $\alpha_5\beta_5$, inducing the Akt/NF-κB signaling pathway and inflammatory cytokines. Periostin has been implicated in enhanced transmigration, chemotaxis, and adhesion of several cell types, including immune cells (reviewed in Ref.[108]). ITGB5 was elevated in PsA serum compared with skin psoriasis-only serum controls.[107] ITGB5 is a ligand for Cyr61. Cyr61 is made by synoviocytes and stimulated IL-6 production through the ITGA5-ITGB5/Akt/NF-κB signaling. Additional studies will provide insights regarding which serum, cellular, and imaging biomarkers will be effective in the identification of arthritis risk in psoriasis patients.

ANIMAL MODELS

The study of PsA has been hampered by the difficulty in obtaining tissues from patients with enthesitis and dactylitis and the lack of representative animal models. Until recently, animal models with the key features of PsA were not identified, but the finding that enthesitis, psoriasis, and dactylitis with axial and peripheral arthritis could be induced with IL-23 greatly advanced the field; these models are discussed under the Enthesitis heading above. Many additional animal models share PsA features and provide insights into disease pathways (see **Table 2**). Inducible targeted deletion of the transcription factors JunB and c-Jun in keratinocytes was associated with psoriasiform lesions and erosive arthritis with periostitis. This model suggested deletion of a keratinocyte transcription factor may trigger arthritis that required a functional acquired immune response.[109] In another model mentioned earlier, male DBA/1 mice housed under crowded conditions, which induced fighting and trauma, developed arthritis, dactylitis, and ankylosing enthesitis. Germ-free environments prevented this phenotype.[69] Transgenic mice lacking endogenous MHC class II develop resorption of the distal phalanx, nail pitting, and hyperkeratosis.[110] Mice lacking β2 microglobulin exhibit paw swelling, joint ankyloses, and nail changes.[111] Introduction of HLA-B27/β2 microglobulin transgenes in the rat caused psoriasiform skin lesions, nail changes, peripheral nonerosive arthritis, and gut lesions.[112] The arthritis did not develop under germ-free conditions. SKG mice with Zap70 mutations injected with mannan or curdlan manifest enthesitis, sacroiliitis, plantar fasciitis, axial disease, and uveitis.[113] Overexpression of human amphiregulin in the epidermis of transgenic mice produced skin lesions and knee synovitis.[66,114] K5.Stat3C transgenic mice, who have with constitutively active Stat3 signaling in their keratinocytes, when crossed with F759, a strain with amplified IL-6 signaling due to impaired SOCS3-negative feedback, develop a scaling skin disease similar to psoriasis and go on to develop enthesitis, nail deformities, paw swelling, and bone erosions.[115] Up to 30% of baboons may exhibit spondyloarthropathy, but psoriasiform lesions have not been identified.[116] These models demonstrate that altered gene expression in skin, repeated trauma, overexpression of IL-23, mutations in T-cell receptors, and constitutively activated signaling pathways can lead to psoriasiform lesions and joint inflammation. The most convincing pathways to date based on animal data and results from clinical trials support a pivotal role for the IL-23/Th17 pathway and TNF in the pathogenesis of PsA.

SUMMARY

The current model of PsA implicates amplification of the IL-23/IL-17 axis and overexpression of TNF as the underlying mechanisms underlying disease pathogenesis. Although specific MHC class I molecules are associated with the psoriatic disease phenotype, no specific antigen has been universally implicated. Instead, susceptible genes are hypothesized to drive an auto-inflammatory loop initiated via mechanical stress and dysbiosis interpreted as danger signals by the innate immune system that ultimately leads to altered bone metabolism. Amplification of the IL-23/IL-17 pathway in response to innate immune signals leads to a diverse array of associated pathologies at distant body sites and potentially explains the association of psoriasis with arthritis, enthesitis, spondylitis, nail disease, dactylitis, and uveitis.

REFERENCES

1. Wright V. Psoriasis and arthritis. Ann Rheum Dis 1956;15(4):348–56.
2. Moll JM, Wright V. Psoriatic arthritis. Semin Arthritis Rheum 1973;3(1):55–78.
3. Moll JM, Johnson G, Wright V. Psoriatic arthritis: a unique family. Rheumatol Rehabil 1974;13(3):154–7.
4. Chandran V, Schentag CT, Brockbank JE, et al. Familial aggregation of psoriatic arthritis. Ann Rheum Dis 2009;68(5):664–7.
5. Rigby AS, Voelm L, Silman AJ. Epistatic modeling in rheumatoid arthritis: an application of the Risch theory. Genet Epidemiol 1993;10(5):311–20.
6. Karason A, Love TJ, Gudbjornsson B. A strong heritability of psoriatic arthritis over four generations–the reykjavik psoriatic arthritis study. Rheumatology 2009;48(11):1424–8.
7. Trembath RC, Clough RL, Rosbotham JL, et al. Identification of a major susceptibility locus on chromosome 6p and evidence for further disease loci revealed by a two stage genome-wide search in psoriasis. Hum Mol Genet 1997;6(5):813–20.
8. Gudjonsson JE, Karason A, Runarsdottir EH, et al. Distinct clinical differences between HLA-Cw*0602 positive and negative psoriasis patients–an analysis of 1019 HLA-C- and HLA-B-typed patients. J Invest Dermatol 2006;126(4):740–5.
9. Okada Y, Han B, Tsoi LC, et al. Fine mapping major histocompatibility complex associations in psoriasis and its clinical subtypes. Am J Hum Genet 2014;95(2):162–72.
10. Bowes J, Budu-Aggrey A, Huffmeier U, et al. Dense genotyping of immune-related susceptibility loci reveals new insights into the genetics of psoriatic arthritis. Nat Commun 2015;6:6046.
11. Castillo-Gallego C, Aydin SZ, Emery P, et al. Magnetic resonance imaging assessment of axial psoriatic arthritis: extent of disease relates to HLA-B27. Arthritis Rheum 2013;65(9):2274–8.
12. Winchester R, Minevich G, Steshenko V, et al. HLA associations reveal genetic heterogeneity in psoriatic arthritis and in the psoriasis phenotype. Arthritis Rheum 2012;64(4):1134–44.
13. Telfer NR, Chalmers RJ, Whale K, et al. The role of streptococcal infection in the initiation of guttate psoriasis. Arch Dermatol 1992;128(1):39–42.
14. Valdimarsson H, Sigmundsdottir H, Jonsdottir I. Is psoriasis induced by streptococcal superantigens and maintained by M-protein-specific T cells that cross-react with keratin? Clinical and experimental immunology. Clin Exp Immunol 1997;107(Suppl 1):21–4.
15. Diluvio L, Vollmer S, Besgen P, et al. Identical TCR beta-chain rearrangements in streptococcal angina and skin lesions of patients with psoriasis vulgaris. J Immunol 2006;176(11):7104–11.
16. Thorleifsdottir RH, Sigurdardottir SL, Sigurgeirsson B, et al. Improvement of psoriasis after tonsillectomy is associated with a decrease in the frequency of

circulating T cells that recognize streptococcal determinants and homologous skin determinants. J Immunol 2012;188(10):5160–5.

17. Besgen P, Trommler P, Vollmer S, et al. Ezrin, maspin, peroxiredoxin 2, and heat shock protein 27: potential targets of a streptococcal-induced autoimmune response in psoriasis. J Immunol 2010;184(9):5392–402.

18. Hsieh J, Kadavath S, Efthimiou P. Can traumatic injury trigger psoriatic arthritis? A review of the literature. Clin Rheumatol 2014;33(5):601–8.

19. Cox MJ, Cookson WO, Moffatt MF. Sequencing the human microbiome in health and disease. Hum Mol Genet 2013;22(R1):R88–94.

20. Naik S, Bouladoux N, Linehan JL, et al. Commensal-dendritic-cell interaction specifies a unique protective skin immune signature. Nature 2015;520(7545): 104–8.

21. Takemoto A, Cho O, Morohoshi Y, et al. Molecular characterization of the skin fungal microbiome in patients with psoriasis. J Dermatol 2015;42(2):166–70.

22. Alekseyenko AV, Perez-Perez GI, De Souza A, et al. Community differentiation of the cutaneous microbiota in psoriasis. Microbiome 2013;1(1):31.

23. Nibali L, Henderson B, Sadiq ST, et al. Genetic dysbiosis: the role of microbial insults in chronic inflammatory diseases. J Oral Microbiol 2014;6. http://dx.doi. org/10.3402/jom.v6.22962.

24. Scarpa R, Manguso F, D'Arienzo A, et al. Microscopic inflammatory changes in colon of patients with both active psoriasis and psoriatic arthritis without bowel symptoms. J Rheumatol 2000;27(5):1241–6.

25. Li WQ, Han JL, Chan AT, et al. Psoriasis, psoriatic arthritis and increased risk of incident Crohn's disease in US women. Ann Rheum Dis 2013;72(7): 1200–5.

26. Scher JU, Ubeda C, Artacho A, et al. Decreased bacterial diversity characterizes the altered gut microbiota in patients with psoriatic arthritis, resembling dysbiosis in inflammatory bowel disease. Arthritis Rheumatol 2015;67(1):128–39.

27. Brestoff JR, Artis D. Immune regulation of metabolic homeostasis in health and disease. Cell 2015;161(1):146–60.

28. Versini M, Jeandel PY, Rosenthal E, et al. Obesity in autoimmune diseases: not a passive bystander. Autoimmun Rev 2014;13(9):981–1000.

29. Wang Y, Chen J, Zhao Y, et al. Psoriasis is associated with increased levels of serum leptin. Br J Dermatol 2008;158(5):1134–5.

30. Coimbra S, Oliveira H, Reis F, et al. Circulating adipokine levels in Portuguese patients with psoriasis vulgaris according to body mass index, severity and therapy. J Eur Acad Dermatol Venereol 2010;24(12):1386–94.

31. Johnston A, Arnadottir S, Gudjonsson JE, et al. Obesity in psoriasis: leptin and resistin as mediators of cutaneous inflammation. Br J Dermatol 2008;159(2): 342–50.

32. Takahashi H, Tsuji H, Honma M, et al. Increased plasma resistin and decreased omentin levels in Japanese patients with psoriasis. Arch Dermatol Res 2013; 305(2):113–6.

33. Setty AR, Curhan G, Choi HK. Obesity, waist circumference, weight change, and the risk of psoriasis in women: nurses' health study II. Arch Intern Med 2007;167(15):1670–5.

34. Armstrong AW, Harskamp CT, Armstrong EJ. The association between psoriasis and obesity: a systematic review and meta-analysis of observational studies. Nutr Diabetes 2012;2:e54.

35. Love TJ, Zhu Y, Zhang Y, et al. Obesity and the risk of psoriatic arthritis: a population-based study. Ann Rheum Dis 2012;71(8):1273–7.

36. Edson-Heredia E, Zhu B, Lefevre C, et al. Prevalence and incidence rates of cardiovascular, autoimmune, and other diseases in patients with psoriatic or psoriatic arthritis: a retrospective study using Clinical Practice Research Datalink. J Eur Acad Dermatol Venereol 2014;29(5):955–63.
37. Naldi L, Conti A, Cazzaniga S, et al. Diet and physical exercise in psoriasis: a randomized controlled trial. Br J Dermatol 2014;170(3):634–42.
38. Jensen P, Zachariae C, Christensen R, et al. Effect of weight loss on the severity of psoriasis: a randomized clinical study. JAMA Dermatol 2013; 149(7):795–801.
39. Farias MM, Achurra P, Boza C, et al. Psoriasis following bariatric surgery: clinical evolution and impact on quality of life on 10 patients. Obes Surg 2012;22(6):877–80.
40. Hossler EW, Wood GC, Still CD, et al. The effect of weight loss surgery on the severity of psoriasis. Br J Dermatol 2013;168(3):660–1.
41. Al-Mutairi N, Nour T. The effect of weight reduction on treatment outcomes in obese patients with psoriasis on biologic therapy: a randomized controlled prospective trial. Expert Opin Biol Ther 2014;14(6):749–56.
42. Mosmann TR, Cherwinski H, Bond MW, et al. Two types of murine helper T cell clone. I. Definition according to profiles of lymphokine activities and secreted proteins. J Immunol 1986;136(7):2348–57.
43. Park H, Li Z, Yang XO, et al. A distinct lineage of CD4 T cells regulates tissue inflammation by producing interleukin 17. Nat Immunol 2005;6(11):1133–41.
44. Harrington LE, Hatton RD, Mangan PR, et al. Interleukin 17-producing CD4+ effector T cells develop via a lineage distinct from the T helper type 1 and 2 lineages. Nat Immunol 2005;6(11):1123–32.
45. Rouvier E, Luciani MF, Mattei MG, et al. CTLA-8, cloned from an activated T cell, bearing AU-rich messenger RNA instability sequences, and homologous to a herpesvirus saimiri gene. J Immunol 1993;150(12):5445–56.
46. Manel N, Unutmaz D, Littman DR. The differentiation of human T(H)-17 cells requires transforming growth factor-beta and induction of the nuclear receptor RORgammat. Nat Immunol 2008;9(6):641–9.
47. Lee YK, Turner H, Maynard CL, et al. Late developmental plasticity in the T helper 17 lineage. Immunity 2009;30(1):92–107.
48. Annunziato F, Cosmi L, Santarlasci V, et al. Phenotypic and functional features of human Th17 cells. J Exp Med 2007;204(8):1849–61.
49. Eyerich S, Eyerich K, Pennino D, et al. Th22 cells represent a distinct human T cell subset involved in epidermal immunity and remodeling. J Clin Invest 2009; 119(12):3573–85.
50. Leipe J, Grunke M, Dechant C, et al. Role of Th17 cells in human autoimmune arthritis. Arthritis Rheum 2010;62(10):2876–85.
51. Menon B, Gullick NJ, Walter GJ, et al. Interleukin-17+CD8+ T cells are enriched in the joints of patients with psoriatic arthritis and correlate with disease activity and joint damage progression. Arthritis Rheumatol 2014;66(5):1272–81.
52. Cai Y, Shen X, Ding C, et al. Pivotal role of dermal IL-17-producing γδ T cells in skin inflammation. Immunity 2011;35(4):596–610.
53. Witte E, Kokolakis G, Witte K, et al. IL-19 is a component of the pathogenetic IL-23/IL-17 cascade in psoriasis. J Invest Dermatol 2014;134(11):2757–67.
54. Li N, Yamasaki K, Saito R, et al. Alarmin function of cathelicidin antimicrobial peptide LL37 through IL-36γ induction in human epidermal keratinocytes. J Immunol 2014;193(10):5140–8.
55. Papp KA, Leonardi C, Menter A, et al. Brodalumab, an anti-interleukin-17-receptor antibody for psoriasis. N Engl J Med 2012;366(13):1181–9.

56. Krueger JG, Ferris LK, Menter A, et al. Anti-IL-23A mAb BI 655066 for treatment of moderate-to-severe psoriasis: safety, efficacy, pharmacokinetics, and biomarker results of a single-rising-dose, randomized, double-blind, placebo-controlled trial. J Allergy Clin Immunol 2015;136(1):116–24.e7.

57. Leonardi C, Matheson R, Zachariae C, et al. Anti-interleukin-17 monoclonal antibody ixekizumab in chronic plaque psoriasis. N Engl J Med 2012;366(13): 1190–9.

58. Tan AL, Benjamin M, Toumi H, et al. The relationship between the extensor tendon enthesis and the nail in distal interphalangeal joint disease in psoriatic arthritis–a high-resolution MRI and histological study. Rheumatology 2007; 46(2):253–6.

59. Carney CK, Cantrell W, Elewski BE. Nail psoriasis: a review of current topical and systemic therapies. Adv Psor Inflamm Skin Dis 2010;1(3):89–97.

60. Radtke MA, Beikert FC, Augustin M. Nail psoriasis—a treatment challenge. J Dtsch Dermatol Ges 2013;11(3):203–19 [quiz: 20].

61. Healy PJ, Groves C, Chandramohan M, et al. MRI changes in psoriatic dactylitis–extent of pathology, relationship to tenderness and correlation with clinical indices. Rheumatology 2008;47(1):92–5.

62. Benjamin M, Moriggl B, Brenner E, et al. The "enthesis organ" concept: why enthesopathies may not present as focal insertional disorders. Arthritis Rheum 2004;50(10):3306–13.

63. Siegel EL, Orbai AM, Ritchlin CT. Targeting extra-articular manifestations in PsA: a closer look at enthesitis and dactylitis. Curr Opin Rheumatol 2015; 27(2):111–7.

64. Paramarta JE, van der Leij C, Gofita I, et al. Peripheral joint inflammation in early onset spondyloarthritis is not specifically related to enthesitis. Ann Rheum Dis 2014;73(4):735–40.

65. Jacques P, Lambrecht S, Verheugen E, et al. Proof of concept: enthesitis and new bone formation in spondyloarthritis are driven by mechanical strain and stromal cells. Ann Rheum Dis 2014;73(2):437–45.

66. Sherlock JP, Joyce-Shaikh B, Turner SP, et al. IL-23 induces spondyloarthropathy by acting on ROR-gammat(+) CD3(+)CD4(−)CD8(−) entheseal resident T cells. Nat Med 2012;18(7):1069–76.

67. Ferguson EG, Coates LC. Optimisation of rheumatology indices: dactylitis and enthesitis in psoriatic arthritis. Clin Exp Rheumatol 2014;32(5 Suppl 85):S-113–7.

68. Braem K, Carter S, Lories RJ. Spontaneous arthritis and ankylosis in male DBA/1 mice: further evidence for a role of behavioral factors in "stress-induced arthritis". Biol Proced Online 2012;14(1):10.

69. Lories RJ, Matthys P, de Vlam K, et al. Ankylosing enthesitis, dactylitis, and onychoperiostitis in male DBA/1 mice: a model of psoriatic arthritis. Ann Rheum Dis 2004;63(5):595–8.

70. Baeten D, Demetter P, Cuvelier C, et al. Comparative study of the synovial histology in rheumatoid arthritis, spondyloarthropathy, and osteoarthritis: influence of disease duration and activity. Ann Rheum Dis 2000;59(12):945–53.

71. van Kuijk AW, Reinders-Blankert P, Smeets TJ, et al. Detailed analysis of the cell infiltrate and the expression of mediators of synovial inflammation and joint destruction in the synovium of patients with psoriatic arthritis: implications for treatment. Ann Rheum Dis 2006;65(12):1551–7.

72. Kruithof E, Baeten D, De Rycke L, et al. Synovial histopathology of psoriatic arthritis, both oligo- and polyarticular, resembles spondyloarthropathy more than it does rheumatoid arthritis. Arthritis Res Ther 2005;7(3):R569–80.

73. Celis R, Planell N, Fernandez-Sueiro JL, et al. Synovial cytokine expression in psoriatic arthritis and associations with lymphoid neogenesis and clinical features. Arthritis Res Ther 2012;14(2):R93.
74. Raychaudhuri SP, Raychaudhuri SK, Genovese MC. IL-17 receptor and its functional significance in psoriatic arthritis. Mol Cell Biochem 2012;359(1–2): 419–29.
75. Hueber AJ, Asquith DL, Miller AM, et al. Mast cells express IL-17A in rheumatoid arthritis synovium. J Immunol 2010;184(7):3336–40.
76. van Baarsen LG, Lebre MC, van der Coelen D, et al. Heterogeneous expression pattern of interleukin 17A (IL-17A), IL-17F and their receptors in synovium of rheumatoid arthritis, psoriatic arthritis and osteoarthritis: possible explanation for nonresponse to anti-IL-17 therapy? Arthritis Res Ther 2014;16(4):426.
77. Finzel S, Ohrndorf S, Englbrecht M, et al. A detailed comparative study of high-resolution ultrasound and micro-computed tomography for detection of arthritic bone erosions. Arthritis Rheum 2011;63(5):1231–6.
78. Herman S, Muller RB, Kronke G, et al. Induction of osteoclast-associated receptor, a key osteoclast costimulation molecule, in rheumatoid arthritis. Arthritis Rheum 2008;58(10):3041–50.
79. Lam J, Takeshita S, Barker JE, et al. TNF-alpha induces osteoclastogenesis by direct stimulation of macrophages exposed to permissive levels of RANK ligand. J Clin Invest 2000;106(12):1481–8.
80. Sato K, Suematsu A, Okamoto K, et al. Th17 functions as an osteoclastogenic helper T cell subset that links T cell activation and bone destruction. J Exp Med 2006;203(12):2673–82.
81. Kikuta J, Wada Y, Kowada T, et al. Dynamic visualization of RANKL and Th17-mediated osteoclast function. J Clin Invest 2013;123(2):866–73.
82. Ritchlin CT, Haas-Smith SA, Li P, et al. Mechanisms of TNF-alpha- and RANKL-mediated osteoclastogenesis and bone resorption in psoriatic arthritis. J Clin Invest 2003;111(6):821–31.
83. Anandarajah AP, Schwarz EM, Totterman S, et al. The effect of etanercept on osteoclast precursor frequency and enhancing bone marrow oedema in patients with psoriatic arthritis. Ann Rheum Dis 2008;67(3):296–301.
84. Freeston JE, Coates LC, Helliwell PS, et al. Is there subclinical enthesitis in early psoriatic arthritis? A clinical comparison with power doppler ultrasound. Arthritis Care Res 2012;64(10):1617–21.
85. Lories RJ, Luyten FP. Bone morphogenetic protein signaling in joint homeostasis and disease. Cytokine Growth Factor Rev 2005;16(3):287–98.
86. Pacheco-Tena C, Perez-Tamayo R, Pineda C, et al. Bone lineage proteins in the entheses of the midfoot in patients with spondyloarthritis. J Rheumatol 2015; 42(4):630 7.
87. Semenov M, Tamai K, He X. SOST is a ligand for LRP5/LRP6 and a Wnt signaling inhibitor. J Biol Chem 2005;280(29):26770–5.
88. Baron R, Kneissel M. WNT signaling in bone homeostasis and disease: from human mutations to treatments. Nat Med 2013;19(2):179–92.
89. Vincent C, Findlay DM, Welldon KJ, et al. Pro-inflammatory cytokines TNF-related weak inducer of apoptosis (TWEAK) and TNFalpha induce the mitogen-activated protein kinase (MAPK)-dependent expression of sclerostin in human osteoblasts. J bone miner Res 2009;24(8):1434–49.
90. Xiong L, Jung JU, Wu H, et al. Lrp4 in osteoblasts suppresses bone formation and promotes osteoclastogenesis and bone resorption. Proc Natl Acad Sci U S A 2015;112(11):3487–92.

91. Mao B, Wu W, Davidson G, et al. Kremen proteins are Dickkopf receptors that regulate Wnt/beta-catenin signalling. Nature 2002;417(6889):664–7.
92. Glass DA 2nd, Bialek P, Ahn JD, et al. Canonical Wnt signaling in differentiated osteoblasts controls osteoclast differentiation. Dev Cel 2005;8(5):751–64.
93. Heiland GR, Zwerina K, Baum W, et al. Neutralisation of Dkk-1 protects from systemic bone loss during inflammation and reduces sclerostin expression. Ann Rheum Dis 2010;69(12):2152–9.
94. Daoussis D, Liossis SN, Solomou EE, et al. Evidence that Dkk-1 is dysfunctional in ankylosing spondylitis. Arthritis Rheum 2010;62(1):150–8.
95. Wanders A, Heijde D, Landewe R, et al. Nonsteroidal antiinflammatory drugs reduce radiographic progression in patients with ankylosing spondylitis: a randomized clinical trial. Arthritis Rheum 2005;52(6):1756–65.
96. Hreggvidsdottir HS, Noordenbos T, Baeten DL. Inflammatory pathways in spondyloarthritis. Mol Immunol 2014;57(1):28–37.
97. Notley CA, Inglis JJ, Alzabin S, et al. Blockade of tumor necrosis factor in collagen-induced arthritis reveals a novel immunoregulatory pathway for Th1 and Th17 cells. J Exp Med 2008;205(11):2491–7.
98. Alzabin S, Abraham SM, Taher TE, et al. Incomplete response of inflammatory arthritis to TNFalpha blockade is associated with the Th17 pathway. Ann Rheum Dis 2012;71(10):1741–8.
99. Hull DN, Williams RO, Pathan E, et al. Anti-TNF treatment increases circulating Th17 cells similarly in different types of inflammatory arthritis. Clin Exp Immunol 2015. http://dx.doi.org/10.1111/cei.12626.
100. Sieper J, Appel H, Braun J, et al. Critical appraisal of assessment of structural damage in ankylosing spondylitis: implications for treatment outcomes. Arthritis Rheum 2008;58(3):649–56.
101. Kavanaugh A, Mease PJ, Gomez-Reino JJ, et al. Treatment of psoriatic arthritis in a phase 3 randomised, placebo-controlled trial with apremilast, an oral phosphodiesterase 4 inhibitor. Ann Rheum Dis 2014;73(6):1020–6.
102. Schafer PH, Parton A, Gandhi AK, et al. Apremilast, a cAMP phosphodiesterase-4 inhibitor, demonstrates anti-inflammatory activity in vitro and in a model of psoriasis. Br J Pharmacol 2010;159(4):842–55.
103. Mease PJ, Genovese MC, Greenwald MW, et al. Brodalumab, an anti-IL17RA monoclonal antibody, in psoriatic arthritis. N Engl J Med 2014;370(24):2295–306.
104. Kavanaugh A, Ritchlin C, Rahman P, et al. Ustekinumab, an anti-IL-12/23 p40 monoclonal antibody, inhibits radiographic progression in patients with active psoriatic arthritis: results of an integrated analysis of radiographic data from the phase 3, multicentre, randomised, double-blind, placebo-controlled PSUMMIT-1 and PSUMMIT-2 trials. Ann Rheum Dis 2014;73(6):1000–6.
105. McInnes IB, Sieper J, Braun J, et al. Efficacy and safety of secukinumab, a fully human anti-interleukin-17A monoclonal antibody, in patients with moderate-to-severe psoriatic arthritis: a 24-week, randomised, double-blind, placebo-controlled, phase II proof-of-concept trial. Ann Rheum Dis 2014;73(2):349–56.
106. Letko E, Yeh S, Foster CS, et al. Efficacy and safety of intravenous secukinumab in noninfectious uveitis requiring steroid-sparing immunosuppressive therapy. Ophthalmology 2015;122(5):939–48.
107. Cretu D, Liang K, Saraon P, et al. Quantitative tandem mass-spectrometry of skin tissue reveals putative psoriatic arthritis biomarkers. Clin Proteomics 2015;12(1):1.

108. Yamaguchi Y. Periostin in skin tissue and skin-related diseases. Allergol Int 2014;63(2):161–70.
109. Zenz R, Eferl R, Kenner L, et al. Psoriasis-like skin disease and arthritis caused by inducible epidermal deletion of Jun proteins. Nature 2005;437(7057):369–75.
110. Bardos T, Zhang J, Mikecz K, et al. Mice lacking endogenous major histocompatibility complex class II develop arthritis resembling psoriatic arthritis at an advanced age. Arthritis Rheum 2002;46(9):2465–75.
111. Khare SD, Luthra HS, David CS. Spontaneous inflammatory arthritis in HLA-B27 transgenic mice lacking beta 2-microglobulin: a model of human spondyloarthropathies. J Exp Med 1995;182(4):1153–8.
112. Yanagisawa H, Richardson JA, Taurog JD, et al. Characterization of psoriasiform and alopecic skin lesions in HLA-B27 transgenic rats. Am J Pathol 1995;147(4):955–64.
113. Ruutu M, Thomas G, Steck R, et al. Beta-glucan triggers spondylarthritis and Crohn's disease-like ileitis in SKG mice. Arthritis Rheum 2012;64(7):2211–22.
114. Cook PW, Brown JR, Cornell KA, et al. Suprabasal expression of human amphiregulin in the epidermis of transgenic mice induces a severe, early-onset, psoriasis-like skin pathology: expression of amphiregulin in the basal epidermis is also associated with synovitis. Exp Dermatol 2004;13(6):347–56.
115. Yamamoto M, Nakajima K, Takaishi M, et al. Psoriatic inflammation facilitates the onset of arthritis in a mouse model. J Invest Dermatol 2015;135(2):445–53.
116. Rothschild BM. Primate spondyloarthropathy. Curr Rheumatol Rep 2005;7(3):173–81.
117. Wang C, Wu L, Bulek K, et al. The psoriasis-associated D10N variant of the adaptor Act1 with impaired regulation by the molecular chaperone hsp90. Nat Immunol 2013;14(1):72–81.
118. Courtenay JS, Dallman MJ, Dayan AD, et al. Immunisation against heterologous type II collagen induces arthritis in mice. Nature 1980;283(5748):666–8.
119. Adamopoulos IE, Tessmer M, Chao CC, et al. IL-23 is critical for induction of arthritis, osteoclast formation, and maintenance of bone mass. J Immunol 2011;187(2):951–9.
120. Keffer J, Probert L, Cazlaris H, et al. Transgenic mice expressing human tumour necrosis factor: a predictive genetic model of arthritis. EMBO J 1991;10(13):4025–31.
121. Hammer RE, Richardson JA, Simmons WA, et al. High prevalence of colorectal cancer in HLA-B27 transgenic F344 rats with chronic inflammatory bowel disease. J Investig Med 1995;43(3):262–8.

Etiology and Pathogenesis of Psoriasis

Wolf-Henning Boehncke, MD[a,b,*]

KEYWORDS

- Psoriasis • Genome-wide association study • Etiology • Pathogenesis • IL-17
- T lymphocytes • Dendritic cells • Keratinocytes

KEY POINTS

- Psoriasis is characterized by the parallel appearance of epidermal hyperproliferation, inflammation, and angioneogenesis.
- Psoriasis is driven by an intimate interplay between the innate and the adaptive immune systems.
- The central axes of psoriatic inflammation comprise the nuclear factor-κB, interferon-γ, and interleukin (IL)-23 signaling pathways as well as antigen presentation.
- Biologic therapies targeting tumor necrosis factor-α, IL-23, or IL-17 are highly effective, underlining the clinical importance of these inflammatory mediators.
- Recent genetic and clinical observations allow differentiation of generalized pustular psoriasis as a distinct entity.

INTRODUCTION

Given the prevalence of around 2% in most populations studied so far, psoriasis is a common disease. In its most typical type, the disease manifests as well-demarcated, red, scaly plaques about the size of a palm. These lesions highlight already clinically the 2 pillars of its pathogenesis, namely epidermal hyperproliferation (scaling) and inflammation (infiltrated, red lesions; **Fig. 1**). Genetic analyses, particularly genome-wide association studies, identified key players in these processes, namely cells as well as mediators. Proof for their relevance in patients arises from the successful use of biologic drugs targeting these crucial components, resulting in unparalleled efficacy in relief of the signs and symptoms of psoriasis.

Disclosures: The author has received honoraria as a speaker or advisor for Abbvie, Biogen Idec, Celgene, Covagen, Galderma, Janssen, Leo, Lilly, MSD, Novartis, Pantec Biosolutions, Pfizer, and UCB.

[a] Department of Dermatology and Venereology, Geneva University Hospitals, Rue Gabrielle-Perret-Gentil 4, Genève 14 CH – 1211, Switzerland; [b] Department of Pathology and Immunology, University of Geneva, Rue Michel-Servet 7, Geneva CH – 1206, Switzerland
* Department of Dermatology and Venereology, Geneva University Hospitals, Rue Gabrielle-Perret-Gentil 4, Genève 14 CH – 1211, Switzerland.
E-mail address: wolf-henning.boehncke@hcuge.ch

Rheum Dis Clin N Am 41 (2015) 665–675
http://dx.doi.org/10.1016/j.rdc.2015.07.013
0889-857X/15/$ – see front matter © 2015 Elsevier Inc. All rights reserved.

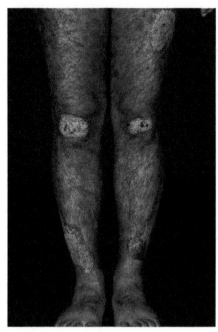

Fig. 1. Chronic plaque-type psoriasis. Well-demarcated, red, scaly plaques symmetrically distributed on the legs of a patient.

Noteworthy, pustular forms of psoriasis also exist. These forms do not respond to many of the drugs proven effective in chronic plaque-type psoriasis. Recent genetic studies suggest that at least generalized pustular psoriasis should be viewed as a distinct entity distinct from what formerly was regarded as "psoriasis."

This review provides an overview of the etiology of psoriasis, followed by a more in-depth discussion of pathogenesis, the need to differentiate between "psoriasis" and "generalized pustular psoriasis," and a discussion of the concept of "psoriatic disease" extending beyond the level of the skin.

ETIOLOGY

Psoriasis is a multifactorial disease with extrinsic as well as intrinsic factors playing major roles, as evidenced by the so-called Koebner phenomenon: nonspecific—extrinsic—triggers induce the manifestation of typical psoriatic lesions locally in the skin of patients, intrinsically "set" to develop such lesions. In addition, numerous triggers for a general aggravation have been described. Among the factors known to induce or worsen psoriasis, are:

- Mild localized trauma, such as scratching, piercings, tattoos, sunburns, chemical irritants ("classical" Koebner phenomenon)
- Drugs,[1] including β-blockers, lithium, antimalarials, and nonsteroidal antiinflammatory drugs
- HIV infection[2]
- Streptococcal pharyngitis.[3]

The climate in general and exposure to natural sun light in particular are discussed as additional extrinsic factors with clinically important impacts on disease activity.

Some researchers suggest the ultraviolet index is of interest based on the known effects of weather patterns on cutaneous psoriasis and psoriatic arthritis, which both worsen during winter and improve during summer.[4,5] Others reported a weak link between latitude and psoriasis prevalence, suggesting that other factors, or combinations of factors may also be important.

One factor of central importance is genetics. The importance of genetic factors is highlighted by the following observations:

- Population studies indicate a greater incidence of psoriasis among first- and second-degree relatives of patients than among the general population.[6]
- Concordance rates between monozygotic twins are up to 3 times higher than among dizygotic twins.[7]
- Patients with an early disease onset exhibit a more severe course and a positive family history, whereas patients with late-onset disease tend to experience a less severe presentation and course and often exhibit a negative family history.[8]
- Although commonly in the order of 2%, the prevalence of psoriasis does differ among different ethnic groups. Ethnicities basically free of psoriasis comprise American Samoa[7] and the Mapuche in Chile.[9]

PSORIASIS SUSCEPTIBILITY LOCI

These studies point toward genetics as an important component in the etiology of psoriasis in general. Indeed, the first chromosomal locus associated with the risk of psoriasis was found on chromosome 6p several decades ago. Since then, most genome-wide linkage analyses have reproduced this association and suggested HLA-Cw6 to be the susceptibility allele within what is now called the psoriasis susceptibility locus 1 (PSORS1). To date, PSORS1 is still by far the most strongly associated locus with psoriasis, thought to account for around 50% of the heritability of the disease.[10,11] Meanwhile, around 40 additional loci have been found to be associated with psoriasis (**Table 1**). Many of the potentially corresponding genes point toward a central role of both the innate as well as the adaptive immune system.[12–14] The importance of T cells in general and T helper (Th)17 lymphocytes in particular is underlined by variants in the genes encoding the interleukin (IL)-23 receptor and IL-12 as indicators of psoriasis risk.[15,16]

PATHOGENESIS

Psoriasis is currently widely regarded as an immune-mediated disease.[17] As discussed, genome-wide association studies identified predominantly immune-related genes to be linked to psoriasis.[18] Psoriatic plaques are thus considered to originate from dysregulated interactions of innate and adaptive components of the immune system with resident cells of the skin (**Fig. 2**).

Cross-Talk Between Innate and Adaptive Immunity

The cross-talk between the innate and the adaptive immune system through cytokines such as tumor necrosis factor (TNF)-α, interferon-γ, and IL-1 is a hot spot of current research in the field.[19] At the cellular level, dendritic cells and T cells are regarded as key effector cells, with important and complex interactive feedback loops with antigen-presenting cells, neutrophilic granulocytes, keratinocytes, vascular endothelial cells, and the cutaneous nervous system. A potential initiating event, triggering the inflammatory cascade and resulting in psoriatic plaque formation, might be the

Table 1
Major gene variants associated with psoriasis

Gene	Protein Function	Pathway	Comment
TNFA1P3	Inhibitor of TNF-α–induced NF-κB signaling	NF-κB signaling	TNF-α inhibitors are clinically effective in treating psoriasis
TNIP1	Inhibitor of TNF-α–induced NF-κB signaling	NF-κB signaling	TNF-α inhibitors are clinically effective in treating psoriasis
IL28RA	IL-29 receptor subunit	IFN signaling	—
IL12B	Shared subunit of IL-12 and IL-23	IL-23 signaling	—
IL23R	IL-23 receptor subunit	IL-23 signaling	—
IL23A	IL-23 subunit	IL-23 signaling	Ustekinumab (inhibiting IL-12 and IL-23) and specific anti–IL-23 antibodies are clinically effective in treating psoriasis
PSORS1 (HLA-C)	HLA class I antigen	Antigen presentation	—
ERAP1	Peptidase processing HLA class I ligands	Antigen presentation	—

Italic: Genes related to the function of the innate immune system.
Bold: Genes related to the function of the adaptive immune system.
Abbreviations: ERAP, endoplasmic reticulum aminopeptidase; IL, interleukin; NF-κB, nuclear factor-κB; PSORS, psoriasis susceptibility locus; TNF, tumor necrosis factor.
Adapted from Capon F, Burden AD, Trembath RC, et al. Psoriasis and other complex trait dermatoses: from Loci to functional pathways. J Invest Dermatol 2012;132(3):918.

stimulation of dermal plasmacytoid dendritic cells by DNA complexed with LL-37 (cathelicidin), an antimicrobial peptide produced by keratinocytes.[20] Among the cytokines produced by activated dendritic cells are TNF-α and IL-23. The former exerts pleiotropic effects on a wide array of cells from different lineages.[21] Among the proinflammatory activities of TNF-α is the induction of several secondary mediators as well as adhesion molecules, all of which are implicated in the psoriatic disease process.

The Interleuikn-23/T Helper 17 Axis

Several years ago, the IL-23/Th17 pathway entered the center stage of scientific attention. Although psoriasis was considered a Th1 cell–mediated disease, it is now clear that a subset of T lymphocytes expressing IL-17 (hence named Th17 cells) and distinct from the "classical" Th1 cells[22] plays a predominant role in the pathogenesis of psoriasis[23] and other inflammatory disorders.[24,25] IL-23, produced by myeloid cells, is a major expansion and survival factor for these T cells. Differentiation into Th17 cells occurs primarily on memory T cells, because naïve T cells lack expression of the IL-23 receptor.[26] Th17 cells are themselves a source of multiple proinflammatory cytokines, such as IL-17A, IL-17F, and IL-22, resulting among others in keratinocyte proliferation as a hallmark of psoriasis. Although CD4+ Th17 cells were initially believed to be the principal source of IL-17, evidence is accumulating that other cell types such as epidermal CD8+ T cells, neutrophils, innate lymphocytes, and macrophages substantially contribute in this regard.[27,28]

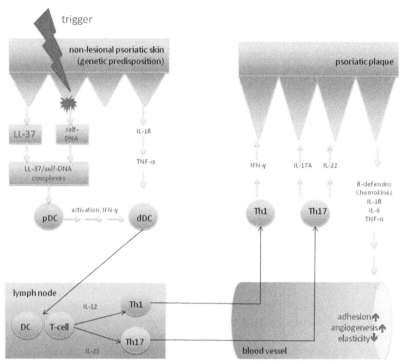

Fig. 2. Pathogenesis of psoriasis. According to a widely accepted hypothesis, psoriatic plaques originate from dysregulated interactions of innate and adaptive components of the immune system with resident cells of the skin. DC, dendritic cells; dDC, dermal dendritic cells; IFN, interferon; IL, interleukin; pDC, plasmacytoid dendritic cells; TNF, tumor necrosis factor; Th, T helper.

Impact on Resident Cells of the Skin

TNF-α and IL-23 exert pleiotropic effects, multiplied by mediators derived from cells responding to activation by these 2 cytokines, and resulting in complex dysregulation of virtually all cutaneous cell types. Keratinocytes are a prominent target, responding with hyperproliferation and cytokine production as well as secretion of antimicrobial peptides. These latter molecules act as chemoattractants for infiltrating immune cells,[29] establishing a positive feedback loop between cells of the immune system and resident epithelial cells in psoriasis.

Beside inflammation and epidermal hyperproliferation, angio(neo)genesis is the third key process in psoriatic pathogenesis. The function of vascular endothelial cells is altered substantially by the inflammatory milieu, because the latter leads to induction and activation of various proangiogenic factors.[30,31] Furthermore, regulatory T cells influence the vascular endothelial growth factor–related angiogenic microenvironment[32] and contribute to epidermal hyperplasia.[33] Another important feature is the induction of adhesion molecules on endothelial cells, which facilitate the recruitment of circulating leukocytes into psoriatic skin.[34] The direct effects of the inflammatory milieu on endothelial (dys)function are discussed separately elsewhere in this article.

Additional feedback loops with other cutaneous cell types, such as nerve fibers, which presumably contribute to the psoriatic pathophysiology.[35] Indeed, a recent study showed that nociceptors in murine psoriasiform lesions induced by imiquimod can induce activation of IL-23 expressing cutaneous dendritic cells under-scoring the interplay between nerve activation and inflammation in the skin.[36]

Clinical Observations

The importance of these findings is underlined by the striking efficacy of innovative therapies targeting key components of the respective pathways. Conventional systemic antipsoriatic drugs such as methotrexate or fumaric acid esters exhibit rather generic modes of action, yielding acceptable therapeutic responses within around 3 to 4 months in about one-half of patients treated.[37] Biologics blocking TNF-α or IL-23 are considerably more effective in most patients.[37] And a novel generation of biologics targeting IL-17A or the IL-17 receptor seem to exhibit an even faster mode of onset along with striking efficacy.[38–40] Preliminary results in early studies of the p19 Ab also demonstrated very high efficacy, further highlighting the pivotal importance of this pathway. In addition, antiangiogenic therapeutic approaches are explored with some success.

TOWARD DEFINING DISTINCT PSORIATIC ENTITIES

Although chronic plaque-type psoriasis is the most common manifestation of psoria-sis, its clinical spectrum is wide (**Table 2**):

- An acute exanthematic manifestation is called guttate psoriasis. It is particularly frequent in children and adolescents and often associated with streptococcal tonsillitis.
- Inverse psoriasis spares the typical predilection sites of chronic plaque-type psoriasis, occurring in skin folds such as the axillae or groin. It lacks the otherwise typical scales.
- Scalp psoriasis is often found behind the ears. When affecting the frontal part, it typically also involves part of the forehead.
- Nail psoriasis causes numerous characteristic changes at the level of the matrix as well as the nail plate.
- Finally, there are localized as well as generalized pustular manifestations.

A first very general hint toward separate pathogenetic mechanisms underlying these manifestations is the clinical experience that they respond differently to distinct

Table 2
Classification of psoriasis based on clinical and genetic criteria

Clinical Criteria	Composite Definition	Genetic Markers
L40 Psoriasis	Type 1	Psoriasis vulgaris
L40.0 Psoriasis vulgaris	• Association with HLA-Cw6	• >30 PSORSs
• Chronic plaque-type	• Positive family history	Guttate psoriasis
• Inverse	• Manifestation <30 y	• PSORS1
• Erythroderma	Type 2	DITRA (minority of cases
L40.1 generalized pustular	• No association with HLA-Cw6	with generalized
psoriasis	• Sporadic	pustular psoriasis
L40.2 Acrodermatitis	• Manifestation >40 y	• Mutations in the
continua suppurativa		IL36RN gene
L40.3 Psoriasis pustulosa		• Lack of association
palmoplantaris		with PSORS1
L40.4 Psoriasis guttata		

Abbreviations: DITRA, deficiency in the interleukin-36 receptor antagonist; PSORS, psoriasis susceptibility locus.

therapies. For example, acitretin is often used in pustular psoriasis, although it is considered not sufficiently effective as a monotherapy in chronic plaque-type psoriasis.[37]

Furthermore, genetics have helped to better understand and reclassify these manifestations:

- PSORS1 is strongly associated with guttate psoriasis, but not with palmoplantar pustulosis.[41]
- Generalized pustular psoriasis has recently been linked to IL-36 receptor antagonist deficiency[42] and mutations or variants of caspase recruitment domain family, member 14 (CARD14).[43]

The need to regard at least generalized pustular psoriasis with IL-36 receptor antagonist deficiency as a distinct entity is underscored by the clinical observation that these patients do not respond to TNF-α inhibitors, but readily to the IL-1β antagonist anakinra.[44]

PSORIASIS AS A CHRONIC SYSTEMIC DISEASE
Genetics of Comorbidity

Psoriasis is associated with numerous other diseases such psoriatic arthritis, Crohn's disease, cancer, depression, nonalcoholic fatty liver disease, the metabolic syndrome or components of it, and cardiovascular disorders.[8] The association of some of these comorbid diseases with psoriasis might be owing to common genetics:

- Numerous genes, including IL-23R, are associated with psoriasis as well as psoriatic arthritis.[45]
- The gene *CDKAL1* is found in association with psoriasis and type 2 diabetes mellitus as well as Crohn's disease.[46]

On the other hand, there are also genetic associations clearly separating psoriasis from psoriatic arthritis. With regard to cardiovascular comorbidity, much less genetic overlap has been observed between psoriasis and cardiovascular disease than between the metabolic syndrome and cardiovascular disease.[47]

Epidemiology of Comorbidity

With regard to malignancies, it is unclear whether lymphoma and skin cancer are related to psoriasis itself, or its treatment.[48] Finally, the increased cardiovascular mortality has long been attributed to cumulating classical cardiovascular risk factors among psoriasis patients.[49] However, this suggestion cannot explain why only patients with severe, but not mild, psoriasis exhibit this increased cardiovascular risk.[50–52] Three recent metaanalyses identified an increased risk for cardiovascular mortality among psoriasis patients.[53–55]

Pathogenesis of Cardiovascular Comorbidity

Although there are still few data addressing potential pathogenetic links between psoriasis and most of its comorbidities, there is some evidence for inflammation-induced insulin resistance driving cardiovascular disease in psoriasis[56,57]:

- Psoriasis is a state of systemic inflammation, because numerous biomarkers for inflammation cannot only readily be detected in the patients' blood, but also correlate with disease activity.[58]
- Systemic inflammation in turn induces insulin resistance, that is, reduced signaling of the insulin receptor upon binding of its ligand.

- At the level of endothelial cells, insulin resistance results in reduced release of vasodilating factors such as nitric oxide.
- The resulting vascular stiffness is known as endothelial dysfunction. It comprises additional features, such as expression of adhesion molecules, and provides the basis for the formation of atherosclerotic plaques.
- Interestingly, dermal endothelial cells (in close vicinity to psoriatic plaques) are particularly susceptible to induction of insulin resistance and endothelial dysfunction by an inflammatory milieu typical for psoriasis.[59]
- Depending on their localization, resulting diseases comprise myocardial infarction or stroke, both known to be associated with psoriasis.

SUMMARY

Over the last couple of years, our understanding of the pathogenesis of psoriasis has deepened substantially in response to new information generated from genetic, pathogenetic, and clinical studies. A major advance resulting from these studies is that, we should no longer regard "psoriasis" as a monolithic entity, but rather as several distinct entities within the spectrum of "psoriasis." Moreover, at the striking prevalence of comorbid disorders and psoriasis comorbidity, there is the concept of "psoriatic disease" as a systemic disorder, comprising manifestations beyond the skin. These associated conditions may in part be linked to psoriatic plaques via insulin resistance and endothelial dysfunction as a consequence of the inflammatory milieu generated by these plaques.

REFERENCES

1. Basavaraj KH, Ashok NM, Rashmi R, et al. The role of drugs in the induction and/or exacerbation of psoriasis. Int J Dermatol 2010;49(12):1351–61.
2. Fry L, Baker BS. Triggering psoriasis: the role of infections and medications. Clin Dermatol 2007;25:606–15.
3. Sigurdardottir SL, Thorleifsdottir RH, Valdimarsson H, et al. The role of the palatine tonsils in the pathogenesis and treatment of psoriasis. Br J Dermatol 2013 Feb;168(2):237–42.
4. Balato N, Di Costanzo L, Patruno C, et al. Effect of weather and environmental factors on the clinical course of psoriasis. Occup Environ Med 2013;70(8):600.
5. Jacobson CC, Kumar S, Kimball AB. Latitude and psoriasis prevalence. J Am Acad Dermatol 2011;65(4):870–3.
6. Farber EM, Nall ML. The natural history of psoriasis in 5,600 patients. Dermatologica 1974;148(1):1–18.
7. Farber EM, Nall L. Epidemiology: natural history and genetics. In: Roenigk HH Jr, Maibach HI, editors. Psoriasis. New York: Dekker; 1998. p. 107–57.
8. Henseler T, Christophers E. Psoriasis of early and late onset: characterization of two types of psoriasis vulgaris. J Am Acad Dermatol 1985;13(3):450–6.
9. Valenzuela F, Valenzuela Y, Zemelman V. Epidemiological survey of psoriasis in the Chilean Mapuche population. Int J Dermatol 2012;51:1005–6.
10. Trembath RC, Clough RL, Rosbotham JL, et al. Identification of a major susceptibility locus on chromosome 6p and evidence for further disease loci revealed by a two stage genome-wide search in psoriasis. Hum Mol Genet 1997;6(5):813–20.
11. Nair RP, Stuart PE, Nistor I, et al. Sequence and haplotype analysis supports HLA-C as the psoriasis susceptibility 1 gene. Am J Hum Genet 2006;78(5): 827–51.

12. Capon F, Burden AD, Trembath RC, et al. Psoriasis and other complex trait dermatoses: from Loci to functional pathways. J Invest Dermatol 2012;132(3): 915–22.
13. Elder JT, Bruce AT, Gudjonsson JE, et al. Molecular dissection of psoriasis: integrating genetics and biology. J Invest Dermatol 2010;130(5):1213–26.
14. Tsoi LC, Spain SL, Knight J, et al. Identification of 15 new psoriasis susceptibility loci highlights the role of innate immunity. Nat Genet 2012;44(12):1341–8.
15. Capon F, Di Meglio P, Szaub J, et al. Sequence variants in the genes for the interleukin-23 receptor (IL23R) and its ligand (IL12B) confer protection against psoriasis. Hum Genet 2007;122(2):201–6.
16. Cargill M, Schrodi SJ, Chang M, et al. A large-scale genetic association study confirms IL12B and leads to the identification of IL23R as psoriasis-risk genes. Am J Hum Genet 2007;80(2):273–90.
17. Schön MP, Boehncke WH. Psoriasis. N Engl J Med 2005;352:1899–912.
18. Elder JT. Genome-wide association scan yields new insights into the immunopathogenesis of psoriasis. Genes Immun 2009;10(3):201–9.
19. Nestle FO, Conrad C, Tun-Kyi A, et al. Plasmacytoid predendritic cells initiate psoriasis through interferon-alpha production. J Exp Med 2005;202(1):135–43.
20. Lande R, Gregorio J, Facchinetti V, et al. Plasmacytoid dendritic cells sense self-DNA coupled with antimicrobial peptide. Nature 2007;449(7162):564–9.
21. Locksley RM, Killeen N, Lenardo MJ. The TNF and TNF receptor superfamilies: integrating mammalian biology. Cell 2001;104(4):487–501.
22. Steinman L. A brief history of T(H)17, the first major revision in the T(H)1/T(H)2 hypothesis of T cell-mediated tissue damage. Nat Med 2007;13:139–45.
23. Lowes MA, Kikuchi T, Fuentes-Duculan J, et al. Psoriasis vulgaris lesions contain discrete populations of Th1 and Th17 T cells. J Invest Dermatol 2008;128(5): 1207–11.
24. Neurath MF. IL-23: a master regulator in Crohn's disease. Nat Med 2007;13(1): 26–8.
25. Kebir H, Kreymborg K, Ifergan I, et al. Human TH17 lymphocytes promote blood-brain barrier disruption and central nervous system inflammation. Nat Med 2007; 13(10):1173–5.
26. Parham C, Chirica M, Timans J, et al. A receptor for the heterodimeric cytokine IL-23 is composed of IL-12Rbeta1 and a novel cytokine receptor subunit, IL-23R. J Immunol 2002;168(11):5699–708.
27. Lin AM, Rubin CJ, Khandpur R, et al. Mast cells and neutrophils release IL-17 through extracellular trap formation in psoriasis. J Immunol 2011;187:490–500.
28. Keijsers RR, Hendriks AG, van Erp PE, et al. In vivo induction of cutaneous inflammation results in the accumulation of extracellular trap-forming neutrophils expressing RORgamma and IL-17. J Invest Dermatol 2014;134:1276–84.
29. Büchau A, Gallo RL. Innate immunity and antimicrobial defense systems in psoriasis. Clin Dermatol 2007;25:616–24.
30. Costa C, Incio J, Soares R. Angiogenesis and chronic inflammation: cause or consequence? Angiogenesis 2007;10(3):149–66.
31. Rosenberger C, Solovan C, Rosenberger AD, et al. Upregulation of hypoxia-inducible factors in normal and psoriatic skin. J Invest Dermatol 2007;127(10): 2445–52.
32. Teige I, Hvid H, Svensson L, et al. Regulatory T cells control VEGF-dependent skin inflammation. J Invest Dermatol 2009;129(6):1437–45.
33. Elias PM, Arbiser J, Brown BE, et al. Epidermal vascular endothelial growth factor production is required for permeability barrier homeostasis, dermal angiogenesis,

and the development of epidermal hyperplasia: implications for the pathogenesis of psoriasis. Am J Pathol 2008;173(3):689–99.

34. Schön MP, Zollner TM, Boehncke WH. The molecular basis of lymphocyte recruitment to the skin: clues for pathogenesis and selective therapies of inflammatory disorders. J Invest Dermatol 2003;121(5):951–62.

35. Madva EN, Granstein RD. Nerve-derived transmitters including peptides influence cutaneous immunology. Brain Behav Immun 2013;34:1–10.

36. Riol-Blanco L, Ordovas-Montanes J, Perro M, et al. Nociceptive sensory neurons drive interleukin-23-mediated psoriasiform skin inflammation. Nature 2014;510:157.

37. Nast A, Boehncke WH, Mrowietz U, et al. German S3-guidelines on the treatment of psoriasis vulgaris (short version). Arch Dermatol Res 2012;304(2):87–113.

38. Leonardi C, Matheson R, Zachariae C, et al. Anti-interleukin-17 monoclonal antibody ixekizumab in chronic plaque psoriasis. N Engl J Med 2012;366(13): 1190–9.

39. Papp KA, Leonardi C, Menter A, et al. Brodalumab, an anti-interleukin-17-receptor antibody for psoriasis. N Engl J Med 2012;366(13):1181–9.

40. Langley RG, Elewski BE, Lebwohl M, et al. Secukinumab in plaque psoriasis–results of two phase 3 trials. N Engl J Med 2014;371(4):326–38.

41. Asumalahti K, Ameen M, Suomela S, et al. Genetic analysis of PSORS1 distinguishes guttate psoriasis and palmoplantar pustulosis. J Invest Dermatol 2003; 120(4):627–34.

42. Marrakchi S, Guigue P, Renshaw BR, et al. Interleukin-36-receptor antagonist deficiency and generalized pustular psoriasis. N Engl J Med 2011;365(7):620–8.

43. Sugiura K. The genetic background of generalized pustular psoriasis: IL36RN mutations and CARD14 gain-of-function variants. J Dermatol Sci 2014;74:187–92.

44. Hüffmeier U, Wätzold M, Mohr J, et al. Successful therapy with anakinra in a patient with generalized pustular psoriasis carrying IL36RN mutations. Br J Dermatol 2014;170(1):202–4.

45. Rahman P, Inman RD, Maksymowych WP, et al. Association of interleukin 23 receptor variants with psoriatic arthritis. J Rheumatol 2009;36(1):137–40.

46. Wolf N, Quaranta M, Prescott NJ, et al. Psoriasis is associated with pleiotropic susceptibility loci identified in type II diabetes and Crohn disease. J Med Genet 2008;45(2):114–6.

47. Gupta Y, Möller S, Zillikens D, et al. Genetic control of psoriasis is relatively distinct from that of metabolic syndrome and coronary artery disease. Exp Dermatol 2013;22(8):552–3.

48. Gelfand JM, Shin DB, Neimann AL, et al. The risk of lymphoma in patients with psoriasis. J Invest Dermatol 2006;126(10):2194–201.

49. Gisondi P, Tessari G, Conti A, et al. Prevalence of metabolic syndrome in patients with psoriasis: a hospital-based case-control study. Br J Dermatol 2007;157(1): 68–73.

50. Gelfand JM, Neimann AL, Shin DB, et al. Risk of myocardial infarction in patients with psoriasis. JAMA 2006;296(14):1735–41.

51. Mallbris L, Akre O, Granath F, et al. Increased risk for cardiovascular mortality in psoriasis inpatients but not in outpatients. Eur J Epidemiol 2004;19(3): 225–30.

52. Ludwig RJ, Herzog C, Rostock A, et al. Psoriasis: a possible risk factor for development of coronary artery calcification. Br J Dermatol 2007;156(2):271–6.

53. Armstrong EJ, Harskamp CT, Armstrong AW. Psoriasis and major adverse cardiovascular events: a systematic review and meta-analysis of cardiovascular studies. J Am Heart Assoc 2013;2:000062.

54. Samarasekera EJ, Neilson JM, Warren RB, et al. Incidence of cardiovascular disease in individuals with psoriasis: a systematic review and meta-analysis. J Invest Dermatol 2013;133:2340–6.
55. Xu T, Zhang YH. Association of psoriasis with stroke and myocardial infarction: meta-analysis of cohort studies. Br J Dermatol 2012;167:1345–50.
56. Boehncke S, Thaci D, Beschmann H, et al. Psoriasis patients show signs of insulin resistance. Br J Dermatol 2007;157(6):1249–51.
57. Boehncke WH, Boehncke S, Schön MP. Managing comorbid disease in patients with psoriasis. Br Med J 2010;340:b5666.
58. Boehncke S, Salgo R, Garbaraviciene J, et al. Effective continuous systemic therapy of severe plaque-type psoriasis is accompanied by amelioration of biomarkers of cardiovascular risk: results of a prospective longitudinal observational study. J Eur Acad Dermatol Venereol 2011;25(10):1187–93.
59. Woth K, Prein C, Steinhorst K, et al. Endothelial cells are highly heterogeneous at the level of cytokine-induced insulin resistance. Exp Dermatol 2013;22(11): 714–8.

Comorbidities in Psoriatic Arthritis

M. Elaine Husni, MD, MPH

KEYWORDS

- Psoriatic arthritis • Comorbidity • Psoriasis • Management • Screening

KEY POINTS

- Providing comprehensive care of patients with psoriatic arthritis includes screening for related comorbidities and taking this into consideration for relevant treatment selection.
- The most common comorbidity among patients with psoriatic arthritis is cardiovascular disease, so there is an emphasis on traditional cardiovascular risk factors such as obesity and diabetes.
- Additional comorbidities include ophthalmic disease, liver disease, inflammatory bowel disease, depression and anxiety, osteoporosis, kidney disease, malignancy, and infection.

INTRODUCTION

Psoriatic arthritis (PsA) is well known to affect the skin and joints and emerging research has identified specific comorbidities related to PsA. More than half of patients with PsA have at least 1 comorbidity (**Table 1**) and this has a significant negative impact on quality of life.[1,7] Recognizing and addressing comorbidities are critical to safely and effectively treating patients with PsA because these comorbidities often have implications not only for impaired function and quality of life but also therapy selection.[8,9] This article summarizes the knowledge to date regarding the most relevant comorbidities in patients with PsA and highlights therapy options for patients with PsA in the setting of comorbid conditions.

Important comorbidities shown to be associated with PsA disease include premature cardiovascular disease (CVD); metabolic syndrome (diabetes, obesity); ophthalmic, liver, kidney, and inflammatory bowel disease (IBD); depression; and anxiety (**Fig. 1**). PsA comorbidities associated with both the disease and the treatments include

Disclosure: Advisory or consulting for Abbvie, Amgen, Bristol Myers Squibb, Celgene, Novartis, and Genentech.
Department of Rheumatic and Immunologic Diseases, Clinical Outcomes Research, Arthritis and Musculoskeletal Center, Cleveland Clinic, Desk A50, 9500 Euclid Avenue, Cleveland, OH 44195, USA
E-mail address: husnie@ccf.org

Table 1			
Incidence of multiple PsA comorbidities			
No of Comorbid Conditions	Salaffi et al,[3] 2009 (n = 101), Peripheral PsA, n (%)[a]	Salaffi et al,[3] 2009 (n = 65), Axial PsA, n (%)[a]	Husted et al,[1] 2013 (Total n = 631), PsA, n (%)[b]
0	45 (44.6)	19 (29.3)	—
1	26 (25.7)	12 (18.5)	—
2	13 (12.9)	21 (32.3)	—
<3	84 (83.2)	52 (80.0)	365 (57.8)
≥3	17 (16.8)	13 (20.0)	266 (42.2)

[a] Based on patient Self-Administered Comorbidity Questionnaire list of 13 comorbidities: heart disease, hypertension, lung disease, diabetes, ulcer or stomach disease, kidney and liver disease, anemia or other blood disease, cancer, depression, osteoarthritis, back pain, and rheumatoid arthritis.
[b] Based on a list of 15 comorbidities: CVD, hypertension, hyperlipidemia, type II diabetes, obesity, respiratory disease, gastrointestinal disease, neurologic disease, autoimmune disease, liver disease, depression/anxiety, cancer, other musculoskeletal conditions, infection, and fibromyalgia.
    Data from Refs.[1–6]

infectious complications, malignancy risk, and osteoporosis. Recently published data on the incidence of specific comorbidities in patients with PsA are listed in **Table 2**.

CARDIOVASCULAR DISEASE
Inflammation and Atherosclerosis

Understanding of atherosclerosis has recently evolved from simply cholesterol deposition to a more complex process that may be a manifestation of a chronic inflammatory disease. It has been shown that systemic inflammation, involving low-grade inflammatory activity in the vascular wall, is pivotal in the pathogenesis of atherosclerosis. Many of the inflammatory cells and cytokines, including tumor necrosis factor (TNF) alpha, that play an active role in synovitis and psoriatic diseases are also active in atherosclerosis. This inflammatory burden is thought to lead to increased insulin resistance, oxidative stress, endothelial cell dysfunction, and the development of atherosclerosis, which may ultimately result in myocardial infarction (MI) or cerebrovascular accidents (CVAs).[10]

The concept of a common pathogenic mechanism for atherosclerosis and systemic rheumatic diseases has resulted in the increasing importance of a multidisciplinary integrated approach to optimize screening and therapy for patients with PsA, with active coordination between primary care and cardiology colleagues. Patients with chronic inflammatory states may interact synergistically with cardiovascular (CV) risk factors or independently to augment vascular dysfunction leading to accelerated atherosclerosis.

Cardiovascular Risk

CVDs, such as an increased prevalence of ischemic heart disease, cerebrovascular disease, diastolic dysfunction, left ventricular dysfunction, abnormal carotid intimal thickness, and CV death, represent a major source of morbidity for patients with PsA.[11–14] Patients with PsA have a higher prevalence and incidence of MI and stroke than the general population.[14,15] Patients with PsA have an increased prevalence of traditional CV risk factors, such as a history of diabetes, hypertension, obesity, dyslipidemia, and smoking. However, this increased prevalence may not fully explain CV

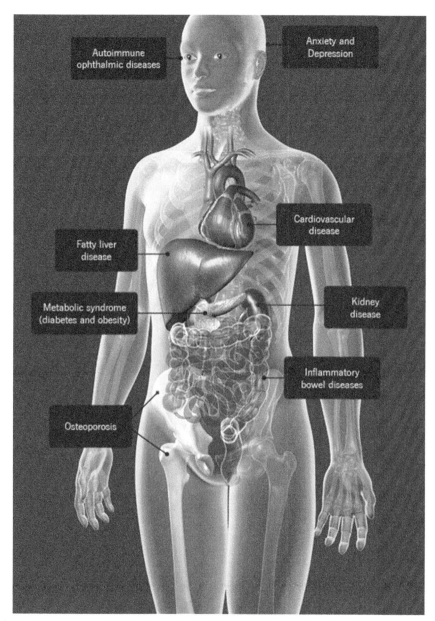

Fig. 1. Common comorbidities in patients with PsA. (*Adapted from* Husni ME. Guidance at last on managing comorbidities of psoriatic arthritis. Rheumatology Connections. 2014–2015. p. 4; with permission; © The Cleveland Clinic Foundation 2014.)

risk in PsA. Recent studies have found that up to 30% to 50% of patients with PsA with atherosclerosis do not have these traditional CV risk factors.[16,17] In several studies this increased risk has been attributed not only to increased traditional risk factors but also to chronic systemic inflammation.[1,18,19] In addition to an increased prevalence of traditional CV risk factors, patients with PsA also have an increased prevalence of

Table 2
Incidence of PsA comorbidity

Comorbidity	Husted et al,[1] 2013 (n = 631), n (%)[a]	Kraishi et al,[4] 2014 (n = 196), n (%)	Edson-Heredia et al,[5] 2015 (n = 1952), n (%)	Feldman et al,[6] 2015 (n = 1230), n (%)[b]	Ogdie et al,[2] 2015 (n = 8706), n (%)
Obesity	204 (32.3)	117 (59.7)	—	—	—
Hypertension	221 (35.0)	64 (32.7)	376 (19.3)	440 (35.8)	—
Infection	216 (34.2)	—	—	—	—
Depression/anxiety	130 (20.6)	27 (13.8)	530 (27.2)	185 (15.0)	—
Hyperlipidemia	124 (19.7)	98 (61.6)[c]	157 (8.0)	425 (34.6)	—
Diabetes	72 (11.4)	27 (13.8)	98 (5.0)	196 (15.9)	—
Cancer	56 (8.9)	—	—	80 (6.5)	—
CVD	48 (7.6)	17 (8.7)	64 (3.3)	118 (9.6)	338 (3.9)
Gastrointestinal disease	37 (5.9)	—	—	16 (1.3)	—
Liver disease	15 (2.4)	—	—	—	—

[a] Based on a list of 15 comorbidities: CVD, hypertension, hyperlipidemia, type II diabetes, obesity, respiratory disease, gastrointestinal disease, neurologic disease, autoimmune disease, liver disease, depression/anxiety, cancer, other musculoskeletal conditions, infection, and fibromyalgia.
[b] Comorbidities in patients with PsA with moderate to severe PsO.
[c] Includes patients on dyslipidemia medications.
Data from Refs.[1–6]

metabolic syndrome, which is a combination of hypertension and hyperlipidemia risk factors and comorbidities such as obesity and diabetes.[20–22] Metabolic syndrome has been associated with increased severity of PsA and increased CVD.[13,23]

Recent studies have suggested that patients with PsA with metabolic syndrome have the highest overall maximum carotid artery intima-media thickness and prevalence of carotid plaques compared with other patients with psoriatic disease.[13] Studies have suggested that the length of disease and exposure to chronic inflammation may play a role in increased carotid plaque burden over time.[24] These observations support the hypothesis that incremental increases in inflammatory pathways in PsA may contribute to an even higher CV risk and metabolic syndrome compared with psoriasis alone.

In a recent controlled study by Han and colleagues[25] prevalence ratios for CVD and their risk factors in 3066 patients with PsA compared with matched controls were increased for the following CVDs: ischemic heart disease (1.3), congestive heart failure (CHF) (1.5), cerebrovascular disease (1.3), atherosclerosis (1.4), peripheral vascular disease (1.6), type II diabetes (1.5), hyperlipidemia (1.2), and hypertension (1.3). Similar increased prevalence ratios were also found in rheumatoid arthritis (RA) (n = 28,208) and ankylosing spondylitis (AS) (n = 1843) cohorts. An increased risk of CVD compared with controls was reported for a large prospective study of 648 patients with PsA followed at The University of Toronto Psoriatic Arthritis Clinic. Of these patients, 23.9% (n = 155) developed at least 1 of the following conditions: hypertension (n = 122), MI (n = 38), angina (n = 21), CHF (n = 11), or a CVA (n = 5). The standardized prevalence ratios (SPRs) for MI (2.57; 95% confidence interval [CI], 1.73–3.80), angina (1.97; 95% CI, 1.24–3.12), and hypertension (1.90; 95% CI, 1.59–2.27) were statistically significant, whereas the SPRs for CHF (1.19; 95% CI, 0.50–2.86) and CVA (0.91; 95% CI, 0.34–2.43) were not.[17]

Given that systemic inflammation has been implicated in accelerated atherosclerosis in patients with rheumatic disease, decreasing inflammation through the use of disease-modifying antirheumatic drugs (DMARDs) has been hypothesized to attenuate CV risk. However 2 recent studies report results that contradict this rationale. Chen and colleagues[26] described a comparable incidence of ischemic heart disease in patients with psoriasis treated with methotrexate (MTX) and those treated with other nonbiologic antipsoriatic drugs. Similarly, recently published data by Ogdie and colleagues[2] on risk of major adverse CV events (MACE) among 8706 patients with PsA from a UK population-based longitudinal cohort study (1994–2010) showed conflicting results on the effects of DMARDs on the incidence of MACE. After adjustment for traditional risk factors, they showed an increased risk for incident MI for both non–DMARD-treated and DMARD-treated patients with PsA (hazard ratio [HR], 1.36; 95% CI, 1.04–1.77; and HR, 1.36; 95% CI, 1.01–1.84 respectively). However, the risk of incident stroke and the composite MACE outcome were significantly increased only in non–DMARD-treated patients with PsA (HR, 1.33; 95% CI, 1.03–1.71; and HR, 1.24; 95% CI, 1.03–1.49 respectively). In addition, CV death was not significantly increased in either non–DMARD-treated or DMARD-treated cohorts (HR, 1.07; 95% CI, 0.79–1.44; and HR, 0.96; 95% CI, 0.64–1.43).[2] These studies stress the need to better understand the mechanism underlying increased CVD in patients with psoriasis and PsA given conflicting results.

The study by Ogdie and colleagues[2] also showed that high Psoriasis Area and Severity Index score was an important factor associated with CVD. Several other studies have supported the increased predictive value of the severity of skin lesions in PsA. A large retrospective cohort study of the General Practice Research Database in the United Kingdom used psoriasis diagnostic codes and any history of systemic therapy to identify patients with mild and severe psoriasis from 1987 to 2002 with the objective of determining the risk of mortality in patients with psoriasis alone and in those with psoriasis and associated inflammatory arthropathies. The investigators reported no overall effect of mild psoriasis on mortality (HR, 1.0; 95% CI, 0.97–1.02), whereas patients with severe psoriasis showed an increased overall mortality risk (HR, 1.5; 95%CI, 1.3–1.7). The association of severe psoriasis with mortality persisted after exclusion of patients with inflammatory arthropathy (HR, 1.5; 95% CI, 1.3–1.8). Male and female patients with severe psoriasis died 3.5 years (95% CI, 1.2–5.8) and 4.4 (95% CI, 2.2–6.6) years younger, respectively, than patients without psoriasis (P<.001).[27] Risk of mortality relative to age was greatest in younger patients with severe psoriasis in this study, and this is supported by another study,[28] which indicated that younger patients (<40 years old) with severe psoriasis had the highest relative risk of CV mortality. These findings point to skin disease severity and age of onset as a tools for predicting increased incidence and severity of CVD in psoriasis and PsA.[16] Some studies report less comparable risks for CV events and CV mortality in psoriasis compared with the general population,[15,29–31] which may suggest a need for further investigation, but nonetheless most data advocate screening and management of CV risk factors in patients with psoriasis.

Cardiovascular Screening and Management

Patients with PsA should be screened at least annually for traditional CV risk factors, such as blood pressure and serum lipids, and more often in patients with added risks.[13,32,33] Screening considerations for CVD and the other comorbidities seen in patients with PsA are listed in **Table 3**. It is important to be aware that typical risk stratification scores for CVD in the general population (eg, Framingham Risk Score and the Systematic Coronary Risk Evaluation algorithm) often underestimate the risk for CV events.[34,35] Identification and subsequent management of traditional risk factors (eg, hypertension, diabetes, hyperlipidemia, and smoking) are important for these patients.[24,36,37] Thus, CV risk factor management should be the same as for the general population in primary prevention CV care.[38]

To date, no prospective studies have specifically examined the effect of aggressive PsA treatment on risk of CV events. Prior studies investigating the hypothesis that CV risk can be attenuated by decreasing inflammation through the use of DMARD therapy have produced conflicting results, as reported earlier. The risk of CV outcomes associated with chronic corticosteroid and nonsteroidal antiinflammatory drug (NSAID) use in patients with PsA has not been studied in a controlled clinical trial. The future results of an ongoing PRECISION (Prospective Randomized Evaluation of Celecoxib Integrated Safety versus Ibuprofen Or Naproxen) trial (clinical trials.gov) investigating the CVD outcomes of 3 different NSAIDs in the treatment of arthritis may help clarify these differential CV risks. In summary, current clinical practice has no definitive pharmacologic treatment recommendations to address future CV risk in patients with PsA or for other systemic rheumatic diseases.

OBESITY

Most patients with PsA are overweight (body mass index [BMI] >25) or obese (BMI>30).[22–24] Several studies have suggested that obese BMI may be a risk factor for psoriasis (PsO) and PsA.[39] An analysis of the CORRONA (Consortium of Rheumatology Researchers of North America) database found patients with PsA to be heavier than patients with RA by an average of 7.7 kg (17 pounds).[20] In a large study comparing BMI in PsA (n = 644), PsO (n = 448), RA (n = 350), and the general population, the percentages with obesity were 37%, 29%, 27%, and 18% respectively

Table 3
Identifying comorbidities in patients with PsA

Comorbidity	Screening Considerations
CVD	Check blood pressure. Check fasting lipid panel (or high-density lipoprotein and total cholesterol). Encourage patients to follow up with primary care physician or preventive cardiologist for management of CV risk factors. Calculate risk score (ie, Framingham or SCORE), recognizing that the 10-year event rate estimate is likely to be an underestimate of the patient's true propensity for CVD. Encourage smoking cessation when applicable. Educate patients about the increased risk for CVD in psoriasis and PsA
Obesity	Measure weight and calculate BMI. Counsel patients on the benefits of weight loss for improvement in CV health and joint health. Normal BMI is associated with achieving disease remission and improved response to therapy
Diabetes	Refer patients with increased random glucose levels of more than 200 mg/dL on routine tests to primary care for diagnosis and management of diabetes. Check fasting glucose or hemoglobin A1c level at least once in patients more than 45 y of age[13] or if symptoms of hyperglycemia occur
IBD	Ask about gastrointestinal symptoms in the review of systems. Refer early to a gastroenterologist if symptoms of IBD are present (eg, hematochezia, chronic diarrhea)
Ophthalmic disease	Ask about ophthalmic symptoms (eg, dryness, redness, pain, vision loss) in the review of systems. Refer early for evaluation
Osteoporosis	Follow general screening recommendations for general population. Calculate a FRAX score[32] based on DEXA results (if applicable). If prescribing glucocorticoids, refer to ACR recommendations for when to consider preventive therapy[33]
Malignancy	Follow screening recommendations for general population. Consider yearly/periodic skin check for patients with a UV light therapy history
Liver and kidney disease	Check liver function tests and creatinine level before initiating therapy. Consider checking HCV Ab, HBV antigen, HBV core antibody, HBV surface antibody
Depression and anxiety	Ask about symptoms of depression and anxiety in the review of systems and refer for management if identified

The above suggestions are the opinion of the author. There are limited data on the effects of ustekinumab and apremilast on comorbidities and the use of these medications is thus not discussed in this table.

Abbreviations: Ab, antibodies; ACR, American College of Rheumatology; BMI, body mass index; DEXA, dual-energy X-ray absorptiometry; FRAX, Fracture Risk Assessment Tool; HBV, hepatitis B virus; HCV, hepatitis C virus; SCORE, systematic coronary risk evaluation; UV, ultraviolet.

From Ogdie A, Schwartzman S, Husni ME. Recognizing and managing comorbidities in psoriatic arthritis. Curr Opin Rheumatol 2015;27:120; with permission.

and the odds of obesity were 61% higher for patients with PsA than for patients with PsO (95% CI, 1.10, 2.37).[40]

Research is needed on the link between PsA and obesity to further examine its relationship with psoriatic disease onset and to determine whether it is a consequence of the disease. Other potential mechanisms linking PsA obesity and CV risk, including dyslipidemia, hypertension, insulin resistance, and smoking, have not been well-defined.

Effect of Body Weight on Therapy

It has been reported that obesity and metabolic syndrome may negatively affect PsA disease activity and response to therapy.[39,41–44] Eder and colleagues[45] found that obesity was associated with a lower probability of achieving sustained remission, irrespective of therapy used. di Minno and colleagues[46] similarly showed that obesity was an independent risk factor (after multivariable adjustment) for not achieving minimal disease activity (MDA) over 24 months of follow-up (HR, 4.90; 95% CI, 3.04 to 7.87). In patients who achieved MDA at 12 months, obesity was a significant risk factor for relapse at 24 months.[45,46] The investigators extended this work to examine the rate of achievement of MDA in overweight/obese patients with PsA who initiated TNF inhibitors.[47] Successful weight loss of 5% or more of total body weight was associated with a higher likelihood of achieving MDA (odds ratio [OR], 4.20; 95% CI, 1.82 to 9.66). In addition, the presence of metabolic syndrome was also a risk factor for not achieving MDA.[48] Therefore, patients who are overweight and/or obese should be encouraged to lose weight, not only for potential increased benefit from therapy but also for decreased risk for other comorbidities associated with obesity, including diabetes and CVD.

DIABETES

PsA has been associated with an increased prevalence and incidence of diabetes mellitus (DM).[49–51] Specifically, type II DM has been observed in 12% to 18.6% of patients with PsA.[52] This finding may be partially explained by increased obesity and unhealthy lifestyles, and possibly related to insulin resistance associated with PsA inflammation.[50,53] DM should always be a consideration when monitoring therapy and appropriate testing should be undertaken when an increased blood glucose level is identified.[54,55]

There are no studies to address management of patients with PsA and diabetes and limited data exist on the effect of therapy on development of DM. Glucocorticoids should naturally be avoided and, when needed, managed carefully in combination with the patient's primary care physician or endocrinologist. The use of oral and topical corticosteroids in an observational study increased the risk of developing DM by 30% in patients with psoriatic disease, whereas the use of a TNF inhibitor was associated with a reduced risk of developing DM (OR, 0.62) compared with the use of other nonbiologic DMARDs (excluding MTX).[51,56]

OPHTHALMIC DISEASE

Although limited evidence exists on ophthalmic disease in patients with PsA, it has been reported that the prevalence and spectrum of autoimmune ophthalmic disease in PsA is significant and the associated potential morbidity is high.[57] Eye symptoms are often missed in a patient's history and direct questions to patients may help increase awareness. Therefore, patients with PsA with eye symptoms should be evaluated early and made aware of the connection. The ophthalmic manifestations of PsA include uveitis, keratitis, blepharitis, conjunctivitis, episcleritis, and scleritis.[58,59] Uveitis has consistently been associated with spondyloarthritis and human leukocyte antigen B27 positivity.[60,61] The association with uveitis seems to be the strongest; with one meta-analysis reporting a 25.1% prevalence of uveitis in PsA,[61] although the estimates vary considerably.[57–59] Autoimmune ophthalmic disease can precede PsA or occur after the onset of PsA. Paiva and colleagues[60] reported a unique clinical phenotype for PsA that, compared with spondyloarthropathy, is more likely to have insidious onset (19% vs 3%), to be simultaneously bilateral (37.5% vs 7%), chronic duration (31% vs 6%), or a posterior (44% vs 17%) uveitis defined as inflammation involving the choroid or retina.

Ophthalmic Disease Therapeutic Options

In patients with both PsA and uveitis, data support the use of corticosteroids (systemic, periocular, and implants), MTX, mycophenolate, cyclosporine, azathioprine, and many of the currently approved biologic agents.[62–64] Rosenbaum[65] reported that very severe, unilateral eye disease with a sudden onset may require locally injected corticosteroids or a brief course of oral prednisone, whereas management options for disease that is bilateral or posterior to the lens might include prednisone, systemic immunosuppression (as with MTX), or rarely a TNF inhibitor. The clinical recommendation depends in part on the severity of the disease and the impact that it is having on activities of daily living.[65] The 2 most frequently used biologic agents are infliximab and adalimumab, and adalimumab was recently granted orphan status for the treatment of some forms of uveitis.[63,66] However, etanercept may not adequately treat uveitis.[67] An ophthalmologist, preferably one with subspecialty training in autoimmune ophthalmic disease, should be involved in the management of patients with autoimmune ophthalmic disease and PsA.

DEPRESSION AND ANXIETY

Depression and anxiety are common among patients with PsA.[68–70] A prevalence study by Gelfand and colleagues[71] indicated that self-reported PsA affects an estimated 520,000 people in the United States and that 39% of these patients considered PsA to be a large problem in their everyday lives. A recent study by McDonough and colleagues[68] suggested that the prevalences of depression and anxiety were 36.6% and 22.2% respectively (compared with 24.4% and 9.6% in patients with psoriasis alone), which is higher than the general population. High actively inflamed joint count, as well as disability, pain, and fatigue, were disease-related variables associated with depression and/or anxiety. Furthermore, in a study by Husted and colleagues[72] that compared RA and PsA and adjusted for disease severity, patients with PsA had significantly worse quality of life, signifying that skin involvement may have greater psychosocial impairments than that of joints alone.[72] Salaffi and colleagues[3] used the Medical Outcome Study Short Form 36 (SF-36) quality-of-life tool to investigate its correlations with the Self-Administered Comorbidity Questionnaire[41] in 166 patients with PsA. The physical component of the SF-36 was influenced by chronic comorbidity ($P<.0001$) and the severity of psoriatic lesions was significantly associated with poor mental functioning scores in peripheral PsA ($P<.0001$).[3] Relative to other rheumatic diseases, their data confirmed PsA Cohort findings from Germany, the United Kingdom, Turkey, and Canada, which found lower health-related quality-of-life measures and more psychosocial problems with PsA than with RA.[3] Mental health limitations caused by emotional health and social functioning were the most typical SF-36 mental health variables affected by PsA. In a 2013 study by Husted and colleagues[1] of 631 patients with PsA, mental health in PsA was more related to the type of comorbidity than the number of comorbidities, with fibromyalgia and depression/anxiety having the greatest effect. Kotsis and colleagues[69] further highlighted the burden of these psychological factors in PsA when their study findings reported that, after adjusting for disease severity and pain, anxiety and perception of bodily symptoms attributed to illness were independent correlates of physical health-related quality of life. These studies unanimously point to the importance of recognition of depression and anxiety and subsequent referral for more debilitating symptoms in patients with PsA. Although treating the symptoms of PsA can help improve depression and anxiety, treating depression and anxiety can improve PsA symptoms. A 2015 study[73] was the first to show that patients with PsA have lower pain thresholds than healthy controls and that pain thresholds in patients with PsA were inversely correlated with their Hamilton Depression Rating scale ($P<.0002$). Treating depression and anxiety has also been shown to influence treatment adherence. This finding was shown by a study in which there was a

10% decrease in adherence in a topical tacrolimus treatment for each 1-point increase in psoriatic skin disease severity on a 9-point sum score scale (*P*<.05).[74] Although the newer class of biologic DMARD treatment has not been shown to significantly affect depression or anxiety symptoms, treatment with apremilast may be associated with worsening depression and thus should be avoided if possible in patients with depression.[75]

INFLAMMATORY BOWEL DISEASE

IBD is associated with spondyloarthritis in general. Given the overlap with the spondyloarthropathies, knowledge about the prevalence and spectrum of IBD is important, particularly because the associated potential morbidity of the co-occurrence of IBD with PsA is high. Data to support the association of IBD with PsA are sparse however, with only some small case reports and series.[76,77] A recent study by Li and colleagues[78] showed an increased risk of Crohn's disease among patients with psoriasis and PsA, but no increased risk of ulcerative colitis. Occasionally, patients develop IBD, uveitis, or psoriasis when being treated with an anti-TNF agent. Because case numbers are so small, a causative role is difficult to determine.[79,80]

Treatment choices for patients with concurrent PsA/IBD should be made carefully, with consideration for the systemic disease; cutaneous, musculoskeletal, and gastrointestinal manifestations; and the risk and benefits of available therapies. Although no data have been published assessing the appropriate therapy for concomitant PsA and IBD, therapy selection often does not differ significantly from patients with PsA alone. Common medications for IBD include aminosalicylates, corticosteroids, metronidazole, ciprofloxacin, 6-mercaptopurine, azathioprine, cyclosporine, tacrolimus, and MTX. Biologics approved for treatment of severe IBD include adalimumab, infliximab, certolizumab (for Crohn's disease), and golimumab (for ulcerative colitis).[81] Etanercept is not used in IBD because of its lack of effectiveness in clinical trials.[82] Vedolizumab, a monoclonal antibody to $\alpha 4\beta 7$ integrins recently approved by the US Food and Drug Administration for treatment of Crohn's disease and ulcerative colitis, is gut selective and should not lessen inflammation in the skin or joints, but studies in subjects with psoriasis or PsA have not been performed.[83] The use of NSAIDs in IBD is controversial because it is unclear whether NSAIDs exacerbate IBD symptoms.[84,85] NSAID use should either be avoided or monitored carefully.[86] The patient's gastroenterologist should be involved in discussions regarding initiating or changing therapies.

LIVER DISEASE

Fatty liver disease, particularly nonalcoholic fatty liver disease (NAFLD), has an increased prevalence in patients with psoriasis.[87–89] Studies examining this relationship in patients with PsA are limited. However, among patients with psoriasis, patients with concomitant PsA have the highest risk for NAFLD.[88,89] Increased prevalence of NAFLD was also associated with metabolic syndrome, hypercholesterolemia, hypertriglyceridemia, obesity, and psoriasis severity.[88,89]

Human and animal studies have shown the significant role that TNF-α plays in NAFLD pathophysiology.[90] Clinical studies have also shown that pentoxifylline, a nonselective phosphodiesterase inhibitor that reduces inflammation in part by TNF inhibition, has beneficial effects on biochemical, metabolic, and histologic parameters in nonarthritic patients with nonalcoholic steatohepatitis.[91–93] A retrospective case-control study in 89 patients with psoriasis, metabolic syndrome, and NAFLD who received 24 weeks of etanercept treatment reported an attenuation of insulin resistance and a significant reduction (*P*<.05) in the aspartate transaminase/alanine transaminase ratio, suggesting that etanercept may play a beneficial role in preventing progression of liver disease in PsO.[94] In general, current clinical practice is to treat NAFLD by addressing lifestyle modifications and dietary recommendations rather than pharmacologic treatments.

Effect of Psoriatic Arthritis Medications on Liver Disease

Liver disease can result from the disease itself as well as the medications used to treat PsA. Some medications can cause liver function test (LFT) abnormalities, and in some cases (eg, MTX and leflunomide) development of nonalcoholic steatohepatitis (NASH)/ NAFLD and/or cirrhosis. Higher rates of NASH/NAFLD may occur in patients with PsA using MTX compared with those with RA,[95] and LFT abnormalities may be similar or slightly higher in PsA.[96–98] However, patients with PsA treated with combination TNF inhibitor/MTX had a lower risk of liver fibrosis than patients treated with MTX alone.[95] In another study, LFTs were not significantly increased in patients with PsA using MTX or TNF inhibitor compared with nonusers, but prior liver disease was associated with LFT abnormalities in all groups.[99]

Effects of Liver Disease on Psoriatic Arthritis Therapy

The presence of liver disease can complicate therapy selection in PsA. In a prospective study, Di Minno and colleagues[100] showed that hepatic steatosis (found in 28.1% of the study population) was an independent predictor of not achieving MDA (HR, 1.91; 95% CI, 1.04–3.38) after adjustment for metabolic syndrome and other clinical/demographic characteristics. Thus, fatty liver disease may play a role in disease activity and/or optimal therapy response. In patients with liver disease, MTX, leflunomide, and sulfasalazine should be avoided.[101] In addition, NSAIDs should be avoided, but monitored carefully if used. TNF inhibitors are frequently used in patients with PsA with hepatitis C virus[102] and have not been associated with a significant increase in transaminase levels or viral load in the short term, but long-term data are lacking.[103] In contrast, patients with rheumatic disease and chronic hepatitis B virus (HBV) infection have increased frequency of reactivation of HBV with biologic treatment.[104,105] A 2011 review of 87 published cases on patients with chronic HBV infection treated with TNF inhibitors reported an HBV reactivation rate of 38%.[106]

OSTEOPOROSIS
Osteoporosis Studies in Psoriatic Arthritis

Although osteoporosis is a well-known comorbidity associated with RA, few studies have addressed the prevalence of systemic osteoporosis among patients with PsA.[107] Some studies have found no significant increase in osteoporosis in PsA,[108–110] whereas others have found the prevalence of osteoporosis in patients with PsA to be similar to that in patients with RA and AS, suggesting a higher prevalence of osteoporosis in PsA than was previously thought.[111,112] Frediani and colleagues[113] used bone mineral density (BMD) and ultrasound densitometry of the heel to study 186 patients with peripheral PsA and found demineralization in more than two-thirds of the patients with PsA. Reddy and colleagues[111] examined BMD data on patients with RA and PsA in the CORRONA registry and found that lumbar spine and femoral neck T scores were significantly lower for 7166 patients with RA compared with 530 patients with PsA in unmatched cohorts; however, differences were no longer significant when cohorts were matched for BMI. This finding suggests the importance of weight in considering BMD screening and appropriate bone health therapy for patients with PsA. A recent review article by Maruotti and colleagues[114] noted conflicting reports on reduced BMD in patients with PsA. A study of 155 patients with PsA showed no differences in BMD compared with the general population in Spain.[108] Maruotti and colleagues[114] cite chronic inflammation and inflammatory cytokines that induce osteoclastogenesis, as well as glucocorticoid and MTX therapies, and also immobilization and reduced physical activity caused by joint pain, as possible causes of osteoporosis in patients with PsA.[115,116] A study of BMD and fragility fracture incidence in 91 patients with PsA showed no significant differences for lumbar spine or femoral neck BMD compared with controls; however, there was a greater prevalence of fragility fractures (14.3% vs 4.3%; $P = .013$) in PsA, with the postmenopausal subgroup being statistically significant.[109]

In spite of these conflicting data, a high index of suspicion for osteopenia and osteoporosis should be maintained in patients with PsA and recommendations for screening and management of osteoporosis for the general population should be followed,[117] because complications of undertreated osteoporosis can be serious. Large, prospective, controlled studies with data on BMD as well as bone turnover and fracture outcome are needed to better define osteoporosis in patients with PsA.

Osteoporosis Therapies in Psoriatic Arthritis

There are limited data on the effect of therapies for osteoporosis on PsA disease activity and likewise limited data on the effect of therapies for PsA on bone quality. In one pilot study, the effect of zoledronic acid on articular bone in patients with PsA showed suppression of bone marrow edema on MRI and improvement in clinical outcomes.[118] One recent study[119] showed no evidence of an increased risk of fracture among patients with psoriasis, PsA, or AS initiating TNF inhibitor therapy. In patients with PsA using glucocorticoids, the American College of Rheumatology standard guidelines for the prevention of glucocorticoid-induced osteoporosis should be followed.[120]

KIDNEY DISEASE

Chronic kidney disease (CKD) has been associated with psoriasis and PsA; however, limited data exist on its prevalence in patients with PsA alone. Patients with moderate to severe psoriasis had a higher risk of CKD than the general population independent of traditional risk factors.[121] Specific to PsA, the prevalence of reduced estimated glomerular filtration rate was 16% in patients with seronegative arthritis (patients with PsA and undifferentiated oligoarthritis), statistically similar to patients with RA (19%). The investigators found a positive independent association between CKD and a history of CVDs but no statistically significant association between CKD and inflammatory disease–specific characteristics such as the use of corticosteroids, DMARDs, and anti-TNF agents.[122] However, routine calculation of estimated glomerular filtration rate can facilitate early diagnosis of cardiorenal disease in this at-risk population.

It is accepted that clinicians should be aware of the potential effect of PsA therapies on renal function when treating patients with psoriatic disease who already have CKD. NSAIDs should generally be avoided because they increase the risk for acute kidney injury,[123] and MTX should not be used in patients with significant renal insufficiency or end-stage renal disease on hemodialysis because this may result in pancytopenia.[124] Limited studies indicate that leflunomide and the TNF inhibitors (data only exist for etanercept) may be more acceptable therapies for patients on hemodialysis.[125,126]

MALIGNANCY

RA and psoriasis have been linked to increased rates of lymphoma and other hematopoietic malignancies, as well as skin cancers.[127] It is uncertain whether the degree of increased risk for cancer is related to uncontrolled disease activity or treatment of PsA. PsA shares similar mechanisms and may share the risks seen in RA; however, evidence-based studies to address this issue in patients with PsA are unclear because the published data are insufficient and conflicting. In a recent population-based study, the average risk of lymphoma in PsA or AS was not increased, in contrast with RA,[131] whereas another study showed that the incidence rates in PsA (5.59 per 1000 patient-years of follow-up) were similar to those in RA.[128]

Although only a few studies have examined risk of malignancy in patients with PsA compared with the general population, the incidence rates do not differ. These studies include a cohort study[129] in Toronto that showed no increased risk compared with an Ontario population; a cohort study[130] in the United Kingdom that found no difference in cancer-specific mortality among patients with PsA; and a cohort study[131] in Sweden that found no increase in risk in patients with lymphoma and PsA. A study[132] in the Consortium of Rheumatology Researchers of North America registry suggested similar rates of malignancy in RA and PsA, with nonmelanoma skin cancer being the most common malignancy in both the groups.

Effects of Therapy on Risk of Malignancy

The introduction of TNF inhibitor for treating PsA has produced some challenges. It remains unclear whether patients with PsA and a history of cancer would be at greater risk of recurrent cancer if placed on chronic anti-TNF therapy. Studies to date have focused on patients with RA or psoriasis and few have specifically examined PsA. In a meta-analysis of randomized controlled trials across all indications, short-term use of TNF inhibitor was not associated with a significantly increased risk of cancer.[133] However, an increase in nonmelanoma skin cancers (70.6% of malignancies in the analysis) was observed in patients using TNF inhibitor (OR, 1.33; 95% CI, 0.58–3.04; incidence rate ratio, 0.72). Stratified by disease, patients with PsA had no increased risk for malignancy (OR, 0.83). Concomitant immunosuppressive therapy use was lower in the 7 included PsA trials (1485 patients) compared with previous RA studies (44.6% on MTX, 5.5% on another DMARD, and 10.5% on corticosteroids at baseline). A recent study[131] in the Swedish National Patient Register found no difference in the risk of lymphoma among patients with PsA and AS exposed or not exposed to TNF inhibitor. Similarly, the HR for incident solid cancer diagnosis was 0.74 (95% CI, 0.20–2.76) for 2498 patients with PsA in an observational study examining the risk for solid malignancy in patients with PsA using TNF inhibitor compared with patients receiving nonbiologics in US-based Medicare and Medicaid databases.[134]

In addition, limited data exist on how to select therapy for patients who have a history of malignancy or an active malignancy. In RA, the American College of Rheumatology suggests avoiding the use of TNF inhibitors in the 5 years following a cancer diagnosis.[102]

Malignancy Screening

Given this information, the issue of cancer screening strategies other than the age-appropriate standards for common cancers has not been routinely developed. Nannini and colleagues[135] conducted a study to help answer whether more intensive cancer screening could help to minimize the incidence of malignancies in patients receiving anti-TNF therapy. A systemic review of randomized controlled trials of patients with RA, AS, and PsA on anti- TNF therapy, as well as a retrospective review of 363 patients compared with 73 historical controls, was performed. About 25% of cancers developed within the first 12 weeks after starting anti-TNF therapy, and the investigators concluded that more intensive screening could help reduce the occurrence of cancers in patients with PsA.[135]

Many of the malignancies were related to RA and not AS or PsA, implicating a more specific disease-related risk. It was also difficult to ascertain some of the preexisting risk factors for these cancers, because this information is not readily available. Given that anti-TNF therapy increases the risk for lymphoma and nonmelanoma skin cancer and that many patients with PsA have had extended courses of ultraviolet light therapy, yearly skin examinations should be considered in patients with PsA.

INFECTION

Although RA is a known risk factor for serious infection (in addition to treatment with immunosuppressive therapy, including corticosteroids, oral DMARDs, and biologics), the rate of serious infection in patients with PsA and psoriasis has not been as well characterized. Some evidence suggests that the risk of serious infection in PsA and psoriasis may be less than that in RA. Rates of serious infections reported in clinical trials across these inflammatory disease indications for which 2 of the anti-TNF agents have been approved were published recently.[136,137] For etanercept, the rates of serious infection per 100 patient-years in RA, PsA, and psoriasis were 3.75, 1.62, and 1.24, respectively. For adalimumab, the corresponding rates were 4.65, 2.81, and 1.32, respectively. This stratification may be the result of the increasing incidence of combination (biologic and nonbiologic DMARD) immunosuppressive therapy use in RA, PsA, and psoriasis respectively.

Epidemiologic studies have offered critical information on infection risks with RA and biologic use. More long-term data and experience are needed to define the role of anti–TNF agents in the management of psoriasis and PsA. In particular, more studies are required to elucidate the mechanisms of synergy in using combination DMARDs. The lack of published guidelines on monitoring implies that clinicians must evaluate individual patients for the risk or presence of any adverse events by standard checkup, with careful assessment for their early detection. Constant attention is needed to balance ongoing effectiveness and avoidance of drug toxicity.

SUMMARY

It is critical that physicians have an appreciation of the common comorbidities associated with PsA so that they can provide optimal management and treatment of patients with PsA. Although a common goal is to eliminate debilitating skin lesions and prevent progressive joint damage, this article highlights the importance of comprehensive disease management. This article highlights the association of PsA with multiple comorbidities and extra-articular/cutaneous manifestations.

Although there is limited evidence correlating the incidence and severity of these comorbidities with the severity of joint disease in PsA, recent publications suggest skin disease severity as a significant causative agent for increased incidence and severity of PsA comorbidities. Psoriatic skin disease severity has been shown to be associated with increased incidence and severity of CVD in PsA,[16] a higher risk of chronic kidney[121] and fatty liver disease,[88,89] poor mental functioning SF-36 scores,[3] and a large psychosocial burden influencing obesity and unhealthy behaviors such as and smoking.[138,139] Much information used in clinical practice with regard to PsA comorbidities is derived from other systemic inflammatory diseases, such as RA, thus limiting its direct validity to the screening and preventive treatment of PsA comorbidities.[140]

Given the spectrum of therapies available for PsA, including traditional DMARDs, anti-TNF, interleukin (IL)-12/IL-23 blockers, and phosphodiesterase-4 inhibitors, clinicians now have many more treatment options and can tailor therapies for individual patients taking into account their comorbidities. Although there is much debate about who should directly manage these comorbidities, it has become more important than ever to receive coordinated input from primary care, rheumatology, and dermatology providers. Communication and collaboration among specialists in cardiology, metabolic, gastrointestinal, and infectious disease specialists as well as mental health care professionals is suggested when comorbidities are present.[75] As disciplines become more subspecialized, it is essential to increase awareness about the prevalence of comorbid conditions in PsA and educate both patients and physicians about their importance.

REFERENCES

1. Husted JA, Thavaneswaran A, Chandran V, et al. Incremental effects of comorbidity on quality of life in patients with psoriatic arthritis. J Rheumatol 2013;40(8): 1349–56.
2. Ogdie A, Yu Y, Haynes K, et al. Risk of major cardiovascular events in patients with psoriatic arthritis, psoriasis and rheumatoid arthritis: a population-based cohort study. Ann Rheum Dis 2015;74(2):326–32.
3. Salaffi F, Carotti M, Gasparini S, et al. The health-related quality of life in rheumatoid arthritis, ankylosing spondylitis, and psoriatic arthritis: a comparison with a selected sample of healthy people. Health Qual Life Outcomes 2009;7:25.
4. Khraishi M, Aslanov R, Rampakakis E, et al. Prevalence of cardiovascular risk factors in patients with psoriatic arthritis. Clin Rheumatol 2014;33(10):1495–500.
5. Edson-Heredia E, Zhu B, Lefevre C, et al. Prevalence and incidence rates of cardiovascular, autoimmune, and other diseases in patients with psoriatic or psoriatic arthritis: a retrospective study using clinical practice research datalink. J Eur Acad Dermatol Venereol 2015;29(5):955–63.
6. Feldman SR, Zhao Y, Shi L, et al. Economic and comorbidity burden among moderate-to-severe psoriasis patients with comorbid psoriatic arthritis. Arthritis Care Res (Hoboken) 2015;67(5):708–17.
7. Sanchez-Carazo JL, Lopez-Estebaranz JL, Guisado C. Comorbidities and health-related quality of life in Spanish patients with moderate to severe psoriasis: a cross-sectional study (Arizona study). J Dermatol 2014;41(8):673–8.
8. Husni ME, Mease PJ. Managing comorbid disease in patients with psoriatic arthritis. Curr Rheumatol Rep 2010;12(4):281–7.
9. Ogdie A, Schwartzman S, Eder L, et al. Comprehensive treatment of psoriatic arthritis: managing comorbidities and extraarticular manifestations. J Rheumatol 2014;41(11):2315–22.
10. Boehncke WH, Boehncke S, Tobin AM, et al. The 'psoriatic march': a concept of how severe psoriasis may drive cardiovascular comorbidity. Exp Dermatol 2011; 20(4):303–7.
11. Shang Q, Tam LS, Sanderson JE, et al. Increase in ventricular-arterial stiffness in patients with psoriatic arthritis. Rheumatology (Oxford) 2012;51(12):2215–23.
12. Eder L, Jayakar J, Shanmugarajah S, et al. The burden of carotid artery plaques is higher in patients with psoriatic arthritis compared with those with psoriasis alone. Ann Rheum Dis 2013;72(5):715–20.
13. Lin YC, Dalal D, Churton S, et al. Relationship between metabolic syndrome and carotid intima-media thickness: cross-sectional comparison between psoriasis and psoriatic arthritis. Arthritis Care Res (Hoboken) 2014;66(1):97–103.
14. Jamnitski A, Symmons D, Peters MJ, et al. Cardiovascular comorbidities in patients with psoriatic arthritis: a systematic review. Ann Rheum Dis 2013;72(2): 211–6.

15. Horreau C, Pouplard C, Brenaut E, et al. Cardiovascular morbidity and mortality in psoriasis and psoriatic arthritis: a systematic literature review. J Eur Acad Dermatol Venereol 2013;27(Suppl 3):12–29.
16. Gelfand JM, Neimann AL, Shin DB, et al. Risk of myocardial infarction in patients with psoriasis. JAMA 2006;296(14):1735–41.
17. Gladman DD, Ang M, Su L, et al. Cardiovascular morbidity in psoriatic arthritis. Ann Rheum Dis 2009;68(7):1131–5.
18. Beinsberger J, Heemskerk JW, Cosemans JM. Chronic arthritis and cardiovascular disease: altered blood parameters give rise to a prothrombotic propensity. Semin Arthritis Rheum 2014;44(3):345–52.
19. Husted JA, Thavaneswaran A, Chandran V, et al. Cardiovascular and other comorbidities in patients with psoriatic arthritis: a comparison with patients with psoriasis. Arthritis Care Res (Hoboken) 2011;63(12):1729–35.
20. Labitigan M, Bahce-Altuntas A, Kremer JM, et al. Higher rates and clustering of abnormal lipids, obesity, and diabetes mellitus in psoriatic arthritis compared with rheumatoid arthritis. Arthritis Care Res (Hoboken) 2014;66(4):600–7.
21. Bostoen J, Van Praet L, Brochez L, et al. A cross-sectional study on the prevalence of metabolic syndrome in psoriasis compared to psoriatic arthritis. J Eur Acad Dermatol Venereol 2014;28(4):507–11.
22. Puig L, Strohal R, Husni ME, et al. Cardiometabolic profile, clinical features, quality of life and treatment outcomes in patients with moderate-to-severe psoriasis and psoriatic arthritis. J Dermatolog Treat 2015;26(1):7–15.
23. Haroon M, Gallagher P, Heffernan E, et al. High prevalence of metabolic syndrome and of insulin resistance in psoriatic arthritis is associated with the severity of underlying disease. J Rheumatol 2014;41(7):1357–65.
24. Eder L, Thavaneswaran A, Chandran V, et al. Increased burden of inflammation over time is associated with the extent of atherosclerotic plaques in patients with psoriatic arthritis. Ann Rheum Dis 2014;0:1–6.
25. Han C, Robinson DW Jr, Hackett MV, et al. Cardiovascular disease and risk factors in patients with rheumatoid arthritis, psoriatic arthritis, and ankylosing spondylitis. J Rheumatol 2006;33(11):2167–72.
26. Chen YJ, Chang YT, Shen JL, et al. Association between systemic antipsoriatic drugs and cardiovascular risk in patients with psoriasis with or without psoriatic arthritis: a nationwide cohort study. Arthritis Rheum 2012;64(6):1879–87.
27. Gelfand JM, Troxel AB, Lewis JD, et al. The risk of mortality in patients with psoriasis: results from a population-based study. Arch Dermatol 2007;143(12): 1493–9.
28. Kimball AB, Gladman D, Gelfand JM, et al. National Psoriasis Foundation clinical consensus on psoriasis comorbidities and recommendations for screening. J Am Acad Dermatol 2008;58(6):1031–42.
29. Parisi R, Rutter MK, Lunt M, et al. Psoriasis and the risk of major cardiovascular events: cohort study using the clinical practice research datalink. J Invest Dermatol 2015;135:2189–97.
30. Seremet S, Genc B, Tastan A, et al. Are all patients with psoriasis at increased risk for coronary artery disease? Int J Dermatol 2015;54(3):355–61.
31. Brauchli YB, Jick SS, Miret M, et al. Psoriasis and risk of incident myocardial infarction, stroke or transient ischaemic attack: an inception cohort study with a nested case–control analysis. Br J Dermatol 2009;160(5):1048–56.
32. US Preventive Services Task Force. USPSTF draft recommendations for screening for abnormal glucose and type 2 diabetes mellitus. US Preventive

Services Task Force. Available at: http://www.uspreventiveservicestaskforce. org/Page/Document/EvidenceReportDraft/screening-for-abnormalglucose- and-type-2-diabetes-mellitus. Accessed October 9, 2014.

33. WHO. FRAX: Fracture risk assessment tool. WHO. Available at: http://www.shef. ac.uk/FRAX/tool.jsp?locationValue=9. Accessed October 9, 2014.

34. Eder L, Chandran V, Gladman DD. The Framingham Risk Score underestimates the extent of subclinical atherosclerosis in patients with psoriatic disease. Ann Rheum Dis 2014;73(11):1990–6.

35. Torres T, Sales R, Vasconcelos C, et al. Framingham Risk Score underestimates cardiovascular disease risk in severe psoriatic patients: implications in cardiovascular risk factors management and primary prevention of cardiovascular disease. J Dermatol 2013;40(11):923–6.

36. Favarato MH, Mease P, Goncalves CR, et al. Hypertension and diabetes significantly enhance the risk of cardiovascular disease in patients with psoriatic arthritis. Clin Exp Rheumatol 2014;32(2):182–7.

37. Puato M, Ramonda R, Doria A, et al. Impact of hypertension on vascular remodeling in patients with psoriatic arthritis. J Hum Hypertens 2014;28(2):105–10.

38. Stone NJ, Robinson JG, Lichtenstein AH, et al. 2013 ACC/AHA guideline on the treatment of blood cholesterol to reduce atherosclerotic cardiovascular risk in adults: a report of the American College of Cardiology/American Heart Association Task Force on Practice Guidelines. J Am Coll Cardiol 2014;63(25 Pt B):2889–934.

39. Love TJ, Zhu Y, Zhang Y, et al. Obesity and the risk of psoriatic arthritis: a population-based study. Ann Rheum Dis 2012;71(8):1273–7.

40. Bhole VM, Choi HK, Burns LC, et al. Differences in body mass index among individuals with PsA, psoriasis, RA and the general population. Rheumatology (Oxford) 2012;51(3):552–6.

41. Li W, Han J, Qureshi AA. Obesity and risk of incident psoriatic arthritis in US women. Ann Rheum Dis 2012;71(8):1267–72.

42. Kumar S, Han J, Li T, et al. Obesity, waist circumference, weight change and the risk of psoriasis in US women. J Eur Acad Dermatol Venereol 2013;27(10):1293–8.

43. Soltani-Arabshahi R, Wong B, Feng BJ, et al. Obesity in early adulthood as a risk factor for psoriatic arthritis. Arch Dermatol 2010;146(7):721–6.

44. Sharma A, Gopalakrishnan D, Kumar R, et al. Metabolic syndrome in psoriatic arthritis patients: a cross-sectional study. Int J Rheum Dis 2013;16(6): 667–73.

45. Eder L, Thavaneswaran A, Chandran V, et al. Obesity is associated with a lower probability of achieving sustained minimal disease activity state among patients with psoriatic arthritis. Ann Rheum Dis 2015;74(5):813–7.

46. Di Minno MN, Peluso R, Iervolino S, et al. Obesity and the prediction of minimal disease activity: a prospective study in psoriatic arthritis. Arthritis Care Res (Hoboken) 2013;65(1):141–7.

47. Di Minno MN, Peluso R, Iervolino S, et al. Weight loss and achievement of minimal disease activity in patients with psoriatic arthritis starting treatment with tumour necrosis factor alpha blockers. Ann Rheum Dis 2014;73(6):1157–62.

48. Di Minno MN, Peluso R, Iervolino S, et al. Hepatic steatosis, carotid plaques and achieving MDA in psoriatic arthritis patients starting TNF-alpha blockers treatment: a prospective study. Arthritis Res Ther 2012;14(5):R211.

49. Dubreuil M, Hee Rho Y, Man D. The independent impact of psoriatic arthritis and rheumatoid arthritis on diabetes incidence: a UK population-based cohort study. Rheumatology (Oxford) 2014;53:346–52.

50. Coto-Segura P, Eiris-Salvado N, Gonzalez-Lara L, et al. Psoriasis, psoriatic arthritis and type 2 diabetes mellitus: a systematic review and meta-analysis. Br J Dermatol 2013;169(4):783–93.

51. Solomon DH, Love TJ, Canning C, et al. Risk of diabetes among patients with rheumatoid arthritis, psoriatic arthritis and psoriasis. Ann Rheum Dis 2010; 69(12):2114–7.

52. Dreiher J, Freud T, Cohen AD. Psoriatic arthritis and diabetes: a population-based cross-sectional study. Dermatol Res Pract 2013;2013:580404.

53. Boehncke S, Salgo R, Garbaraviciene J, et al. Effective continuous systemic therapy of severe plaque-type psoriasis is accompanied by amelioration of biomarkers of cardiovascular risk: results of a prospective longitudinal observational study. J Eur Acad Dermatol Venereol 2011;25(10):1187–93.

54. World Health Organization. Definition and diagnosis of diabetes mellitus and intermediate hyperglycaemia. http://www.who.int/diabetes/publications/diagnosis.diabetes2006/en/. Accessed April 16, 2014.

55. US Preventive Services Task Force. Screening for type 2 diabetes in adults. Available at: http://www.uspreventiveservicestaskforce.org/Page/Topic/recommendation-summary/diabetes-mellitus-type-2-in-adults-screening. Accessed April 3, 2014.

56. Solomon DH, Massarotti E, Garg R, et al. Association between disease-modifying antirheumatic drugs and diabetes risk in patients with rheumatoid arthritis and psoriasis. JAMA 2011;305(24):2525–31.

57. Lambert JR, Wright V. Eye inflammation in psoriatic arthritis. Ann Rheum Dis 1976;35(4):354–6.

58. Altan-Yaycioglu R, Akova YA, Kart H, et al. Posterior scleritis in psoriatic arthritis. Retina 2003;23(5):717–9.

59. Lima FB, Abalem MF, Ruiz DG, et al. Prevalence of eye disease in Brazilian patients with psoriatic arthritis. Clinics (Sao Paulo) 2012;67(3):249–53.

60. Paiva ES, Macaluso DC, Edwards A, et al. Characterisation of uveitis in patients with psoriatic arthritis. Ann Rheum Dis 2000;59(1):67–70.

61. Zeboulon N, Dougados M, Gossec L. Prevalence and characteristics of uveitis in the spondyloarthropathies: a systematic literature review. Ann Rheum Dis 2008;67(7):955–9.

62. Servat JJ, Mears KA, Black EH, et al. Biological agents for the treatment of uveitis. Expert Opin Biol Ther 2012;12(3):311–28.

63. Martel JN, Esterberg E, Nagpal A, et al. Infliximab and adalimumab for uveitis. Ocul Immunol Inflamm 2012;20(1):18–26.

64. Kruh J, Foster CS. The philosophy of treatment of uveitis: past, present and future. Dev Ophthalmol 2012;51:1–6.

65. Rosenbaum JT. Uveitis in spondyloarthritis including psoriatic arthritis, ankylosing spondylitis, and inflammatory bowel disease. Clin Rheumatol 2015;34:999–1002.

66. Zannin ME, Birolo C, Gerloni VM, et al. Safety and efficacy of infliximab and adalimumab for refractory uveitis in juvenile idiopathic arthritis: 1-year followup data from the Italian registry. J Rheumatol 2013;40(1):74–9.

67. Smith JA, Thompson DJ, Whitcup SM, et al. A randomized, placebo-controlled, double-masked clinical trial of etanercept for the treatment of uveitis associated with juvenile idiopathic arthritis. Arthritis Rheum 2005;53(1):18–23.

68. McDonough E, Ayearst R, Eder L, et al. Depression and anxiety in psoriatic disease: prevalence and associated factors. J Rheumatol 2014;41(5):887–96.

69. Kotsis K, Voulgari PV, Tsifetaki N, et al. Anxiety and depressive symptoms and illness perceptions in psoriatic arthritis and associations with physical health-related quality of life. Arthritis Care Res (Hoboken) 2012;64(10):1593–601.

70. Husted JA, Tom BD, Farewell VT, et al. Longitudinal study of the bidirectional association between pain and depressive symptoms in patients with psoriatic arthritis. Arthritis Care Res (Hoboken) 2012;64(5):758–65.
71. Gelfand JM, Gladman DD, Mease PJ, et al. Epidemiology of psoriatic arthritis in the population of the United States. J Am Acad Dermatol 2005;53(4):573.
72. Husted JA, Gladman DD, Farewell VT, et al. Health-related quality of life of patients with psoriatic arthritis: a comparison with patients with rheumatoid arthritis. Arthritis Rheum 2001;45(2):151–8.
73. Bagnato G, De Andres I, Sorbara S, et al. Pain threshold and intensity in rheumatic patients: correlations with the Hamilton Depression Rating Scale. Clin Rheumatol 2015;34(3):555–61.
74. Montaudie H, Sbidian E, Paul C, et al. Methotrexate in psoriasis: a systematic review of treatment modalities, incidence, risk factors and monitoring of liver toxicity. J Eur Acad Dermatol Venereol 2011;25(Suppl 2):12–8.
75. OTEZLA1 (apremilast) prescribing information. Available at: http://www.otezlapro. com/wp-content/uploads/2014/09/otezla-prescribing-information.pdf. Accessed October 07, 2014.
76. Bernstein CN, Wajda A, Blanchard JF. The clustering of other chronic inflammatory diseases in inflammatory bowel disease: a population-based study. Gastroenterology 2005;129(3):827–36.
77. Yates VM, Watkinson G, Kelman A. Further evidence for an association between psoriasis, Crohn's disease and ulcerative colitis. Br J Dermatol 1982;106(3):323–30.
78. Li WQ, Han JL, Chan AT, et al. Psoriasis, psoriatic arthritis and increased risk of incident Crohn's disease in US women. Ann Rheum Dis 2013;72(7):1200–5.
79. Cleynen I, Vermeire S. Paradoxical inflammation induced by anti-TNF agents in patients with IBD. Nat Rev Gastroenterol Hepatol 2012;9(9):496–503.
80. Fiorino G, Danese S, Pariente B, et al. Paradoxical immune-mediated inflammation in inflammatory bowel disease patients receiving anti-TNF-alpha agents. Autoimmun Rev 2014;13(1):15–9.
81. Cohen LB, Nanau RM, Delzor F, et al. Biologic therapies in inflammatory bowel disease. Transl Res 2014;163(6):533–56.
82. Sandborn WJ, Hanauer SB, Katz S, et al. Etanercept for active Crohn's disease: a randomized, double-blind, placebo-controlled trial. Gastroenterology 2001; 121(5):1088–94.
83. Garnock-Jones KP. Vedolizumab: a review of its use in adult patients with moderately to severely active ulcerative colitis or Crohn's disease. BioDrugs 2015;29(1):57–67.
84. Bonner GF, Walczak M, Kitchen L, et al. Tolerance of nonsteroidal antiinflammatory drugs in patients with inflammatory bowel disease. Am J Gastroenterol 2000;95(8):1946–8.
85. Felder JB, Korelitz BI, Rajapakse R, et al. Effects of nonsteroidal antiinflammatory drugs on inflammatory bowel disease: a case-control study. Am J Gastroenterol 2000;95(8):1949–54.
86. Crohn's and Colitis Foundation. Maintenance therapy. Available at: http://www. ccfa.org/resources/maintenance-therapy.html. Accessed April 16, 2014.
87. Madanagobalane S, Anandan S. The increased prevalence of non-alcoholic fatty liver disease in psoriatic patients: a study from south India. Australas J Dermatol 2012;53(3):190–7.
88. Miele L, Vallone S, Cefalo C, et al. Prevalence, characteristics and severity of non-alcoholic fatty liver disease in patients with chronic plaque psoriasis. J Hepatol 2009;51(4):778–86.

89. Gisondi P, Targher G, Zoppini G, et al. Non-alcoholic fatty liver disease in patients with chronic plaque psoriasis. J Hepatol 2009;51(4):758–64.
90. Braunersreuther V, Viviani GL, Mach F, et al. Role of cytokines and chemokines in non-alcoholic fatty liver disease. World J Gastroenterol 2012;18(8):727–35.
91. Sharma BC, Kumar A, Garg V, et al. Randomized controlled trial comparing efficacy of pentoxifylline and pioglitazone on metabolic factors and liver histology in patients with non-alcoholic steatohepatitis. J Clin Exp Hepatol 2012;2: 333–7.
92. Satapathy SK, Sakhuja P, Malhotra V, et al. Beneficial effects of pentoxifylline on hepatic steatosis, fibrosis and necroinflammation in patients with non-alcoholic steatohepatitis. J Gastroenterol Hepatol 2007;22(5):634–8.
93. Satapathy SK, Garg S, Chauhan R, et al. Beneficial effects of tumor necrosis factor-alpha inhibition by pentoxifylline on clinical, biochemical, and metabolic parameters of patients with nonalcoholic steatohepatitis. Am J Gastroenterol 2004;99:1946–52.
94. Campanati A, Ganzetti G, Di Sario A, et al. The effect of etanercept on hepatic fibrosis risk in patients with non-alcoholic fatty liver disease, metabolic syndrome, and psoriasis. J Gastroenterol 2013;48:839–46.
95. Seitz M, Reichenbach S, Moller B, et al. Hepatoprotective effect of tumour necrosis factor alpha blockade in psoriatic arthritis: a cross-sectional study. Ann Rheum Dis 2010;69(6):1148–50.
96. Amital H, Arnson Y, Chodick G, et al. Hepatotoxicity rates do not differ in patients with rheumatoid arthritis and psoriasis treated with methotrexate. Rheumatology (Oxford) 2009;48(9):1107–10.
97. Curtis JR, Beukelman T, Onofrei A, et al. Elevated liver enzyme tests among patients with rheumatoid arthritis or psoriatic arthritis treated with methotrexate and/or leflunomide. Ann Rheum Dis 2010;69(1):43–7.
98. Tilling L, Townsend S, David J. Methotrexate and hepatic toxicity in rheumatoid arthritis and psoriatic arthritis. Clin Drug Investig 2006;26(2):55–62.
99. Kavanaugh A, Greenberg J, Lee S, et al. Incidence of elevated liver enzymes (LFTS) in psoriatic arthritis (PsA) patients: effect of TNF-inhibitors (TNF-I). Ann Rheum Dis 2010;69:579.
100. Di Minno MN, Iervolino S, Peluso R, et al. Hepatic steatosis and disease activity in subjects with psoriatic arthritis receiving tumor necrosis factor-alpha blockers. J Rheumatol 2012;39(5):1042–6.
101. Saag KG, Teng GG, Patkar NM, et al. American College of Rheumatology 2008 recommendations for the use of nonbiologic and biologic disease-modifying antirheumatic drugs in rheumatoid arthritis. Arthritis Rheum 2008;59(6):762–84.
102. Singh JA, Furst DE, Bharat A, et al. 2012 update of the 2008 American College of Rheumatology recommendations for the use of disease-modifying antirheumatic drugs and biologic agents in the treatment of rheumatoid arthritis. Arthritis Care Res (Hoboken) 2012;64(5):625–39.
103. Pompili M, Biolato M, Miele L, et al. Tumor necrosis factor-alpha inhibitors and chronic hepatitis C: a comprehensive literature review. World J Gastroenterol 2013;19(44):7867–73.
104. Nard FD, Todoerti M, Grosso V, et al. Risk of hepatitis B virus reactivation in rheumatoid arthritis patients undergoing biologic treatment: extending perspective from old to newer drugs. World J Hepatol 2015;7(3):344–61.
105. Lee YH, Bae SC, Song GG. Hepatitis B virus reactivation in HBsAg-positive patients with rheumatic diseases undergoing anti-tumor necrosis factor therapy or DMARDs. Int J Rheum Dis 2013;16(5):527–31.

106. Perez-Alvarez R, Diaz-Lagares C, Garcia-Hernandez F, et al. Hepatitis B virus (HBV) reactivation in patients receiving tumor necrosis factor (TNF)-targeted therapy: analysis of 257 cases. Medicine (Baltimore) 2011;90(6):359–71.
107. Del Puente A, Esposito A, Parisi A, et al. Osteoporosis and psoriatic arthritis. J Rheumatol Suppl 2012;89:36–8.
108. Busquets N, Vaquero CG, Moreno JR, et al. Bone mineral density status and frequency of osteoporosis and clinical fractures in 155 patients with psoriatic arthritis followed in a university hospital. Reumatol Clin 2014;10(2):89–93.
109. Riesco M, Manzano F, Font P, et al. Osteoporosis in psoriatic arthritis: an assessment of densitometry and fragility fractures. Clin Rheumatol 2013;32(12):1799–804.
110. Pedreira PG, Pinheiro MM, Szejnfeld VL. Bone mineral density and body composition in postmenopausal women with psoriasis and psoriatic arthritis. Arthritis Res Ther 2011;13(1):R16.
111. Reddy SM, Anandarajah AP, Fisher MC, et al. Comparative analysis of disease activity measures, use of biologic agents, body mass index, radiographic features, and bone density in psoriatic arthritis and rheumatoid arthritis patients followed in a large U.S. disease registry. J Rheumatol 2010;37(12):2566–72.
112. Teichmann J, Voglau MJ, Lange U. Antibodies to human tissue transglutaminase and alterations of vitamin D metabolism in ankylosing spondylitis and psoriatic arthritis. Rheumatol Int 2010;30(12):1559–63.
113. Frediani B, Allegri A, Falsetti P, et al. Bone mineral density in patients with psoriatic arthritis. J Rheumatol 2001;28(1):138–43.
114. Maruotti N, Corrado A, Cantatore FP. Osteoporosis and rheumatic diseases. Reumatismo 2014;66(2):125–35.
115. Ding C, Parameswaran V, Udayan R, et al. Circulating levels of inflammatory markers predict change in bone mineral density and resorption in older adults: a longitudinal study. J Clin Endocrinol Metab 2008;93(5):1952–8.
116. Hofbauer LC, Schoppet M, Christ M, et al. Tumour necrosis factor-related apoptosis-inducing ligand and osteoprotegerin serum levels in psoriatic arthritis. Rheumatology (Oxford) 2006;45(10):1218–22.
117. Kling JM, Clarke BL, Sandhu NP. Osteoporosis prevention, screening, and treatment: a review. J Womens Health (Larchmt) 2014;23(7):563–72.
118. McQueen F, Lloyd R, Doyle A, et al. Zoledronic acid does not reduce MRI erosive progression in PsA but may suppress bone oedema: the Zoledronic Acid in Psoriatic Arthritis (ZAPA) study. Ann Rheum Dis 2011;70(6):1091–4.
119. Kawai VK, Grijalva CG, Arbogast PG, et al. Initiation of tumor necrosis factor alpha antagonists and risk of fractures in patients with selected rheumatic and autoimmune diseases. Arthritis Care Res (Hoboken) 2013;65(7):1085–94.
120. Grossman JM, Gordon R, Ranganath VK, et al. American College of Rheumatology 2010 recommendations for the prevention and treatment of glucocorticoid-induced osteoporosis. Arthritis Care Res (Hoboken) 2010;62(11):1515–26.
121. Wan J, Wang S, Haynes K, et al. Risk of moderate to advanced kidney disease in patients with psoriasis: population based cohort study. BMJ 2013;347:f5961.
122. Haroon M, Adeeb F, Devlin J, et al. A comparative study of renal dysfunction in patients with inflammatory arthropathies: strong association with cardiovascular diseases and not with anti-rheumatic therapies, inflammatory markers or duration of arthritis. Int J Rheum Dis 2011;14(3):255–60.
123. Fine M. Quantifying the impact of NSAID-associated adverse events. Am J Manag Care 2013;19(14 Suppl):s267–72.

124. Al-Hasani H, Roussou E. Methotrexate for rheumatoid arthritis patients who are on hemodialysis. Rheumatol Int 2011;31(12):1545–7.

125. Bergner R, Peters L, Schmitt V, et al. Leflunomide in dialysis patients with rheumatoid arthritis–a pharmacokinetic study. Clin Rheumatol 2013;32(2):267–70.

126. Don BR, Spin G, Nestorov I, et al. The pharmacokinetics of etanercept in patients with end-stage renal disease on haemodialysis. J Pharm Pharmacol 2005;57(11):1407–13.

127. Askling J, van Vollenhoven RF, Granath F, et al. Cancer risk in patients with rheumatoid arthritis treated with anti-tumor necrosis factor alpha therapies: does the risk change with the time since start of treatment? Arthritis Rheum 2009;60(11): 3180–9.

128. Gross R, Schwartzman-Morris J, Krathen M, et al. The risk of malignancy in a large cohort of patients with psoriatic arthritis. Arthritis Rheum 2011;63:S195.

129. Rohekar S, Tom BD, Hassa A, et al. Prevalence of malignancy in psoriatic arthritis. Arthritis Rheum 2008;58(1):82–7.

130. Ogdie A, Maliha S, Love T. Cause-specific mortality in patients with psoriatic arthritis. Ann Rheum Dis 2013;72:519.

131. Hellgren K, Smedby KE, Backlin C, et al. Ankylosing spondylitis, psoriatic arthritis, and risk of malignant lymphoma: a cohort study based on nationwide prospectively recorded data from Sweden. Arthritis Rheumatol 2014;66(5): 1282–90.

132. Gross RL, Schwartzman-Morris JS, Krathen M, et al. A comparison of the malignancy incidence among patients with psoriatic arthritis and patients with rheumatoid arthritis in a large US cohort. Arthritis Rheumatol 2014;66(6):1472–81.

133. Dommasch ED, Abuabara K, Shin DB, et al. The risk of infection and malignancy with tumor necrosis factor antagonists in adults with psoriatic disease: a systematic review and meta-analysis of randomized controlled trials. J Am Acad Dermatol 2011;64(6):1035–50.

134. Haynes K, Beukelman T, Curtis JR, et al. Tumor necrosis factor alpha inhibitor therapy and cancer risk in chronic immune-mediated diseases. Arthritis Rheum 2013;65(1):48–58.

135. Nannini C, Cantini F, Niccoli L, et al. Single-center series and systematic review of randomized controlled trials of malignancies in patients with rheumatoid arthritis, psoriatic arthritis, and ankylosing spondylitis receiving anti-tumor necrosis factor alpha therapy: is there a need for more comprehensive screening procedures? Arthritis Rheum 2009;61(6):801–12.

136. Gottlieb AB, Dann F. Comorbidities in patients with psoriasis. Am J Med 2009; 122(12):1150.e1–9.

137. Burmester GR, Mease P, Dijkmans BA, et al. Adalimumab safety and mortality rates from global clinical trials of six immune-mediated inflammatory diseases. Ann Rheum Dis 2009;68(12):1863–9.

138. Laas K, Roine R, Rasanen P, et al, HUS QoL Study Group. Health-related quality of life in patients with common rheumatic diseases referred to a university clinic. Rheumatol Int 2009;29(3):267–73.

139. Mease PJ, Menter MA. Quality-of-life issues in psoriasis and psoriatic arthritis: outcome measures and therapies from a dermatological perspective. J Am Acad Dermatol 2006;54(4):685–704.

140. Lucke M, Kim S, Husni M. The joint effect of carotid ultrasound and preventive cardiology referral on cardiovascular risk factor modification in psoriatic arthritis patients. Arthritis Rheum 2013;65(10):334.

Outcome Measures in Psoriatic Arthritis

Laura Coates, MBChB, MRCP, PhD[a,b],*

KEYWORDS

- Psoriatic arthritis • Outcome measures • Disease activity • Composite measures
- Function • Quality of life • Impact of disease

KEY POINTS

- Validated outcome measures are now available for the key psoriatic arthritis (PsA) domains of arthritis, skin, enthesitis, and dactylitis.
- New composite measures such as the PsA disease activity score (PASDAS) and Group for Research and Assessment of Psoriasis and Psoriatic Arthritis (GRAPPA) Composite Exercise (GRACE) allow assessment of multiple domains in 1 score with validated response measures and absolute cutoffs for disease activity.
- Involvement of patient research partners is resulting in revision of the core set of domains for PsA and development of new outcome measures that accurately reflect patient experience.

INTRODUCTION

Selection of appropriate outcome measures in clinical trials and observational studies is key to improving the understanding of PsA and effective management. In many cases, specific outcome measures are translated into clinical practice and may guide therapeutic decisions for individuals. Outcome measurement in PsA developed rapidly during the last decade fueled by deeper insights into the diverse domains that comprise PsA and a rigorous collaborative program of validation to define more appropriate instruments and outcome measures.

In many cases, outcome measures in PsA were borrowed from rheumatoid arthritis (RA) based on the notion that the disease shared overlapping pathogenetic and

Disclosures: Dr L. Coates is funded by the NIHR as a Clincial Lecturer. Dr L. Coates has received research funding and/or honoraria from Abbvie, Pfizer, UCB, Celgene, Janssen, and MSD.
[a] Leeds Institute of Rheumatic and Musculoskeletal Medicine, University of Leeds and Leeds Musculoskeletal Biomedical Research Unit, Leeds Teaching Hospitals NHS Trust, Chapel Allerton Hospital, Chapeltown Road, Leeds LS7 4SA, UK; [b] Division of Allergy, Immunology and Rheumatology, University of Rochester Medical Center, Rochester, NY, USA
* Leeds Institute of Rheumatic and Musculoskeletal Medicine, University of Leeds and Leeds Musculoskeletal Biomedical Research Unit, Leeds Teaching Hospitals NHS Trust, Chapel Allerton Hospital, Chapeltown Road, Leeds LS7 4SA.
E-mail address: l.c.coates@leeds.ac.uk

clinical features. Although some measures can be applied across multiple diseases, it is essential that PsA instruments and outcome measures are validated in patients who have the disease and not another inflammatory arthritis. PsA is a complex disease with inflammation that spans a wide spectrum to include peripheral joints, skin, entheses, spine, and other adjacent tissues. Outcome measures commonly evaluate individual features or domains, but the impact of the disease on a patient depends on the cumulative interaction of these domain variables.

DOMAINS

In 2007, the GRAPPA and Outcome Measures in Rheumatology Clinical Trials (OMERACT) group published consensus on a core set of PsA domains that should be assessed in clinical trials (**Fig. 1**).[1] The core set included in the inner circle includes activities of global disease, peripheral joint disease, and skin disease, along with measures of impact such as physical function, quality of life, and pain. Items in the outer circle were designated as useful domains to measure but were not to be included in all clinical trials or observational studies. Some outcome measures were not deemed relevant to all studies, and in other cases, outcome measures were not available or validated at the time.[1] These core measures were approved in 2006, but at the most recent OMERACT meeting in 2014, it was agreed that the core set should be revised with additional patient input. This revision is underway and will be discussed at the OMERACT Meeting in 2016. Fatigue will likely be included in the core set given its impact on patient well-being and function.

ARTHRITIS

Measures of peripheral joint disease activity are based on tender and swollen joint counts and can be combined with other measures in a composite fashion. The key issue in PsA is that a full 68/66 joint count should be performed, as reduced joint counts designed for RA are not appropriate.[1] This issue is particularly crucial in oligoarthritis whereby disease is not accurately assessed using reduced joint counts.[2] However,

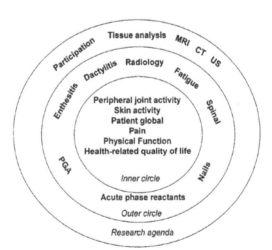

Fig. 1. The 2007 core set for PsA. CT, computed tomography; PGA, physician global assessment; US, ultrasonography. (*From* Gladman DD, Mease PJ, Strand V, et al. Consensus on a core set of domains for psoriatic arthritis. J Rheumatol 2007;34(5):1169; with permission.)

even in patients with polyarthritis, significant proportions of active disease can be missed because of involvement of the distal joints of the hands and all joints in the feet.

The PsA response criteria are based on a 68/66 joint count and were developed for a PsA sulfasalazine trial by a process that was not data driven.[3] Unfortunately, a high placebo response is commonly seen with this measure.[4] Most drug trials in PsA report outcomes in terms of disease activity score and European League Against Rheumatism (EULAR) and/or American College of Rheumatology outcomes (usually modified with a 68/66 joint count). These end points are responsive in PsA clinical trials based on retrospective analysis, but these trials predominantly involve patients with polyarticular RA-like disease.[5] Patients with oligoarticular disease are less likely to fulfill these response criteria, so caution is advised in this subset. The disease activity in PsA (DAPSA) measure is based on the disease activity in reactive arthritis (DAREA) scale following principle component analysis of data from patients with PsA.[6] The DAREA is a data-driven composite joint measure that incorporates full joint counts but does not assess other aspects of the disease.

SKIN

The body surface area (BSA) was the first measure devised to assess psoriasis, and it is based on the rule of nines for burns.[7] Many subsequent measures are partially based on this instrument, including the psoriasis area and severity index (PASI), in common use to assess skin involvement. PASI includes scores for erythema, induration, and scaling, as well as the BSA on different parts of the body (head, trunk, upper limbs, and lower limbs).[8] The PASI is the most widely used outcome for psoriasis in PsA studies, although it is less discriminative at low levels of disease and is therefore not usually applied in patients with less than 3% BSA. The other measures of psoriasis observed in PsA trials include a target lesion score using severity assessments similar to the PASI but limited to 1 focal lesion and the physician global assessment (PGA), which records an overall scale from 0 (clear) to 6 (very severe). The target lesion score and PGA probably show better validity in cohorts with mild skin disease, particularly a target lesion score.

NAILS

Several different measures are available to assess nail involvement in psoriasis. In particular, the nail psoriasis severity index (NAPSI) and a modified version (mNAPSI) are the 2 most popular in PsA studies. Both instruments score each nail individually for features of nail bed changes (onycholysis, oil drop, splinter hemorrhages, and nail bed hyperkeratosis) and nail matrix psoriasis (pitting, leukonychia, red spots in lunula, and nail plate crumbling).[9] The mNAPSI scores the most common features from 0 to 3 (pitting, onycholysis, and crumbling) depending on the area of the nail involved and the other features as present or absent in each nail (possible score, 0–14 per nail).

In some studies, more simplified indices are preferred, including a visual analog scale (VAS) for nail disease severity or a count of nails with any psoriasis involvement. Although these assessment tools provide much less detailed information regarding nail involvement, they are more feasible in practice.

ENTHESITIS

The Mander enthesitis index (MEI) was the first instrument to assess enthesitis and includes 66 potential sites graded for tenderness from 0 to 3. These sites were identified from examination of patients with ankylosing spondylitis (AS) and subsequently validated in a group comprising mainly patients with AS.[10] The Leeds enthesitis index (LEI) was developed to simplify the MEI and provide a more feasible tool specific to patients with PsA. Researchers used dichotomous scoring for pain rather than the 0-to-3 scale at the full 66 sites and then performed stepwise data reduction to identify and retain only those sites with the most common involvement. They analyzed data from 28 patients and aimed to identify enthesitis present in at least 80% of individuals. This process created a 6-site index (bilateral Achilles tendons, bilateral lateral epicondyles of the elbows, and bilateral medial condyles of the knee). This index has been tested in patients with PsA and shown to be sensitive to change. It also has a low floor effect meaning that it identifies most patients with entheseal disease.[11]

The other scale developed for use in patients with PsA is the Spondyloarthritis Research Consortium of Canada (SPARCC) enthesitis measure.[12] The sites included were identified as the most commonly involved entheseal sites from imaging studies of both patients with PsA and AS. This study resulted in 16 sites for assessment, although a reduced score of just 8 sites is also available. This measure was sensitive to change in a small AS trial to assess efficacy of tumor necrosis factor (TNF) inhibitors and also showed a good effect size in a small open-label disease-modifying antirheumatic drug study in PsA.[11] Both the LEI and the SPARCC measures have excellent interrater reliability in patients with PsA assessed by trained rheumatologists and dermatologists.[13] The entheseal sites included in these measures are shown in **Fig. 2**.

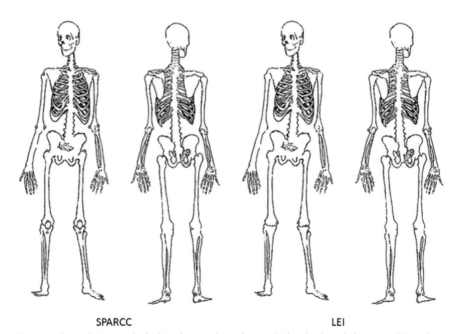

SPARCC   LEI

Fig. 2. Entheseal sites included in the Leeds enthesitis index (LEI) and the Spondyloarthritis Research Consortium of Canada (SPARCC) enthesitis index. (*From* Coates LC, Helliwell PS. Disease measurement—enthesitis, skin, nails, spine and dactylitis. Best Pract Res Clin Rheumatol 2010;24(5):663; with permission.)

DACTYLITIS

Dactylitis or fusiform swelling of an entire digit is a typical feature of PsA. In most clinical trials measuring dactylitis, a simple count of dactylitis digits sometimes with a grading of tenderness from 0 to 3 has been used.[3,14–16] Both these measures show responsiveness in trials of TNF inhibitors and are feasible in clinical practice. A more quantitative scoring system, the Leeds dactylitis index (LDI), is also available for use in clinical trials.[17] This scoring system uses a dactylometer to measure the circumference of affected digits at the level of the web space and compares this result in a ratio to the circumference of the contralateral unaffected digit. In the case of bilateral involvement, charts of average finger circumferences are available. The ratio can be multiplied by a tenderness score (0–3) or a simple presence or absence of tenderness (LDI basic). The LDI is responsive in clinical trials with a good effect size. It also provides the first quantitative definition of dactylitis: an increase in circumference of more than 10% compared with the contralateral unaffected digit.[17]

AXIAL DISEASE

Just as many measures of peripheral joint involvement were borrowed from RA, potential measures for axial disease activity are typically borrowed from AS. For many years, the Bath AS disease activity index (BASDAI) was the predominant and in some cases the only instrument to assess axial disease.[18] This 6-item patient questionnaire has been tested in multiple axial PsA cohorts and correlates well with other measures of disease activity. Based on these findings, some groups recommend its use in axial PsA. Unfortunately, it has been shown that the BASDAI correlates equally well with other measures of disease activity in both axial and peripheral PsA.[19,20] Thus, although the BASDAI can reflect global DAPSA, it cannot differentiate between axial and peripheral disease.

More recently, the AS disease activity score (ASDAS) was developed and validated for AS. This composite measure includes some of the questions from the BASDAI along with an acute phase reactant such as C-reactive protein (CRP).[21] Responses and cutoffs were developed and validated in AS and nonradiographic axial spondyloarthritis (SpA).[22] Two studies show similar discrimination between high and low disease activity states in axial PsA using both BASDAI and ASDAS.[23,24] To date no publications examine whether the ASDAS can discriminate between axial and peripheral PsA, but given that the score includes only BASDAI questions and a CRP, it seems unlikely that this is the case. One open-label study specifically examined response to TNF inhibitors in axial PsA, which used the BASDAI and showed a significant response. It is therefore likely that the BASDAI and ASDAS would reflect changes in disease activity in patients with pure axial PsA, but investigators and clinicians must be aware that they do not differentiate from responses in peripheral involvement.

Similarly, the Bath AS functional index[25] correlates with other functional measures in PsA but does not differentiate axial involvement.[26] Although it may be measured in patients with axial PsA, it does not show any advantages over generic measures of functional ability, which are well validated in PsA such as the health assessment questionnaire (HAQ).

PATIENT-REPORTED OUTCOMES: QUALITY OF LIFE, FUNCTION, FATIGUE, IMPACT OF DISEASE

Both function and quality of life are included in the core set for PsA. Measurements of the impact of the disease on these aspects of a patient's life are commonly reported in interventional trials and cohort studies. The most common measure of physical function is the HAQ, a generic measure used across many forms of arthritis.[27] It consists of 20 items measuring impairment of function in 8 domains, and each task is rated from 0 (no difficulty) to 3 (unable to do). The final score ranges from 0 to 3 as an average of the 8 domains. An effort to develop a specific HAQ for patients with SpA was attempted, but it was not shown to be superior and has not replaced the standard HAQ.[28] The minimal clinically important difference (MCID) for the HAQ does, however, vary between diseases and has been suggested as 0.35 in PsA based on data within a randomized controlled trial (RCT) of etanercept.[29]

Measuring the impact on a patient's quality of life can be performed using generic or disease-specific tools, and each has specific advantages. Quality of life can be measured across multiple diseases using generic tools, such as the medical outcomes study short form 36 (SF-36)[30] or the EuroQol 5 domain (EQ5D).[31] The SF-36 consists of 8 domains but can be subdivided into 2 component scores: physical and mental. The SF-36 is well validated in PsA, with correlations shown between SF-36 and functional impairment, pain, and disease activity.[32] The EQ5D consists of 5 domains assessing mobility, self-care, usual activities, pain, and anxiety/depression and has also been shown to be responsive in PsA trials.[33]

In contrast, measures developed for psoriasis and PsA may provide more insight into the specific problems encountered by patients. The PsA quality of life measure was developed from PsA patient interviews[34] and has been shown to be reliable and responsive to change in clinical trials.[35] This instrument consists of 20 questions answered as true/false covering items that patients reported were important in qualitative interviews. Another specific measure commonly used is the dermatology life quality index developed for multiple skin conditions.[36] It is well validated in psoriasis and also used in PsA trials.[33] This measure allows a specific assessment of the impact of active skin disease.

Fatigue is becoming increasingly recognized in inflammatory arthritis, including PsA, as patients' opinions are further represented. In RA, the core set of domains to be measured in flare now includes fatigue predominantly as a result of increased patient research participation in the OMERACT process.[37] As stated earlier, the PsA core set is under revision, and it seems likely that fatigue will be included in the future.

Several fatigue measures were tested in PsA with good results, but there is no clear evidence to support the optimal instrument. The fatigue severity scale was validated in PsA[38] with changes in fatigue correlating with changes in disease activity.[39] The functional assessment of chronic illness therapy—fatigue scale was also responsive in PsA both in interventional trial data[40] and in observational cohorts.[41] Indeed, these 2 scales correlate closely with each other.[41]

The patient-reported outcomes assessing function and quality of life mentioned earlier do go some way to establishing the patient perspective, but there is evidence that other dimensions of health may be considered important by the patient and should be assessed. To counteract this and ensure a robust assessment of the impact of PsA on individual patients, EULAR convened a group to develop a new specific patient-reported outcome: the psoriatic arthritis impact of disease (PsAID) score. This measure covers a wide variety of domains of impact identified with significant input from patient research partners. The most important 12 domains (pain, fatigue, skin problems, work/leisure activities, functional capacity, discomfort, sleep disturbance, coping, anxiety, embarrassment/shame, social participation, and depression) were identified following a survey of 140 patients, and together the health care professionals and patient research partners developed a question with a 0 to 10 numerical rating scale for each of these 12 domains.[42] Two versions of the PsAID have been developed, the PsAID 9 for clinical trials and the PsAID 12 for clinical practice, and these were validated according to the OMERACT filter and have a proposed MCID of 3 and a cutoff of 4 for the patient acceptable symptom state.[42]

COMPOSITE MEASURES

The easiest global measure of PsA is a global disease activity VAS. This measure can be completed by both physician and patient and aim to encapsulate a global picture of psoriatic disease. However, there has historically been a variety of ways to phrase the question given to the patient, leading to a GRAPPA project to standardize this. The concern was that the patient may not be clear on whether they are being asked about their arthritis only, all musculoskeletal symptoms, or the entire disease burden, including skin and nail disease. The standardized wording validated by the GRAPPA study asks "In all the ways that your psoriasis and arthritis, as a whole, affect you, how would you rate the way you felt over the past week?"[43] There are also validated VAS questions that can be used for skin and arthritis individually.[43] When the patient and physician global disease activity measures were analyzed within the GRACE, they accounted for a massive 90% of the variability, showing how well these patient-reported measures encapsulate disease activity.[44]

The first composite measure to include measures of activity in multiple domains of psoriatic disease was the minimal disease activity (MDA) criteria. These criteria are for a specific disease state rather than a true measure of disease activity. The criteria state that a patient is in MDA if they fulfill 5 of 7 of the following criteria: tender joint count less than or equal to 1; swollen joint count less than or equal to 1; PASI less than or equal to 1 or BSA less than or equal to 3; patient pain VAS less than or equal to 15; patient global disease activity VAS less than or equal to 20; HAQ less than or equal to 0.5; tender entheseal points less than or equal to 1.[45] The criteria can therefore identify specific disease activity in peripheral joints, skin, entheses, and dactylitis (via joint counts), as well as patient-reported indicators such as global disease activity, pain, and physical function. In addition to these validated cutoffs, analysis in the ADEPT (adalimumab effectiveness in psoriatic arthritis trial) data set has suggested that a psoriasis PGA of clear or almost clear could be used instead of the existing skin criteria with similar results. These criteria were validated both in an observational real-life cohort[46] and in interventional trial data[47] and have now been used in an RCT of tight control in PsA.[48]

The first true disease activity composite measure in PsA was the composite psoriatic disease activity index (CPDAI),[49] which was based on the GRAPPA treatment grid system[50] (**Table 1**). Each domain of PsA (peripheral joints, skin, entheses, dactylitis, and axial disease) is assessed using a measure of disease activity and a measure of disease Impact, and these are summed together to create a total score of 0 to 15. The CPDAI correlates well with patient and physician global scores[49] and was able to differentiate between different etanercept doses in the PRESTA (psoriasis randomised etanercept study in subjects with psoriatic arthritis) study,[51] showing that it identifies other aspects of disease beyond the peripheral arthritis.

Given the interest in novel composite measures, GRAPPA set up the GRACE project to collect data on patients worldwide and derive new evidence-based measures. A total of 503 patients were recruited and assessed at baseline, 3, 6, and 12 months. The gold standard for disease activity was the decision of the physician to change or escalate treatment excluding those whose treatment changes related only to an adverse event. Two potential measures were developed in the GRACE project: the PASDAS, which is a weighted index including 7 components identified on principle

Table 1
The CPDAI

	Not Involved (0)	Mild (1)	Moderate (2)	Severe (3)
Peripheral arthritis	No peripheral arthritis	≤4 active joints and normal function (HAQ <0.5)	≤4 active joints with impaired function or >4 active joints, normal function	>4 joints and function impaired
Skin disease	No psoriasis	PASI ≤10 and DLQI ≤10	PASI ≤10 but DLQI >10 or PASI >10 but DLQI ≤10	PASI >10 and DLQI >10
Enthesitis	No enthesitis	≤3 sites and normal function (HAQ <0.5)	≤3 sites with impaired function or >3 sites normal function	>3 sites and function impaired
Dactylitis	No dactylitis	≤3 digits and normal function (HAQ <0.5)	≤3 digits with impaired function or >3 digits normal function	>3 digits and function impaired
Axial disease	No axial involvement	BASDAI <4 and normal function (ASQoL <6)	BASDAI <4 with impaired function or BASDAI >4 with normal function	BASDAI >4 and function impaired

Abbreviations: ASQoL, ankylosing spondylitis quality of life; DLQI, dermatology life quality index.
From Mumtaz A, Gallagher P, Kirby B, et al. Development of a preliminary composite disease activity index in psoriatic arthritis. Ann Rheum Dis 2011;70(2):273; with permission.

component analysis with weighting using logistic regression coefficients, and the GRACE index, which is based on an arithmetical mean of 8 domain measures transformed using desirability functions.[44] Both these new measures performed well in the GRACE data set[44] and in the retrospective analysis of golimumab RCT data.[52] The effect sizes of the PASDAS and GRACE indexes were greater than those for the CPDAI, DAPSA, and disease activity score in 28 joints (DAS28). Candidate cutoffs for different levels of disease activity and response criteria have also been developed for the PASDAS, GRACE, and CPDAI, as well as DAPSA and DAS28 in PsA, using patient and physician global scores as the gold standard.[53] These measures require further validation in other cohorts but potentially provide validated composite measures for future trials. The larger effect sizes of these measures mean that trials could answer questions with smaller sample sizes.

FUTURE CONSIDERATIONS/SUMMARY

Over the last decade, the evaluation of clinical response in PsA was transformed by the rapid development and validation of specific outcome measures. Tools required to dramatically advance clinical research in this disease are now available. The emergence of new composite measures and definitive treatment targets lay the groundwork for future trials that focus on targeted strategies that hold great promise in PsA based on the experience in RA and the recent Tight Control of Psoriatic Arthritis (TICOPA) trial. Furthermore, the inclusion of measures with defined response criteria will facilitate a better understanding of the impact of therapies on multiple PsA domains assessed with 1 instrument. Marked advances in patient-reported outcome measures culminated in the PsAID, developed using a fully integrated approach with patients, which accurately reflects the impact of the disease from the patient and not the physician perspective.

Despite the marked advances, many challenges remain to be addressed in the area of outcome assessment in this disease. In particular, how does one assess and quantify oligoarthritis? Joint counts and related measures will likely underestimate the burden of the disease, and response measures are less sensitive in this subgroup. Given the high prevalence of this subset in clinical practice, it is essential to include patients with oligoarthritis in clinical trials assessed with accurate and validated outcome instruments. The other key issue is translating these validated outcome measures from interventional trials to clinical practice. Ensuring that composite measures are feasible in clinical practice can optimize care in the clinic and will be of great impact for the treating clinician as they utilise treat-to –target strategies for patients with PsA.

REFERENCES

1. Gladman DD, Mease PJ, Strand V, et al. Consensus on a core set of domains for psoriatic arthritis. J Rheumatol 2007;34(5):1167–70.
2. Coates LC, FitzGerald O, Gladman DD, et al. Reduced joint counts misclassify patients with oligoarticular psoriatic arthritis and miss significant numbers of patients with active disease. Arthritis Rheum 2013;65(6):1504–9.
3. Clegg DO, Reda DJ, Mejias E, et al. Comparison of sulfasalazine and placebo in the treatment of psoriatic arthritis. A Department of Veterans Affairs Cooperative Study. Arthritis Rheum 1996;39(12):2013–20.
4. Jones G, Crotty M, Brooks P. Interventions for psoriatic arthritis. Cochrane Database Syst Rev 2000;(3):CD000212.
5. Fransen J, Antoni C, Mease PJ, et al. Performance of response criteria for assessing peripheral arthritis in patients with psoriatic arthritis: analysis of data from randomised controlled trials of two tumour necrosis factor inhibitors. Ann Rheum Dis 2006;65(10):1373–8.
6. Schoels M, Aletaha D, Funovits J, et al. Application of the DAREA/DAPSA score for assessment of disease activity in psoriatic arthritis. Ann Rheum Dis 2010; 69(8):1441–7.
7. Wallace AB. The exposure treatment of burns. Lancet 1951;1(6653):501–4.
8. Fredriksson T, Pettersson U. Severe psoriasis–oral therapy with a new retinoid. Dermatologica 1978;157(4):238–44.
9. Rich P, Scher RK. Nail psoriasis severity index: a useful tool for evaluation of nail psoriasis. J Am Acad Dermatol 2003;49(2):206–12 [see comment].
10. Mander M, Simpson JM, McLellan A, et al. Studies with an enthesis index as a method of clinical assessment in ankylosing spondylitis. Ann Rheum Dis 1987; 46(3):197–202.
11. Healy PJ, Helliwell PS. Measuring clinical enthesitis in psoriatic arthritis: assessment of existing measures and development of an instrument specific to psoriatic arthritis. Arthritis Rheum 2008;59(5):686–91.
12. Maksymowych WP, Mallon C, Morrow S, et al. Development and validation of the Spondyloarthritis Research Consortium of Canada (SPARCC) enthesitis index. Ann Rheum Dis 2009;68(6):948–53.
13. Gladman DD, Inman RD, Cook RJ, et al. International spondyloarthritis interobserver reliability exercise–the INSPIRE study: II. Assessment of peripheral joints, enthesitis, and dactylitis. J Rheumatol 2007;34(8):1740–5.
14. Salvarani C, Cantini F, Olivieri I, et al. Efficacy of infliximab in resistant psoriatic arthritis. Arthritis Rheum 2003;49(4):541–5.

15. Kaltwasser JP, Nash P, Gladman D, et al. Efficacy and safety of leflunomide in the treatment of psoriatic arthritis and psoriasis: a multinational, double-blind, randomized, placebo-controlled clinical trial. Arthritis Rheum 2004;50(6):1939–50.

16. Antoni C, Krueger GG, de Vlam K, et al. Infliximab improves signs and symptoms of psoriatic arthritis: results of the IMPACT 2 trial. Ann Rheum Dis 2005;64(8): 1150–7.

17. Healy PJ, Helliwell PS. Measuring dactylitis in clinical trials: which is the best instrument to use? J Rheumatol 2007;34(6):1302–6.

18. Garrett S, Jenkinson T, Kennedy LG, et al. A new approach to defining disease status in ankylosing spondylitis: the Bath ankylosing spondylitis disease activity index. J Rheumatol 1994;21(12):2286–91.

19. Taylor WJ, Harrison AA. Could the Bath ankylosing spondylitis disease activity index (BASDAI) be a valid measure of disease activity in patients with psoriatic arthritis? Arthritis Rheum 2004;51(3):311–5.

20. Fernandez-Sueiro JL, Willisch A, Pertega-Diaz S, et al. Validity of the Bath ankylosing spondylitis disease activity index for the evaluation of disease activity in axial psoriatic arthritis. Arthritis Care Res (Hoboken) 2010;62(1):78–85.

21. Lukas C, Landewe R, Sieper J, et al. Development of an ASAS-endorsed disease activity score (ASDAS) in patients with ankylosing spondylitis. Ann Rheum Dis 2009;68(1):18–24.

22. Machado P, Landewe R, Lie E, et al. Ankylosing spondylitis disease activity score (ASDAS): defining cut-off values for disease activity states and improvement scores. Ann Rheum Dis 2011;70(1):47–53.

23. Eder L, Chandran V, Shen H, et al. Is ASDAS better than BASDAI as a measure of disease activity in axial psoriatic arthritis? Ann Rheum Dis 2010;69(12):2160–4.

24. Kilic G, Kilic E, Nas K, et al. Comparison of ASDAS and BASDAI as a measure of disease activity in axial psoriatic arthritis. Clin Rheumatol 2015;34(3):515–21.

25. Calin A, Garrett S, Whitelock H, et al. A new approach to defining functional ability in ankylosing spondylitis: the development of the Bath ankylosing spondylitis functional index. J Rheumatol 1994;21(12):2281–5.

26. Leung YY, Tam LS, Kun EW, et al. Comparison of 4 functional indexes in psoriatic arthritis with axial or peripheral disease subgroups using Rasch analyses. J Rheumatol 2008;35(8):1613–21.

27. Fries JF, Spitz P, Kraines RG, et al. Measurement of patient outcome in arthritis. Arthritis Rheum 1980;23(2):137–45.

28. Blackmore MG, Gladman DD, Husted J, et al. Measuring health status in psoriatic arthritis: the Health Assessment Questionnaire and its modification. J Rheumatol 1995;22(5):886–93.

29. Mease PJ, Woolley JM, Bitman B, et al. Minimally important difference of Health Assessment Questionnaire in psoriatic arthritis: relating thresholds of improvement in functional ability to patient-rated importance and satisfaction. J Rheumatol 2011;38(11):2461–5.

30. Ware JE Jr, Sherbourne CD. The MOS 36-item short-form health survey (SF-36). I. Conceptual framework and item selection. Med Care 1992;30(6):473–83.

31. EuroQol Group. EuroQol–a new facility for the measurement of health-related quality of life. Health Policy 1990;16(3):199–208.

32. Husted JA, Gladman DD, Farewell VT, et al. Validating the SF-36 health survey questionnaire in patients with psoriatic arthritis. J Rheumatol 1997;24(3):511–7.

33. Mease PJ. Measures of psoriatic arthritis: tender and swollen joint assessment, psoriasis area and severity index (PASI), nail psoriasis severity index (NAPSI), modified nail psoriasis severity index (mNAPSI), Mander/Newcastle enthesitis

index (MEI), Leeds enthesitis index (LEI), Spondyloarthritis Research Consortium of Canada (SPARCC), Maastricht ankylosing spondylitis enthesis score (MASES), Leeds dactylitis index (LDI), patient global for psoriatic arthritis, dermatology life quality index (DLQI), psoriatic arthritis quality of life (PsAQOL), functional assessment of chronic illness therapy-fatigue (FACIT-F), psoriatic arthritis response criteria (PsARC), psoriatic arthritis joint activity index (PsAJAI), disease activity in psoriatic arthritis (DAPSA), and composite psoriatic disease activity index (CPDAI). Arthritis Care Res (Hoboken) 2011;63(Suppl 11):S64–85.

34. McKenna SP, Doward LC, Whalley D, et al. Development of the PsAQoL: a quality of life instrument specific to psoriatic arthritis. Ann Rheum Dis 2004; 63(2):162–9.

35. Healy PJ, Helliwell PS. Psoriatic arthritis quality of life instrument: an assessment of sensitivity and response to change. J Rheumatol 2008;35(7):1359–61.

36. Finlay AY, Khan GK. Dermatology life quality index (DLQI)–a simple practical measure for routine clinical use. Clin Exp Dermatol 1994;19(3):210–6.

37. Bykerk VP, Lie E, Bartlett SJ, et al. Establishing a core domain set to measure rheumatoid arthritis flares: report of the OMERACT 11 RA flare Workshop. J Rheumatol 2014;41(4):799–809.

38. Schentag C, Cichon J, MacKinnon A, et al. Validation and normative data for the 0-10 point scale version of the fatigue severity scale (FSS). Arthritis Rheum 2000; 2000(43 Suppl):S177.

39. Schentag C, Gladman D. Changes in fatigue in psoriatic arthritis: disease activity of fibromyalgia. Arthritis Rheum 2002;46(Suppl):S177.

40. Mease PJ, Gladman DD, Ritchlin CT, et al. Adalimumab for the treatment of patients with moderately to severely active psoriatic arthritis: results of a double-blind, randomized, placebo-controlled trial. Arthritis Rheum 2005;52(10):3279–89.

41. Chandran V, Bhella S, Schentag C, et al. Functional assessment of chronic illness therapy-fatigue scale is valid in patients with psoriatic arthritis. Ann Rheum Dis 2007;66(7):936–9.

42. Gossec L, de Wit M, Kiltz U, et al. A patient-derived and patient-reported outcome measure for assessing psoriatic arthritis: elaboration and preliminary validation of the Psoriatic Arthritis Impact of Disease (PsAID) questionnaire, a 13-country EULAR initiative. Ann Rheum Dis 2014;73(6):1012–9.

43. Cauli A, Gladman D, Mathieu A, et al. Patient and physician perception of disease in psoriatic arthritis (PsA). A multicentre GRAPPA and OMERACT study. Arthritis Rheum 2007;56(9S):610 [abstract].

44. Helliwell PS, Fitzgerald O, Fransen J, et al. The development of candidate composite disease activity and responder indices for psoriatic arthritis (GRACE project). Ann Rheum Dis 2013;72(6):986–91 (online first 17/07/2012).

45. Coates LC, Fransen J, Helliwell PS. Defining minimal disease activity in psoriatic arthritis: a proposed objective target for treatment. Ann Rheum Dis 2010;69(1): 48–53.

46. Coates LC, Schentag CT, Lee K, et al. Frequency and predictors of minimal disease activity in an observational psoriatic arthritis cohort. Ann Rheum Dis 2009; 68(3):137 [abstract].

47. Coates LC, Helliwell PS. Validation of minimal disease activity for psoriatic arthritis using interventional trial data. Arthritis Care Res 2010;62(2):965–9.

48. Coates LC, Navarro-Coy N, Brown SR, et al. The TICOPA protocol (TIght COntrol of Psoriatic Arthritis): a randomised controlled trial to compare intensive management versus standard care in early psoriatic arthritis. BMC Musculoskelet Disord 2013;14:101.

49. Mumtaz A, Gallagher P, Kirby B, et al. Development of a preliminary composite disease activity index in psoriatic arthritis. Ann Rheum Dis 2011;70(2):272–7.
50. Ritchlin CT, Kavanaugh A, Gladman DD, et al. Treatment recommendations for psoriatic arthritis. Ann Rheum Dis 2009;68(9):1387–94.
51. Fitzgerald O, Helliwell P, Mease P, et al. Application of composite disease activity scores in psoriatic arthritis to the PRESTA data set. Ann Rheum Dis 2011;71(3): 358–62.
52. Helliwell PS, Kavanaugh A. Comparison of composite measures of disease activity in psoriatic arthritis using data from an interventional study with golimumab. Arthritis Care Res (Hoboken) 2014;66(5):749–56.
53. Helliwell PS, FitzGerald O, Fransen J. Composite disease activity and responder indices for psoriatic arthritis: a report from the GRAPPA 2013 meeting on development of cutoffs for both disease activity states and response. J Rheumatol 2014;41(6):1212–7.

Management of Psoriatic Arthritis

Traditional Disease-Modifying Rheumatic Agents and Targeted Small Molecules

Enrique R. Soriano, MD, MSc

KEYWORDS

- Traditional disease-modifying antirheumatic drugs • Small molecules
- Treatment psoriatic arthritis • Psoriatic arthritis

KEY POINTS

- Traditional disease-modifying antirheumatic drugs (DMARDs) remain first-line treatment for psoriatic arthritis in many centers.
- New targeted small molecules are alternative choices for patients that do not tolerate or do not respond to conventional DMARDs or tumor necrosis factor inhibitors.
- Additional research and drug development is needed to address unmet needs in the treatment of PsA.

INTRODUCTION

Traditional disease-modifying antirheumatic drugs (DMARDs) are the first line for the treatment of psoriatic arthritis (PsA) around the world.[1,2] Despite findings in several reviews and metaananalyses that demonstrated sparse high-quality evidence in support of the efficacy of these drugs in PsA,[3–6] they are still recommended as first choice for peripheral arthritis in published guidelines and recommendations.[7,8] Several factors may explain the paradox between evidence and clinical use, a practice not unique to PsA[9] and include:

1. The lack of large, well-designed clinical trials
2. The perception of many rheumatologists that DMARDs are effective at least in some patients
3. General knowledge and comfort with the side effect profiles of these agents

Disclosure: E.R. Soriano participated in advisory boards, gave conferences or received grants from: Pfizer; Abbvie; Novartis; Bristol-Myers Squibb; Janssen; UCB and Roche.
Rheumatology Unit, Internal Medical Services, Hospital Italiano de Buenos Aires, Instituto Universitario, y Fundcion PM. Catoggio, Peron 4190, Buenos Aires (1181) CABA, Argentina
E-mail address: enrique.soriano@hospitalitaliano.org.ar

Rheum Dis Clin N Am 41 (2015) 711–722
http://dx.doi.org/10.1016/j.rdc.2015.07.012
0889-857X/15/$ – see front matter © 2015 Elsevier Inc. All rights reserved.

rheumatic.theclinics.com

4. The relatively low cost in most countries; particularly compared with biologics
5. The perception that delay in starting a biologic to determine if DMARDs are effective will not negatively impact function and quality of life.

Tumor necrosis factor inhibitors (TNFi) are very effective in the treatment of not only peripheral arthritis, but also other manifestations such as skin, enthesitis, dactylitis, and axial involvement as well, and greatly altered the expectations of patients and physicians on the long-term outcomes of this disabling disease.[5,6,10–12] With the increased understanding of immunopathogenesis of PsA, new therapeutic agents targeting different biologic pathways are in development or approved for psoriasis and/or PsA, such as the interleukin (IL)-12 and IL-23 inhibitor ustekinumab, IL-17 inhibitors secukinumab and ixekizumab, and the anti–IL-17R agent brodalumab.[13] In addition to biologics, novel targeted small molecules, orally available, are currently in clinical development for the treatment of psoriasis and PsA, including the phosphodiesterase 4 inhibitor apremilast and Janus kinase (JAK) inhibitors.[13] Targeted small molecules have theoretic advantages over biologics: they are less complex, easier and cheaper to produce, can be administered orally, have broader target selectivity, and inhibit intracellular signaling.[14] In this review, we focus on the efficacy and safety of traditional DMARDs and new targeted small molecules for the treatment of PsA.

TRADITIONAL DISEASE-MODIFYING RHEUMATIC AGENTS

The DMARDs methotrexate (MTX), sulfasalazine (SSZ), leflunamide, and cyclosporine are prescribed in PsA. High-quality experimental evidence to support the use of these agents in PsA is scarce. Studies that address the efficacy and safety of DMARDs in PsA are summarized in **Table 1**. We focus attention in more recent clinical trials and observational studies not included in most of the systematic reviews, with special attention to reports that provide evidence to support the efficacy and safety of traditional DMARDs in PsA therapy.

Methotrexate

Since 2003, 2 randomized, control trials (RCT) have been published.[15,16] In the first, Scarpa and colleagues[15] randomized 35 patients with early oligoarthritis (<12 weeks' disease duration) to nonsteroidal antiinflammatory drugs (NSAIDs) alone or NSAIDs plus MTX for 3 months; thereafter, all patients continued with the combination. A significant improvement was noted at 3 and 6 months compared with baseline in both groups. However, at 3 months, patients on the MTX/NSAIDs combination had a significantly better joint response than patients with NSAIDs alone, although no differences were noted between the 2 groups at 6 on MTX/NSAIDs. In this study, patients with early oligoarthritis demonstrated an improved response to MTX compared with NSAIDs, and that delay of 3 months in the administration of MTX did not significantly lower treatment response at 6 months, although differences in radiographic progression were not addressed in the study.

In the Methotrexate In Psoriatic Arthritis (MIPA) trial, 221 patients were randomized to MTX (target dose 15 mg/wk) or placebo and outcomes assessed at 6 months with the PsA response criteria (PsARC) as the primary one.[16] At 6 months, no differences in any of the individual outcomes (PsARC, American College of Rheumatology 20/50/70 Response [ACR20/50/70], Disease Activity Score C-reactive protein) were noted, except for patient global and physician global assessments, which were higher in the MTX compared with the placebo group.[16] The results of this trial indicate that MTX is not effective for PsA, but several flaws in this trial emerged. First, despite the study's short duration, only 65% and 69% of patients in the active and placebo

Table 1
Summary of randomized control trials with DMARDs and targeted small molecules

Study or First Author	Population	Intervention	Comparator	Patients (n) on Active Treatment/Controls	Primary Outcome	Outcome Reached at 12 wk	Outcome Reached at 24 wk
Willkens[49]	Active (>3 SWJ) PsA DMARD naïve	MTX (7.5–15 mg)	Placebo	16/21	Swollen joint score	No	—
Scarpa[15]	Active oligoarthritis	MTX 10 mg IM	NSAIDs	16/19	SWJ	—	No
MIPA[16]	Active (>1 SWJ) PsA MTX naïve	MTX up to 15 mg/wk	Placebo	109/112	PsARC	No	No
TOPAS[26]	Active (>3 SWJ) PsA DMARD naïve or I-R	Leflunamide 20 mg/d	Placebo	98/92	PsARC	—	Yes
Clegg[31]	Active (>3 SWJ) PsA DMARD naïve	Sulfasalazine 2 g/d	Placebo	109/112	PsARC	—	Yes
PALACE 1[40]	Active (>3 SWJ) PsA DMARDs or TNFi I-R	Apremilast 20 or 30 mg bid	Placebo	324/165	ACR20	Yes	—
PALACE 2[39]	Active (>3 SWJ) PsA DMARDs or TNFi I-R	Apremilast 20 or 30 mg bid	Placebo	325/159	ACR20	Yes	—
PALACE 3[41]	Active (>3 SWJ) PsA DMARDs or TNFi -R	Apremilast 20 or 30 mg bid	Placebo	322/164	ACR20	Yes	—
PALACE 4[42]	Active (>3 SWJ) PsA DMARDs naïve	Apremilast 20 or 30 mg bid	Placebo	271/NA	ACR20	Yes	—
Tofacitinib[48]	Active (>3 SWJ) PsA DMARDs naïve or DMARDS I-R	Tofacitinib 5 bid or 10 mg bid	No controls	12	ACR20	NA	NA

Abbreviations: ACR20, American College of Rheumatology 20 Response; bid, twice daily; DMARD, disease-modifying antirheumatic drug; IM, intramuscular; I-R, inadequate responders; MIPA, Methotrexate In Psoriatic Arthritis; MTX, methotrexate; NA, not applicable/not available; NSAIDs, nonsteroidal antiinflammatory drugs; PsA, psoriatic arthritis; PALACE, Psoriatic Arthritis Long-term Assessment of Clinical Efficacy; PsARC, psoriatic arthritis response criteria; SWJ, swollen joint count; TNFi, tumor necrosis factor inhibitors; TOPAS, Treatment of Psoriatic Arthritis Study.

groups, respectively, completed the trial, which might bias results toward a null effect. Second, patient recruitment lasted 5 years, which might reflect an element of selection bias. Third around 35% of the patients included had oligoarticular disease and the maximum dose of MTX was 15 mg/wk a dose achieved by only 78% of patients.

Most of the evidence to support use of MTX in PsA is based on observational study data.[17] In the reevaluation of the efficacy of MTX in the University of Toronto PsA registry, they reported that patients in the 1994 to 2004 cohort had shorter disease duration and received higher MTX doses (16.2 vs 10.8 mg/wk) compared with the 1978 to 1993 cohort.[18] In this cohort, 68% had 40% or greater decrease in swollen joint counts and less radiographic progression, compared with the earlier cohort (1.5 [SD, 1.8] vs 2.3 [SD, 1.2] increase in radiographic damage score as assessed by the modified Steinbrocker method, respectively), suggesting that, with higher MTX doses, there may be better response with less progression of damage.[18] Cantini and colleagues[19,20] reported a remission rate (using very strict remission criteria) of 19%, and ACR20/50/70 responses in 34%, 23%, and 10%, respectively, in 121 patients with peripheral PsA treated with MTX monotherapy. In the Norwegian DMARD registry, effectiveness and retention rate of MTX was compared in 430 patients with PsA and 1280 patients with rheumatoid arthritis (RA).[21] After 6 months of MTX treatment, both PsA and RA patients improved in most disease activity measures and patient-reported outcomes. MTX retention rates at 2 years, providing indirect evaluation of efficacy and toxicity, were 65% and 66% in PsA and RA patients, respectively.[21]

In an open-label study, 115 patients with mild PsA were randomized to MTX or MTX plus infliximab.[22] Although patients on combination therapy achieved significantly better response, ACR20/50/70 responses were observed in 67%, 40%, and 19%, respectively of patients treated with MTX monotherapy.[22] Recently, a study in Japanese patients was published.[23] Fifty-one PsA patients treated with TNFi plus MTX or MTX alone were investigated retrospectively. Both treatments were equally effective in reducing clinical activity.[23]

One of the intriguing issues with MTX is the difference in toxicities observed between patients with RA compared with patients with psoriasis or PsA.[24] A recent cross-sectional study confirmed that pulmonary toxicity was more common in RA patients compared with patients with PsA, and that hepatotoxicity was more common in PsA patients.[2] A metaanalysis of long-term MTX treatment studies in RA and psoriatic disease showed a 3-fold greater risk of hepatic fibrosis in patients with psoriatic disease.[25] The reasons for such differences may be related to higher rates of obesity and fatty liver, and these results may justify different toxicity monitoring protocols for patients with psoriatic disease.[24] This subject was discussed at the 2007 Group for Research and Assessment of Psoriasis and Psoriatic Arthritis (GRAPPA) meeting related to MTX toxicity.[24] The attendees reached the following consensus. Insufficient data exist to recommend or not recommend serial liver biopsies, but the presence of other risk factors may help to guide decision making. Although data are insufficient to form strong recommendations, in practice small amounts of alcohol are probably safe. Three months off treatment before conception for both female and male partner is appropriate. The combination of MTX with SSZ or with an anti-TNF agent is safe; much less consensus existed regarding the combination of MTX with leflunomide or with cyclosporine.[24]

Leflunamide

Leflunamide was significantly superior to placebo in a 24 week RCT in 186 patients based on improvements in PsARC, tender and swollen joint scores, Health Assessment Questionnaire, and Dermatology Life Quality Index.[26] More recently, the results on a multinational observational study in 440 patients with active PsA treated with leflunamide were reported.[27] At 24 weeks, 86% of patients achieved a PsARC response with significant improvements also seen in tender and swollen joint count, patient and physician global assessments, fatigue, skin disease, dactylitis, and nail lesions.[27] Results on 85 patients followed at the University of Toronto PsA Clinic who received leflunamide (43 patients) alone or in combination with MTX (42 patients) were published.[28] Of the 55 patients who continued the drug, 38%, 48%, and 56% achieved a 40% or greater reduction of actively inflamed joint count at 3, 6, and 12 months, respectively.[28] Although MTX did not modify arthritis response, psoriasis did improve. Patients taking MTX in combination with leflunomide were more likely to achieve a Psoriasis Area and Severity Index (PASI50) response than patients taking leflunomide alone.[28]

Sakellariou and colleagues[29] found that, among 11 patients who received leflunamide in combination with MTX owing to inadequate MTX response, 7 demonstrated moderate improvement and 1 was a nonresponder based on the European League Against Rheumatism (EULAR) response criteria.

Related to safety, withdrawal owing to toxicity was almost 4 times more frequent with leflunomide than with placebo in a published metaanalysis.[4] In the European study, 13% of patients experienced adverse events; the more frequent ones included diarrhea (16.3% of all ADR), alopecia (9.2%), hypertension (8.2%), and pruritus (5.1%). Only 3 adverse events were serious, affecting 2 patients, and none of the unexpected adverse events was considered serious by the investigator. Importantly, addition of leflunomide to concomitant DMARDs (93 patients, most of them with leflunamide plus MTX, followed for 24 weeks) did not lead to an increase in adverse events.[27]

Sulfasalazine

In a systematic review, 6 RCT compared SSZ with placebo. SSZ demonstrated efficacy in PsA,[3] although effect size was very low, and there is no effect on other manifestations such as enthesitis.

SSZ does not seem to halt radiographic progression in PsA. In a case-control study, 20 patients who received SSZ for more than 3 months were compared with 20 control patients.[30] The mean change in the radiographic score at 24 months between the 2 groups was not significant.[30] A trend has been observed in most of the RCT toward higher withdrawal rates in the SSZ group compared with the placebo group, mostly related to adverse events, such as gastrointestinal intolerance, dizziness, and liver toxicity, which have been observed in up to one-third of patients receiving SSZ.[31]

Cyclosporine is rarely used for the treatment of PsA and is not included in this review.

TRADITIONAL DISEASE-MODIFYING ANTIRHEUMATIC DRUGS IN COMBINATION WITH TUMOR NECROSIS FACTOR INHIBITORS

Another potential role for traditional DMARDs is their use in combination with TNFi. In RA, it is clear that the combination of TNFi with traditional DMARDs improves efficacy. Whether combining MTX with a TNFi benefits patients with PsA remains controversial. The randomized, placebo-controlled trials of the 5 commercially available TNF antagonists involved stratification on whether MTX was used concomitantly and showed no differences regarding the effect on the rheumatic manifestations.[32] Data from registries also showed no differences on efficacy between TNFi monotherapy or combined with MTX, although some of them showed better TNFi survival with the combination.

The Swedish registry (SSATG) showed that concomitant MTX (hazard ratio [HR], 0.64; 95% CI, 0.39–0.95; $P = .03$), etanercept (HR, 0.49; 95% CI, 0.28–0.86; $P = .01$), and high C-reactive protein levels (HR, 0.77; 95% CI, 0.61–0.97; $P = .03$) at treatment initiation are related to higher TNFi survival.[33]

In the Danish DANBIO registry, the drug continuation rates were not different with and without MTX, except fort the subgroup of infliximab-treated patients, in which concomitant MTX therapy improved biotherapy continuation.[34] The Norwegian (NOR-DMARD) registry showed similar 6-month EULAR response rates in patients treated with TNFi in the presence or absence of MTX, although drug continuation rates at 1 and 2 years were higher with combination therapy, with the difference being greatest in the infliximab-treated subgroup.[35] In summary, none of the RCT or the registries have provided evidence that MTX should be combined with TNFi to improve efficacy. Some data from registries suggest that the combination might improve drug survival, in particular with infliximab. There is no evidence that adding a traditional DMARD to a patient that failed TNFi monotherapy would improve efficacy.[32] In the TIght COntrol of Psoriatic Arthritis (TICOPA) study, 206 patients with early PsA were randomized to receive either standard care (12 weekly review) or intensive management (4 weekly review) for 48 weeks.[36] Patients assigned to the intensive management group followed a strict treatment protocol whereby dose continuation/escalation was determined through the objective assessment of the minimal disease activity criteria. Treatment with DMARDs was escalated initiating with MTX up to 25 mg/wk, adding SZS, and then switching to MTX + cyclosporin or MTX + leflunamide, or MTX + TNFi (according to the number of swollen joints), in the intensive management group.[36] At 48 weeks, significantly more patients in the intensive group than in the standard care group received combination DMARDs (22.8% vs 12%, respectively) or combination with biologics (37% vs 7.6%, respectively). In a similar way, significantly more patients in the intensive management group achieved ACR20/50/70 and PASI75 response at week 48 (62%, 51%, 38%, and 72% vs 45%, 25%, 17%, and 56%, respectively). There were no differences in the number or severity of adverse events. This well-designed trial showed that combination therapy with DMARDs and MTX plus TNFi is effective and well-tolerated in patients with active early PsA.

Two other important issues related to traditional DMARDs are that there is

- No evidence that DMARDs inhibit radiographic progression
- No evidence that DMARDS are effective for treatment of enthesitis, dactylitis, or axial disease.

TARGETED SYNTHETIC DISEASE-MODIFYING ANTIRHEUMATIC DRUGS (SMALL MOLECULES)

The definition of "small molecule" is by no means unambiguous, but in general refers to a molecule produced by chemical synthesis of low molecular weight, typically less than 500 MW. Small, chemically manufactured molecules are the classic active substances and still make up more than 90% of the drugs on the market today and all traditional DMARDs fulfill this definition. The difference with the "new" small molecules is that, unlike traditional DMARDs, they have unique and well-characterized mechanisms of action. Our understanding of the inflammatory process and the molecular pathways involved profoundly influenced drug development, whereby therapies are pursued that directly target molecules involved in the inflammatory process. Based on this concept, a more appropriate label for these compounds have been suggested as "targeted synthetic DMARDs."[37]

Apremilast

Apremilast is a targeted synthetic DMARD that specifically inhibits phosphodiesterase 4, resulting in increase cyclic adenosine monophosphate in immune cells. Increase cyclic adenosine monophosphate inhibits expression of inflammatory cytokines and increases expression of antiinflammatory mediators such as IL-10.[38] The US Food and Drug Administration approved apremilast for the treatment of adults with active PsA in March 2014. The Psoriatic Arthritis Long-term Assessment of Clinical Efficacy (PALACE) 1, 2, and 3 studies are the pivotal phase III multicenter RCTs. PALACE 1 (504 patients), PALACE 2 (484 patients), and PALACE 3 (505 patients) compared the efficacy and safety of apremilast with placebo in PsA patients previously treated with DMARDs and/or biologic therapy; PALACE 4 (527 patients) evaluated apremilast in DMARDs-naive PsA patients.[39–41] Patients in the PALACE 1, 2, and 3 trials were stratified by prior DMARD use and were allowed to continue receiving stable DMARD therapy in addition to study medication. The primary endpoint of the PALACE studies was the proportion of patients achieving ACR20 response at week 16.[39–41] At week 16, apremilast was associated with significantly higher ACR20 response rates than placebo in PALACE 1, 2, and 3 trials (see **Table 1**).[39–41] In all 3 studies, ACR20 responses were maintained through week 52 for patients randomized to apremilast at baseline. Response rates were similar for patients switched to apremilast after the blinded period at week 16 (early escape, were placebo patients not achieving 20% or greater improvement in joint counts were re-randomized to one of the apremilast groups) or week 24 (were all patients remaining on placebo were re-randomized to one of the apremilast groups). Other secondary outcomes, such as improvement in the Maastricht Ankylosing Spondylitis Enthesitis Score, dactylitis count, Short Form-36 Physical Function and Physical Component Summary scores, Health Assessment Questionnaire Disability Index, Disease Activity Score, and PASI scores were also demonstrated in PALACE 1, 2, and 3 trials. PALACE 1 study included 119 patients with prior biologic exposure and 47 who were considered biologic therapeutic failures.[40] Significantly, more patients in both apremilast groups (20 mg and 30 mg bid) achieved an ACR20 response versus placebo among patients with prior biologic exposure. Differences were numerically better, but not statistically significant among the small number of patients classified as biologic therapeutic failures.[40] Importantly, apremilast was effective in DMARD-naive patients in the PALACE 4 study,[42] although results are published only in abstract. ACR20 response rates at week 16 were 29.2%, 32.3%, and 16.9% for apremilast 20, apremilast 30 mg bid, and placebo, respectively. This differences seems small for a DMARD-naïve population were greater responses are expected, so we would need to wait until the paper is fully published with a better characterization of the population included to draw more firm conclusions.

Apremilast was generally well-tolerated in phase III trials. Pooled data on safety on 1493 patients from the PALACE 1, 2, and 3 trials were reported.[43,44] The most common adverse events were gastrointestinal and generally occurred early, were self-limiting, and infrequently led to discontinuation.[43] Nausea and headache, upper respiratory tract infection (3.9% vs 1.8% for placebo), vomiting, nasopharyngitis, and upper abdominal pain were also reported. During clinical trials, 1.0% of patients treated with apremilast reported depression or depressed mood compared with 0.8% treated with placebo.[44] Body weight loss of 5% to 10% was reported in 10% of patients taking apremilast and this was not confined to the patients with the gastrointestinal side effects outlined. No clinically significant changes in laboratory parameters were noted in any of the 3 PALACE trials.[43]

Janus kinase Inhibitors

Kinases such as JAK are intracellular molecules that play a pivotal role in signal transduction of ILs. The Janus family consists of four members: tyrosine protein kinase 2 (TYK2), JAK1, JAK2, and JAK3. These molecules interact with various members of the signal transducers and activators of transcription family to modulate gene transcription downstream of a variety of cell surface cytokine and growth factor receptors.[13] JAKs are associated with the different cytokine receptors, briefly: JAK1 and 3 associate with the IL-2Rg chain (IL-2, -4, -7, -9, -15 and -21), JAK1 and JAK2 associate with the gp130 subunit (IL-6, -11, -33, LIF, OSM, CT-1, CNTF, CLC) and interferon receptors; JAK2 also associates with receptors of erythropoietin, growth hormone, prolactin, and thrombopoietin, whereas TYK2 has been implicated in interferon-α, IL-6, -10, and -12 signaling (**Fig. 1**).[45]

Tofacitinib

Tofacitinib is an oral inhibitor of JAK3, JAK1, and, to a lesser degree, JAK2. Tofacitinib was evaluated in psoriasis phase II studies.[46,47] One hundred ninety-seven patients were included.[46] At week 12, PASI 75 response rates were significantly higher for all tofacitinib twice-daily groups: 25.0% (2 mg; P<.001), 40.8% (5 mg; P<.0001), and 66.7% (15 mg; P<.0001) compared with placebo (2.0%).[46] Significant increases in the proportion of PASI 75 responses was observed by week 4 and were maintained

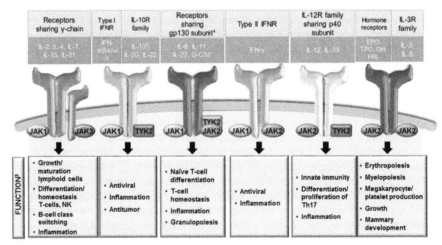

Fig. 1. The biologic significance of signaling through different Janus kinase (JAK) combinations. [a] Type II cytokine receptors such as those for interleukin (IL)-10, IL-19, IL-20, and IL-22 as well as gp 130 subunit sharing receptors for IL-6 and IL-11 mainly signal through JAK1, but also associate with JAK2 and TYK2.[2] [b] IL-10/IL-22 may have proinflammatory or antiinflammatory activities depending on the cellular environment and/or disease state. EPO, erythropoietin; G-CSF, granulocyte colony stimulating factor; GH, growth hormone; IFN, interferon; IFNR, interferon receptor; NK, natural killer; PRL, prolactin; Th17, T helper 17; TPO, thrombopoietin; TYK, tyrosine protein kinase. (*From* Clark JD, Flanagan ME, Telliez JB. Discovery and development of Janus kinase (JAK) inhibitors for inflammatory diseases. J Med Chem 2014;57(12):5023–38; with permission. Copyright © 2014 American Chemical Society.)

at week 12. The most frequently reported adverse effects were upper respiratory tract infection, nasopharyngitis, and headache.[13,46,47] Three unpublished studies examined the efficacy of tofacitinib in PsA: 2 of them (including the open-label extension) are still in progress and one has been completed, and some information is available through www.clinicaltrials.gov. This last study is a phase 3, multisite, randomized, double-blind study of the long-term safety, tolerability, and efficacy of 2 oral doses of tofacitinib in subjects with moderate to severe plaque psoriasis and/or PsA in Japanese population.[48] No controls were included and both doses were not compared among them. Only 12 patients with PsA were included (4 in the 5 mg bid dose and 8 in the 10 mg bid dose). By week 16 (primary outcome), 100%, 83%, and 58% achieved ACR20/50/70 response respectively. This response was achieved by week 52 (open label) in 83%, 75%, and 73% of patients. Owing to the small number of patients and the fact that there was no control group, no conclusions can be drawn at this point in time.

SUMMARY

Traditional DMARDs remain first-line agents for PsA despite a paucity of randomized controlled trial evidence. Although TNFi remain the first choice of biologic treatment for moderate to severe PsA, an unmet need has clearly been identified in those PsA patients who are not suitable, do not tolerate, or do not respond to conventional DMARDs and/or TNFi. Targeted small molecules such as apremilast or tofacitinib may fill a portion of the treatment gap. Apremilast, depending on its cost outside the United States, may be prescribed early in the treatment paradigm although it may not be appropriate recommended after TNFi failure, given the efficacy in that population remains to be established. The TICOPA trial demonstrated that combination therapy combined with a tight control strategy is effective for control of signs and symptoms although the impact on radiographic progression and the safety of this strategy remains to be established. It is important to underscore the fact that PsA often involves numerous domains in a single patient and no convincing data are available to demonstrate that conventional DMARDs are effective for dactylitis, enthesitis, or axial disease. Thus, if these agents are prescribed as monotherapy, they should be restricted to patients with nonerosive peripheral arthritis until further data become available.

The treatment of PsA advanced rapidly over the last several years with the addition of agents that block IL-12 and IL-23 along with agents that effectively target in the IL-17 pathway. It is apparent from these studies, however, that a single agent is not effective for a significant population of PsA patients, particularly the subset that is TNFi nonresponsive. Thus, it is imperative that we gain improved understanding regarding the efficacy and safety of conventional DMARDS and small molecule DMARDs, both as solo agents and in combination regimens for the various domains of PsA. It is anticipated that, as knowledge regarding the physiopathology of psoriatic disease unfolds, additional targets will emerge that will facilitate drug development. The future looks promising for patients who suffer from this debilitating disease.

REFERENCES

1. Soriano ER. The actual role of therapy with traditional disease-modifying antirheumatic drugs in psoriatic arthritis. J Rheumatol Suppl 2012;89:67–70.
2. Helliwell PS, Taylor WJ, Group CS. Treatment of psoriatic arthritis and rheumatoid arthritis with disease modifying drugs – comparison of drugs and adverse reactions. J Rheumatol 2008;35(3):472–6.

3. Soriano ER, McHugh NJ. Therapies for peripheral joint disease in psoriatic arthritis. A systematic review. J Rheumatol 2006;33(7):1422–30.
4. Ravindran V, Scott DL, Choy EH. A systematic review and meta-analysis of efficacy and toxicity of disease modifying anti-rheumatic drugs and biological agents for psoriatic arthritis. Ann Rheum Dis 2008;67(6):855–9.
5. Ash Z, Gaujoux-Viala C, Gossec L, et al. A systematic literature review of drug therapies for the treatment of psoriatic arthritis: current evidence and meta-analysis informing the EULAR recommendations for the management of psoriatic arthritis. Ann Rheum Dis 2012;71(3):319–26.
6. Acosta Felquer ML, Coates LC, Soriano ER, et al. Drug therapies for peripheral joint disease in psoriatic arthritis: a systematic review. J Rheumatol 2014; 41(11):2277–85.
7. Soriano ER. Treatment guidelines for psoriatic arthritis. Int J Clin Rheumatol 2009; 4:329–42.
8. Gossec L, Smolen JS, Gaujoux-Viala C, et al, European League Against Rheumatism. European League Against Rheumatism recommendations for the management of psoriatic arthritis with pharmacological therapies. Ann Rheum Dis 2012; 71(1):4–12.
9. Ramos-Casals M, Diaz-Lagares C, Khamashta MA. Rituximab and lupus: good in real life, bad in controlled trials. Comment on the article by Lu et al. Arthritis Rheum 2009;61(9):1281–2.
10. Rose S, Toloza S, Bautista-Molano W, et al. Comprehensive treatment of dactylitis in psoriatic arthritis. J Rheumatol 2014;41(11):2295–300.
11. Nash P, Lubrano E, Cauli A, et al. Updated guidelines for the management of axial disease in psoriatic arthritis. J Rheumatol 2014;41(11):2286–9.
12. Boehncke WH, Alvarez Martinez D, Solomon JA, et al. Safety and efficacy of therapies for skin symptoms of psoriasis in patients with psoriatic arthritis: a systematic review. J Rheumatol 2014;41(11):2301–5.
13. Hansen RB, Kavanaugh A. Novel treatments with small molecules in psoriatic arthritis. Curr Rheumatol Rep 2014;16(9):443.
14. Mocsai A, Kovacs L, Gergely P. What is the future of targeted therapy in rheumatology: biologics or small molecules? BMC Med 2014;12:43.
15. Scarpa R, Peluso R, Atteno M, et al. The effectiveness of a traditional therapeutical approach in early psoriatic arthritis: results of a pilot randomised 6-month trial with methotrexate. Clin Rheumatol 2008;27(7):823–6.
16. Kingsley GH, Kowalczyk A, Taylor H, et al. A randomized placebo-controlled trial of methotrexate in psoriatic arthritis. Rheumatology 2012;51(8):1368–77.
17. Ceponis A, Kavanaugh A. Use of methotrexate in patients with psoriatic arthritis. Clin Exp Rheumatol 2010;28(5 Suppl 61):S132–7.
18. Chandran V, Schentag CT, Gladman DD. Reappraisal of the effectiveness of methotrexate in psoriatic arthritis: results from a longitudinal observational cohort. J Rheumatol 2008;35(3):469–71.
19. Cantini F, Niccoli L, Nannini C, et al. Frequency and duration of clinical remission in patients with peripheral psoriatic arthritis requiring second-line drugs. Rheumatology 2008;47(6):872–6.
20. Cantini F, Niccoli L, Nannini C, et al. Criteria, frequency, and duration of clinical remission in psoriatic arthritis patients with peripheral involvement requiring second-line drugs. J Rheumatol Suppl 2009;83:78–80.
21. Lie E, van der Heijde D, Uhlig T, et al. Effectiveness and retention rates of methotrexate in psoriatic arthritis in comparison with methotrexate-treated patients with rheumatoid arthritis. Ann Rheum Dis 2010;69(4):671–6.

22. Baranauskaite A, Raffayova H, Kungurov NV, et al, RESPOND investigators. Inflix-imab plus methotrexate is superior to methotrexate alone in the treatment of pso-riatic arthritis in methotrexate-naive patients: the RESPOND study. Ann Rheum Dis 2012;71(4):541–8.

23. Mori Y, Kuwahara Y, Chiba S, et al. Efficacy of methotrexate and tumor necrosis factor inhibitors in Japanese patients with active psoriatic arthritis. Mod Rheuma-tol 2014;25(3):431–4.

24. Taylor WJ, Korendowych E, Nash P, et al. Drug use and toxicity in psoriatic dis-ease: focus on methotrexate. J Rheumatol 2008;35(7):1454–7.

25. Whiting-O'Keefe QE, Fye KH, Sack KD. Methotrexate and histologic hepatic ab-normalities: a meta-analysis. Am J Med 1991;90(6):711–6.

26. Kaltwasser JP, Nash P, Gladman D, et al, Treatment of Psoriatic Arthritis Study Group. Efficacy and safety of leflunomide in the treatment of psoriatic arthritis and psoriasis: a multinational, double-blind, randomized, placebo-controlled clin-ical trial. Arthritis Rheum 2004;50(6):1939–50.

27. Behrens F, Finkenwirth C, Pavelka K, et al. Leflunomide in psoriatic arthritis: re-sults from a large European prospective observational study. Arthritis Care Res 2013;65(3):464–70.

28. Asiri A, Thavaneswaran A, Kalman-Lamb G, et al. The effectiveness of lefluno-mide in psoriatic arthritis. Clin Exp Rheumatol 2014;32(5):728–31.

29. Sakellariou GT, Sayegh FE, Anastasilakis AD, et al. Leflunomide addition in pa-tients with articular manifestations of psoriatic arthritis resistant to methotrexate. Rheumatol Int 2013;33(11):2917–20.

30. Rahman P, Gladman DD, Cook RJ, et al. The use of sulfasalazine in psoriatic arthritis: a clinic experience. J Rheumatol 1998;25(10):1957–61.

31. Clegg DO, Reda DJ, Mejias E, et al. Comparison of sulfasalazine and placebo in the treatment of psoriatic arthritis. A Department of Veterans Affairs Cooperative Study. Arthritis Rheum 1996;39(12):2013–20.

32. Paccou J, Wendling D. Current treatment of psoriatic arthritis: update based on a systematic literature review to establish French Society for Rheumatology (SFR) rec-ommendations for managing spondyloarthritis. Joint Bone Spine 2014;82(2):80–5.

33. Kristensen LE, Gulfe A, Saxne T, et al. Efficacy and tolerability of anti-tumour ne-crosis factor therapy in psoriatic arthritis patients: results from the South Swedish Arthritis Treatment Group register. Ann Rheum Dis 2008;67(3):364–9.

34. Glintborg B, Ostergaard M, Dreyer L, et al. Treatment response, drug survival, and predictors thereof in 764 patients with psoriatic arthritis treated with anti-tumor necrosis factor alpha therapy: results from the nationwide Danish DANBIO registry. Arthritis Rheum 2011;63(2):382–90.

35. Fagerli KM, Lie E, van der Heijde D, et al. The role of methotrexate co-medication in TNF-inhibitor treatment in patients with psoriatic arthritis: results from 440 pa-tients included in the NOR-DMARD study. Ann Rheum Dis 2013;73(1):132–7.

36. Coates LC, Navarro-Coy N, Brown SR, et al. The TICOPA protocol (TIght COntrol of Psoriatic Arthritis): a randomised controlled trial to compare intensive manage-ment versus standard care in early psoriatic arthritis. BMC Musculoskelet Disord 2013;14:101.

37. Smolen JS, van der Heijde D, Machold KP, et al. Proposal for a new nomenclature of disease-modifying antirheumatic drugs. Ann Rheum Dis 2014;73(1):3–5.

38. Schafer P. Apremilast mechanism of action and application to psoriasis and pso-riatic arthritis. Biochem Pharmacol 2012;83(12):1583–90.

39. Cutolo MM, Fleischmann R, Liote F, et al. Long-term (52-week) results of a phase 3, randomized, controlled trial of apremilast, an oral phosphodiesterase 4

inhibitor, in patients with psoriatic arthritis (PALACE 2). Arthritis Rheum 2013; 65(Suppl):S346.

40. Kavanaugh A, Mease PJ, Gomez-Reino JJ, et al. Treatment of psoriatic arthritis in a phase 3 randomised, placebo-controlled trial with apremilast, an oral phospho-diesterase 4 inhibitor. Ann Rheum Dis 2014;73(6):1020–6.

41. Schett G, Wollenhaupt J, Papp K, et al. Oral apremilast in the treatment of active psoriatic arthritis: results of a multicenter, randomized, double-blind, placebo-controlled study. Arthritis Rheum 2012;64(10):3156–67.

42. Wells A, Adebajo AO, Aelion AJ, et al. Apremilast, an Oral Phosphodiesterase 4 Inhibitor, Is Associated with Long-Term (52-Week) Improvement in the Signs and Symptoms of Psoriatic Arthritis in DMARD-Naive Patients: Results from a Phase 3, Randomized, Controlled Trial. Arthritis Rheum 2014;66(Suppl):S680.

43. Mease P, Kavanaugh A, Adebajo AO, et al. Laboratory abnormalities in patients with psoriatic arthritis receiving apremilast, an oral phosphodiesterase 4 inhibitor: pooled safety analysis of three phase 3, randomized, controlled trials. Arthritis Rheum 2013;65(Suppl):S151.

44. Mease P, Kavanaugh J, Gladman DD, et al. Long-term safety and tolerability of apremilast, an oral phospho- diesterase 4 inhibitor, in patients with psoriatic arthritis: pooled safety analysis of three Phase 3, randomized, controlled trials. Arthritis Rheum 2013;65(Suppl):S131.

45. Meier FM, McInnes IB. Small-molecule therapeutics in rheumatoid arthritis: scientific rationale, efficacy and safety. Best Pract Res Clin Rheumatol 2014;28(4):605–24.

46. Papp KA, Menter A, Strober B, et al. Efficacy and safety of tofacitinib, an oral Janus kinase inhibitor, in the treatment of psoriasis: a Phase 2b randomized placebo-controlled dose-ranging study. Br J Dermatol 2012;167(3):668–77.

47. Mamolo C, Harness J, Tan H, et al. Tofacitinib (CP-690,550), an oral Janus kinase inhibitor, improves patient-reported outcomes in a phase 2b, randomized, double-blind, placebo-controlled study in patients with moderate-to-severe psoriasis. J Eur Acad Dermatol Venereol 2014;28(2):192–203.

48. A Phase 3, Multi Site, Randomized, Double Blind Study of the Long-Term Safety, Tolerability and Efficacy of 2 Oral Doses of CP 690,550 in Subjects with Moderate to Severe Plaque Psoriasis and/or Psoriatic Arthritis. Available at: https://clinicaltrials.gov/ct2/show/NCT01519089?term=A3921137&rank=1. Accessed August 17, 2015.

49. Willkens RF, Williams HJ, Ward JR, et al. Randomized, double-blind, placebo controlled trial of low-dose pulse methotrexate in psoriatic arthritis. Arthritis Rheum 1984;27(4):376–81.

Biologic Therapy for Psoriatic Arthritis

Philip J. Mease, MD[a,b,]*

KEYWORDS

- Psoriatic arthritis • Psoriasis • Biologics • TNF inhibition • IL-12–23 inhibition
- IL-17 inhibition • IL-23 inhibition

KEY POINTS

- Biologic medicines target specific cells and cytokines in the immunologic pathway of inflammation, inhibiting and modulating proinflammatory processes.
- Tumor necrosis factor (TNF) alpha is a key proinflammatory cytokine that drives inflammation and tissue destruction in autoimmune diseases, including psoriatic arthritis (PsA). Medicines that target and diminish the activity of this cytokine show significant benefit in curtailing arthritis, enthesitis, dactylitis, spondylitis, and skin and nail disease; inhibiting progressive structural damage; and improving function and quality of life.
- TNF inhibitors may not work in all patients and may lose effectiveness over time, partly because of immunogenicity. Agents with different mechanisms of action, including the interleukin (IL)-12/23 inhibitor ustekinumab, IL-17 inhibitors such as secukinumab, ixekizumab, and brodalumab, and potentially other emerging therapies such as abatacept and IL-23 inhibitors, show effectiveness in clinical domains of PsA.
- Adoption of treatment strategies such as treatment early in the course of disease, tight control, and treating to target, and the emerging use of biosimilars to reduce cost of therapy may improve outcomes and broaden availability of these medicines for patients.
- Serious safety issues can arise with biologic therapy, so cost-benefit risk must be weighed in decision making about use of biologic medications.

INTRODUCTION

Biologic therapies are parenteral (administered subcutaneously or intravenously) complex proteins biologically manufactured in mammalian or yeast cell lines that typically function by binding to proinflammatory cytokines or cell receptor sites to diminish

Disclosures: Research grant from, and consultant and/or speaker for AbbVie, Amgen, Biogen Idec, Bristol-Myers Squibb, Celgene, Covagen, Crescendo, Genentech, Janssen, Lilly, Merck, Novartis, Pfizer, and UCB.
[a] Clinical Rheumatology Research, Swedish Medical Center, 601 Broadway, Seattle, WA 98122, USA; [b] University of Washington School of Medicine, 1959 NE Pacific Street, Seattle, WA 98195, USA
* Seattle Rheumatology Associates, 601 Broadway, Suite 600, Seattle, WA 98122.
E-mail address: pmease@philipmease.com

immunologic cell function. Before the introduction of biologic therapy in the late 1990s, therapy for psoriatic arthritis (PsA) consisted primarily of synthetic medicinals such as methotrexate, sulfasalazine, nonsteroidal antiinflammatory medications, along with adjunctive approaches, including physical and occupational therapy.[1,2] Although partially effective, these medicines were not able to achieve low disease activity or remission states and often were not well tolerated. The first biologic therapies approved for the treatment of PsA were the tumor necrosis factor alpha (TNFα) inhibitors.[1,2] These agents have revolutionized the ability to effectively treat all of the clinical manifestations of PsA, including arthritis, enthesitis, dactylitis, spondylitis, skin and nail disease, as well as associated inflammatory bowel disease and uveitis. PsA treatment recommendations developed by international groups such as the Group for Research and Assessment of Psoriasis and Psoriatic Arthritis (GRAPPA) and the European League Against Rheumatism (EULAR) recommend biologic agents as therapy for patients with moderate to severe disease, noting that the biologics are highly effective in all disease domains of PsA, including arthritis, enthesitis, dactylitis, spondylitis, and skin and nail disease.[3,4] Sustained remission or a low disease activity state is now achievable with these agents. With time, effectiveness may diminish and be lost, necessitating cycling between TNFα inhibitors or switching to agents with a different mechanism of action. This article addresses all biologic therapies for PsA, albeit with a greater emphasis on newer therapies.

TUMOR NECROSIS FACTOR INHIBITION

TNFα was one of the first proinflammatory cytokines implicated in the pathogenesis of numerous inflammatory/autoimmune diseases. It is produced by several types of immune cells and activates several key effector cells involved in tissue inflammation and destruction in psoriasis and PsA, including lymphocytes, macrophages, chondroctyes, osteoclasts, and keratinoctyes. Five agents that inhibit TNFα are now US Food and Drug Administration (FDA) approved, including etanercept, infliximab, adalimumab, golimumab, and certolizumab. These agents were first shown to be effective in the treatment of rheumatoid arthritis, and subsequently showed effectiveness in PsA and ankylosing spondylitis (AS). With the exception of etanercept, these agents are monoclonal antibodies with demonstrated effectiveness in inflammatory bowel disease, whereas etanercept has not. Etanercept, infliximab, and adalimumab are approved for the treatment of psoriasis. The effects of these agents in PsA are reviewed later and American College of Rheumatology (ACR) 20/50/70 responses are summarized in **Table 1**.

Table 1
Anti-TNF therapies in PsA: ACR responses

Trial	n	ACR20%		ACR50%		ACR70%	
		Rx	P	Rx	P	Rx	P
Adalimumab[a,10]	315	58	14	36	4	20	1
Certolizumab[a,16]	409	58	24	36	11	25	3
Etanercept[a,6]	205	59	15	38	4	11	0
Golimumab[b,13]	405	52	8	32	3.5	18	0.9
Infliximab[b,9]	200	58	11	36	3	15	1

Abbreviations: Rx, Treatment Arm; P, placebo.
   [a] 12 weeks.
   [b] 14 weeks.

Etanercept

Etanercept is a soluble receptor antibody administered subcutaneously at 50 mg per week. Its efficacy in PsA was first shown in an investigator-initiated trial of 60 patients,[5] later confirmed in a phase 3 trial in 205 patients (see **Table 1**).[6] Dosing in PsA is 50 mg subcutaneously weekly. This anti-TNFα agent was the first to be approved for PsA and was the first of this class to show the ability to inhibit progressive joint damage as measured by serial radiographs of hands and feet.[6] Ability to improve enthesitis and dactylitis with this agent was shown in the PRESTA (Psoriasis Randomized Etanercept Study in Patients with Psoriatic Arthritis) study,[7] an observational study in which the 50-mg weekly regimen was compared with 50 mg twice weekly for 12 weeks followed by 50 mg weekly in patients with moderate to severe arthritis and severe skin disease. The latter regimen is the approved regimen for this agent in psoriasis. Improvement of musculoskeletal domains (arthritis, enthesitis, and dactylitis) was similar between these two dosage regimens. However, skin manifestations of psoriasis were more effectively treated in the initial higher-dose arm of the study. Etanercept can be administered with or without background methotrexate and durability of effectiveness does not seem to be affected by background methotrexate use, implying a lesser tendency to immunogenicity.[8]

Infliximab

Infliximab, an intravenously administered anti-TNFα agent, showed effectiveness in a 200-patient study using 5 mg/kg every 2 months after a loading dose regimen.[9] As with other anti-TNFα agents, the multiple clinical domains of PsA improve significantly, including inhibition of structural damage (see **Table 1**). This agent has murine sequences, and may generate more immunogenicity with subsequent neutralization of effect over time. Thus, although it can be administered without background methotrexate, its efficacy may be more sustained if methotrexate is used concomitantly.[8]

Adalimumab

Adalimumab is a fully human subcutaneously administered anti-TNFα antibody given at a dose of 40 mg every other week. Its efficacy in PsA was established in the Adalimumab Effectiveness in Psoriatic Arthritis Trial (ADEPT) trial of 313 patients (see **Table 1**).[10] Sustained effectiveness has been shown in various PsA clinical domains, including inhibition of structural damage and patient-reported outcomes of function, quality of life, and fatigue, as it has for other anti-TNFα agents.[11] Durability of effectiveness has been shown with or without background methotrexate.[8] Antidrug antibodies have been noted in patients with PsA treated with adalimumab, which may decrease drug levels and effectiveness of the agent, and may be abrogated with concomitant use of methotrexate.[12]

Golimumab

Golimumab is an anti-TNFα antibody with a prolonged half-life, allowing monthly subcutaneous administration, approved for PsA, in 50-mg doses based on a 405-patient study.[13] It is also available in intravenous formulation, although that is only approved for rheumatoid arthritis (RA). Effectiveness in all clinical domains of PsA, including inhibition of structural damage, as well as long-term efficacy through 5 years has been noted[13,14] (see **Table 1**). In RA, 1 study with golimumab showed its efficacy after previous anti-TNF therapy.[15]

Certolizumab

Certolizumab is a unique antibody composed of the Fab portion of an immunoglobulin molecule attached to 2 polyethylene glycol moieties to prolong half-life. It is administered subcutaneously at a dose of 200 mg every 2 weeks or 400 mg every 4 weeks. In the RAPID (RA Prevention of structural Damage)-PsA trial, at 12 and 24 weeks, 405 patients were evaluated with both doses versus placebo, showing statistically significant benefit in ACR responses (see **Table 1**) as well as significant improvement in Disease Activity Score (DAS28), Health Assessment Questionnaire (HAQ)-DI, enthesitis, dactylitis, skin and nail measures, inhibition of radiologic damage progression, as well as improvement in Short Form 36 and work productivity measures.[16] Uniquely, in this study 20% of patients had previously been exposed to anti-TNFα therapy and similar degrees of response were seen in this group compared with anti-TNFα–naïve patients. Safety results were similar to other agents of this class.

COSTIMULATORY BLOCKADE MODULATING T-LYMPHOCYTE FUNCTION
Abatacept

Abatacept is a costimulatory blockade agent that inhibits T-cell activation through second signal inhibition and is approved for RA. A phase 2 study of 170 patients with PsA, using various doses of its intravenous formulation, showed significant improvement of ACR20 response.[17] MRI study of hands or feet at 24 weeks showed improved synovitis, erosion, and osteitis scores. Skin psoriasis responses were low. In patients who had previously taken anti-TNF agents, responses in ACR scores were lower than in patients naive to anti-TNF therapy. This agent is now in phase 3 development in its subcutaneous form in PsA.

INTERLEUKIN-6 INHIBITION

Like TNFα, interleukin (IL)-6 is a pleiotropic proinflammatory cytokine that has a significant role in RA and has been shown to be at increased levels in psoriasis skin lesions and PsA synovium.[18] Tocilizumab is an IL-6 receptor blocker approved for RA. There have been mixed results from case reports about its efficacy in PsA.[19]

Clazakizumab

Clazakizumab is a direct IL-6 inhibitor that has shown efficacy in RA.[20] This agent was studied in a phase 2 dose ranging trial with 165 patients with PsA, 70% of whom were on background methotrexate.[21] ACR20 response was observed in 29%, 46%, 52%, and 39% of patients in the placebo, 25-mg, 100-mg, and 200-mg monthly groups, respectively, at the week 16 primary end point, which was statistically significant in the 100-mg group. A reduction of 75% in the Psoriasis Area and Severity Index (PASI75) responses were observed in 12%, 15%, 17%, and 5% of placebo, 25-mg, 100-mg, and 200-mg groups. Improvements in enthesitis and dactylitis were most noted in the 100-mg group. The safety profile was that expected for an IL-6–inhibiting agent. Thus, this trial did show an effect in musculoskeletal inflammation domains, supporting the concept that IL-6 inhibition may be helpful for this set of domains, but it showed minimal effect for treatment of psoriasis lesions. The trial also lacked a true dose effect given the underperformance of the 200-mg group, partly because of the use of nonresponder imputation analysis and a greater number of adverse effects and dropouts in the higher-dose group.

B-LYMPHOCYTE INHIBITION

Rituximab, a B-lymphocyte ablating agent, has been approved for the treatment of RA and vasculitis. In RA, B lymphocytes play a prominent role and subsets of patients with RA have significant B-cell aggregation in synovial tissue, denoting a more severe phenotype. Although some B-cell aggregation has been noted in PsA symovium,[22] in general B cells are not considered to be important players in psoriasis or PsA pathogenesis. Small series of patients have been treated with rituximab[23,24] and, in general, although modest efficacy in arthritis has been shown in such open-label use, not enough efficacy has been shown in joints or psoriasis skin lesions to lead to placebo-controlled studies of this agent in PsA.

TARGETING THE T-HELPER 17 CELL AXIS IN PSORIATIC ARTHRITIS

The cytokine IL-17A was discovered in 1993.[25] Since then, a family of related cytokines, IL-17A-F, has been characterized, which led to the discovery, in 2005, of a distinct form of T cells, T-helper (TH) 17, distinguished by their ability to produce a distinct repertoire of cytokines, including IL-17s, IL-21, and IL-22, and not interferon-gamma (IFN γ) or IL-4, which are reflective of TH1 and TH2 lineage cells[26–28] (**Fig. 1**). Since then, new discoveries regarding the functional and immunologic significance of this T-cell lineage have been published, including front-line antimicrobial defense via the innate immune response as well as a prominent role in several immunologic diseases, such as psoriasis; the spondyloarthritides, including PsA and axial spondyloarthritis; inflammatory bowel disease (IBD); and RA.

TH17 cell differentiation is induced by IL-1β plus IL-23, and possibly transforming growth factor beta, in the presence of inflammatory cytokines such as IL-6, IL-21, and IL-23.[26] Human TH17 cells produce IL-17A through IL-17F, IL-22, IL-26, and the chemokine CCL20. IL-17A is more potent than IL-17F, IL-17E (also known as IL-25) is involved in TH2 responses, and IL-17B, IL-17C, and IL-17D are less well characterized in terms of their biological significance.[26] In the quiescent state, IL-17A and F are primarily observed in spleen and small intestine lamina propria cells. In inflammatory states, activated T cells, particularly TH17 cells, are the main producers of both isoforms of IL-17, but CD8+, natural killer T cells, gamma and delta T cells, neutrophils, myeloid cells, and type 3 innate lymphoid cells may synthesize and release these cytokines.[28]

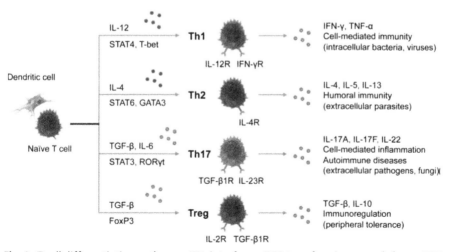

Fig. 1. T-cell differentiation pathways. IFN, interferon; TGF, transforming growth factor; TNF, tumor necrosis factor; T_reg, T regulatory cell. (*From* Patel DD, Lee DM, Kolbinger F, et al. Effect of IL-17A blockade with secukinumab in autoimmune diseases. Ann Rheum Dis 2013;72(Suppl 2):ii116–23; with permission.)

The IL-17 receptor is broadly expressed in the immune cell pathway by a wide array of cell types, including endothelium, epithelium, fibroblasts, keratinocytes, osteoblasts, monocytes, and macrophages.[28] In a pioneering murine study, Sherlock and colleagues[29] found that IL-23 encased in minicircles preferentially gravitated to entheseal insertion sites and the aortic root, where a local inflammatory reaction occurred involving a unique group of resident lymphocytes (CD3+CD-CD8-ROR-γt+IL-23R+). The enthesitis inflammatory response was primarily driven by IL-17 produced by these cells, whereas IL-22 expression activated signal transducer and activator of transcription 3 (STAT3)-dependent osteoblast-mediated bone remodeling. Lories and McInnes[30] subsequently proposed the model that, in humans, a variety of factors such as microbial antigens, alterations in the gut microbiome, the human leukocyte antigen (HLA)-B27 unfolded protein response, and biomechanical stress may lead to expression of IL-23 (Fig. 2). IL-23 then incites differentiation and activation of specific populations of T cells, including TH17 cells, which in turn produce cytokines such as IL-17 and IL-22, with IL-17 driving an inflammatory response that may result in such consequences as bone erosion, in addition to clinical features such as inflammation in synovium and skin, whereas IL-22 may, among other inflammatory activities, lead to osteoproliferation, as is seen in the periostitis and ankylosis of PsA and ankylosis of AS. Such a model could help explain why both osteolysis and osteoproliferation, seemingly opposite processes, are both seen in parallel in the spondyloarthritis conditions, including PsA. This model also posits a greater role for the innate immune system relative to the adaptive immune system, distinct from some other autoimmune diseases, such as RA.

Numerous studies have shown that IL-23, IL-17, and IL-22 are richly expressed in the psoriatic skin lesions and the synovium of patients with PsA, and participate in the pathophysiologic aspects of these diseases, including hyperproliferation of keratinocytes and promotion of synovitis.[28,31–34] Inhibition of key cytokines in this pathway, including IL-23 and IL-17, results in clinical improvement in diseases such as psoriasis and the spondyloarthritides, as discussed later.

INTERLEUKIN-12 TO INTERLEUKIN-23 INHIBITORS
Ustekinumab

Ustekinumab is a fully human monoclonal immunoglobulin (Ig) G1 antibody that binds to the common p40 subunit of IL-12 and IL-23, thus inhibiting their activity and,

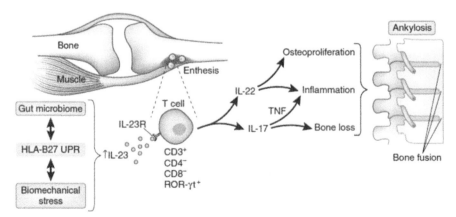

Fig. 2. IL-23 and resident T cells promote enthesitis and osteoproliferation. HLA, human leukocyte antigen; UPR, unfolded protein response. (*From* Lories RJ, McInnes IB. Primed for inflammation: enthesis-resident T cells. Nat Med 2012;18(7):1018–9; with permission.)

presumably, the T-cell pathways that they influence: TH1 and TH17 respectively. Ustekinumab is now approved by the FDA for the treatment of psoriasis and PsA in a weight-based regimen: 45 mg for patients less than 100 kg and 90 mg for those who are heavier. The drug is administered subcutaneously at baseline, at 4 weeks, then every 12 weeks thereafter.

Ustekinumab was assessed in 2 phase 3 trials in psoriasis. In the first study, 766 patients treated with 45 mg, 90 mg, or placebo achieved PASI75 responses of 67.1%, 66.4%, and 3.1% respectively at the primary end point of 12 weeks.[35] In the second study, PASI75 responses in the 1230 subjects were 66.7%, 75.7%, and 3.7% in the 45-mg, 90-mg, and placebo arms respectively.[36] Other key measures of response, including nail disease and quality of life, also showed significant improvement. No major serious side effect issues emerged in these trials.

Ustekinumab was assessed in 2 phase 3 trials in PsA. In PSUMMIT 1, 615 patients who had inadequate response to methotrexate were randomized to receive 45 or 90 mg of ustekinumab versus placebo.[37] Ustekinumab was given at week 0, 4, and every 12 weeks thereafter subcutaneously. At the primary end point, week 24, 42.4% and 49.5% of the patients treated with 45 and 90 mg achieved ACR20 response compared with 22.8% of placebo-treated patients, which was statistically significant. Other key measures of enthesitis, dactylitis, skin and nail disease, function, and quality of life also improved. Similar rates of adverse events were noted between the groups and there were no opportunistic infections or major cardiovascular events. PSUMMIT 2 was similar in design but 55% to 60% of the subjects had prior exposure to 1 or more anti-TNF agents.[38] ACR20 response was observed in 43.7%, 43.8%, and 20.2% of the patients treated with 45 mg, 90 mg, and placebo in the overall population, and 36.7%, 34.5%, and 14.5% of the anti-TNF–experienced population. In a separate report in which radiographic data from the two trials were pooled, inhibition of structural damage was observed, although this benefit was driven by the methotrexate-inadequate response population from PSUMMIT 1 rather than the subjects from PSUMMIT 2 who had previously been exposed to anti-TNF therapy.[39]

It is anticipated that development of this drug for the treatment of AS/axial spondyloarthritis will occur based on promising results from an open-label trial in ankylosing spondylitis.[40] There are no published data for ustekinumab in RA.

INTERLEUKIN-17 INHIBITORS

Two IL-17 inhibitors, secukinumab and ixekizumab, are in development and/or are approved for the treatment of psoriasis, PsA, and axial spondyloarthritis/AS, as well as other conditions (secukinumab, ixekizumab). A third agent, an IL-17 receptor inhibitor, brodalumab, has also shown effectiveness in psoriasis and PsA, but its further development, at the time of this writing, is uncertain, as discussed later.

Secukinumab

Secukinumab is a human monoclonal IgG1k antibody that targets IL-17A, which has recently gained FDA approval for psoriasis. Two phase 3, 52-week trials, ERASURE (Efficacy of Response and Safety of Two Fixed Secukinumab Regimens in Psoriasis) and FIXTURE (Full-Year Investigative Examination of Secukinumab vs Etanercept Using Two Dosing Regimens to Determine Efficacy in Psoriasis). In ERASURE, 738 patients and, in FIXTURE, 1306 patients were randomized to subcutaneous secukinumab at doses of 300 mg or 150 mg administered once weekly for 5 weeks then every 4 weeks thereafter, versus placebo.[41] In the ERASURE study, PASI75 was met at week 12 by 81.6%, 71.6%, and 4.5% with 300 mg, 150 mg, and placebo respectively. PASI90 was met by 59.2%, 39.1%, and 1.2% respectively. In the FIXTURE study, PASI75 was met by 77.1%, 67.0%, 44%, and 4.9% with 300 and 150 mg of secukinumab, etanercept 50 mg twice weekly, and placebo respectively. PASI90 was met by 54.2%, 41.9%, 20.7%, and 1.5% respectively. All responses statistically separated from placebo. Improvements in nail disease, itch, and quality of life were also significant. Serious adverse events were infrequent and similar in frequency across all groups. There were no deaths. Rates of infections were similar across all 3 treatment arms, including etanercept, and were numerically greater than in the placebo arm. Candida infections, of specific interest because of the potential for IL-17 inhibition to increase the rate of these infections, occurred in a mild to moderate form in 4.7% of the 300-mg and 2.35% of the 150-mg secukinumab groups, and 1.2% in the etanercept group, half of which were considered severe in the FIXTURE study. Grade 3 neutropenia occurred in 9 patients (1.0%) in all secukinumab groups and none in the etanercept or placebo groups. Rates for these adverse events were similar between the two studies.

Two phase 3 trials in PsA were recently reported.[42,43] FUTURE 1 enrolled 606 patients who were randomized to an intravenous loading dose of secukinumab, 10 mg/kg at baseline, week 2, and week 4, and then either 150 mg or 75 mg every 4 weeks from week 8 versus placebo. Thirty percent had received prior anti-TNF therapy and 60% were on concomitant methotrexate, randomized equally. At 24 weeks, the 150-mg dose arm showed 50.0%, 34.7%, and 18.8% ACR20/50/70 responses, whereas the 75-mg arm showed 50.5%, 30.7%, and 16.8% responses, and the placebo arm 17.3%, 7.4%, and 2.0% responses respectively. Key secondary measures of enthesitis, dactylitis, skin disease, radiographic evidence of inhibition of progression, function, and quality of life all separated statistically from placebo in the treatment arms compared with placebo. FUTURE 2[44] enrolled 397 patients to receive subcutaneous secukinumab 300 mg, 150 mg, 75 mg, and placebo at weeks 1, 2, 3, 4, and every 4 weeks thereafter. Thirty-five percent had received previous anti-TNF therapy. ACR, enthesitis, dactylitis, skin, function, and quality of life responses were similar to those seen in FUTURE 1. However, analysis of the TNF inadequate response subgroup showed lower responses in the 75-mg and 150-mg groups compared with the 300-mg group. Overall serious adverse events were few and similar in frequency between the treatment and placebo arms through week 16 in both studies. In FUTURE 1, overall infection rate was slightly greater in the secukinumab arm than in the placebo arm; there were no opportunistic infections, including tuberculosis.

Two phase 3 trials in AS have been recently reported as well. In MEASURE 1, 371 patients with AS were randomized to receive secukinumab 75 or 150 mg subcutaneously every 4 weeks after a loading dose of 10 mg/kg weekly for 4 weeks or placebo. At 16 weeks, the Assessment of SpondyloArthritis international Society (ASAS20) responses were 59.7%, 60.8%, and 28.7% respectively.[45] In MEASURE 2, subjects received either 75-mg or 150-mg secukinumab subcutaneously weekly for 4 weeks followed by this dose every 4 weeks or placebo. ASAS20 responses were 41.1%, 61.1%, and 28.4% respectively.[46] Other key measures, such as ASAS40, ASAS partial remission, and function measures, also improved. No new safety issues emerged.

Results with secukinumab in RA have not been as robust. In a phase 2 trial in 237 patients with RA with an inadequate response to methotrexate, subjects receiving 25, 75, 150, and 300 mg of secukinumab showed 36.0% to 53.7% ACR20 response versus 34% in the placebo group; no dose arm statistically separated from placebo.[13] In contrast, it was noted that the continuous measure, DAS28, did show statistical separation, as did high-sensitivity C-reactive protein (CRP) level reduction.

Ixekizumab

Another IL-17A inhibitor, ixekizumab, is in development for psoriasis and PsA. In a phase 2 study of 142 subjects with psoriasis, at 12 weeks, PASI75 responses in those treated with 25, 75, or 150 mg of ixekizumab at weeks 0, 2, 4, 8, and 12 were 76.7%, 82.8%, and 82.1% respectively compared with 7.7% in the placebo arm.[47] A 10-mg dose arm did not achieve statistical significance. In the highest 2 dose groups, 150 mg and 75 mg, PASI100 response was noted in 39.3% and 37.3% respectively. Separation from placebo was seen as early as 1 week. No new safety issues were noted compared with the secukinumab data, thus this agent seems to have overall similar good effect in psoriasis. A phase 3 trial program in PsA is being conducted and results are pending.

Ixekizumab has been studied in a phase 2 study in RA.[48] In this trial, 260 biologic-naive patients and 188 patients with inadequate response to anti-TNF therapy were studied. Subcutaneous doses of 3, 10, 30, 80, and 180 mg of ixekizumab versus placebo were studied in the former group and 80 or 180 mg versus placebo in the latter group. At week 12 in the biologic-naive group, ACR20 responses of 45%, 43%, 70%, 51%, and 54% were seen in the 5 different drug doses versus placebo response of 35%. Of these, only the 30-mg response, seen in 70%, achieved statistical signifi-cance. In the anti-TNF inadequate response group, ACR20 responses of 40% and 39% were seen versus placebo response of 23%. These values were statistically sig-nificant. As was seen in the secukinumab RA study, significant response was seen in DAS28 improvement and CRP reduction, thus supporting the concept that there was some treatment effect of the agent even though a true dose response was not seen and most doses failed to achieve statistically significant ACR20 response. No new safety signals were seen. It is not clear whether ixekizumab or secukinumab will undergo additional evaluation in phase III RA clinical trials.

Brodalumab

Brodalumab is a fully human monoclonal antibody that blocks the IL-17A receptor. Because this receptor joins with other IL-17R subunits to form the receptor complex for IL-17A to IL-17-F, it has the capability to broadly block IL-17 signaling. As in the trials of the direct IL-17A inhibitors, brodalumab has shown significant efficacy in psoriasis. In a phase 2 study, 198 patients receiving 70, 140, 210, and 280 mg of brodalumab subcutaneously experienced PASI75 responses of 45%, 85.9%, 86.3%, and 76% compared with 16% of those receiving placebo at 12 weeks.[49] PASI100 responses were observed in 38% and 62% of the 140-mg and 210-mg doses. Grade 3 neutropenia was observed in 2 cases, resolved with drug withdrawal, and did not result in infection. Cases of suicidal ideation and suicide were noted in the psoriasis trials. Although it is known that there is a higher rate of depression and suicidality in patients with psoriasis than in the general population, the rate of this problem in the brodalumab program was such that the future development of this agent is in question at the time of this writing.

A phase 2 study in 168 patients with PsA has been conducted with brodalumab.[50] At the prespecified 12-week primary end point, ACR20 response was experienced by 37% and 39% of subjects treated with 140 and 280 mg versus 18% in the placebo group, which was statistically superior for both treatment arms. As these same patients continued into open-label use of brodalumab on these same doses, ACR20 responses were observed in 51% and 64% respectively of the patients treated with 140 and 280 mg. As a result of this observation, the primary end point in the phase 3 program will be extended beyond 12 weeks, because it seemed that, in multiple clinical domains, responses were still increasing at that point in time. During the open-label extension, 2 events of grade 2 neutropenia occurred.

Brodalumab has also been studied in RA. In a phase 1B ascending dose study in 40 subjects with RA, statistical separation of brodalumab-treated subjects versus placebo was not showed, a finding mirrored in phase 2 study in patients with RA who had had an inadequate response to methotrexate therapy.[51,52]

Brodalumab and the direct IL-17 inhibitors will not be studied in IBD. Pilot work suggests that there is no benefit for this disease and there could possibly be a signal of potential flare of IBD with IL-17 inhibition, which is a caution.

INTERLEUKIN-23 INHIBITORS

As previously discussed, IL-23 is a key cytokine involved in the differentiation and proliferation of TH17 cells, thus acting upstream from IL-17 expression and potentially capable of inhibiting the production of several different types of cytokines from TH17 cells and other immune cells, including both IL-17 and IL-22. Preliminary results have been reported for 2 IL-23 inhibitors in the treatment of psoriasis and there is contemplation of their development in PsA and axial spondyloarthritis.

Guselkumab

Guselkumab is a human monoclonal antibody directed against the p19 subunit of IL-23. In a phase 1 single ascending-dose study, patient response was evaluated at 12 weeks after single doses of 10, 30, 100, or 300 mg of guselkumab.[53] PASI75 responses were shown in 50%, 60%, 60%, and 100% respectively compared with 0% in the placebo group. Adverse effect frequency was similar between the treatment and placebo groups.

Tildrakizumab

Tildrakizumab is a humanized IgG1/x antibody targeting the p19 subunit of IL-23. A phase 2 study was reported at the American Academy of Dermatology in 2013. In 355 patients at 12 weeks, PASI75 response was reported in 33%, 64%, 66%, and 74% of patients receiving 5, 25, 100, and 200 mg of tildrakizumab versus 2% of patients receiving placebo. A low rate of adverse effects was noted.[54,55]

THERAPEUTIC STRATEGIES WITH BIOLOGIC THERAPY
Early Treatment

In an open-label trial of methotrexate versus methotrexate plus infliximab in early treatment-naive patients with PsA, the RESPOND (Remicade Study in Psoriatic Arthritis Patients Of Methotrexate-Naïve Disease) trial, significantly higher ACR and PASI responses were noted in the combination group.[56] A more substantial controlled trial is now initiating, which will compare clinical and radiographic outcomes in patients with early PsA randomized to methotrexate alone, anti-TNFα biologic alone, and combination of the two. This trial should provide a better understanding of the potential value of monotherapy versus combination treatment in the treatment of early PsA.

Avoidance of Immunogenicity

Because biologic agents are therapeutic proteins with varying degrees of foreignness to the human body, it is theoretically possible that antibodies to the therapeutic protein may be formed and have a potential effect of neutralizing or diminishing therapeutic efficacy. This effect has generally been seen most frequently with the chimeric antibody, infliximab, and with lesser frequencies with the human or humanized antibody constructs. Some observational registries have shown decreased durability of anti-TNFα agents, presumably partly because of diminished efficacy with time, when prescribed as monotherapy versus combination with methotrexate. One explanation for this observation is that methotrexate may diminish immunogenicity, thereby lessening the likelihood of losing clinical response. The development of antidrug antibodies has most commonly been observed with infliximab and is lowest with etanercept, of the 3 agents most studied in these registries (infliximab, adalimumab, and etanercept).[8,57] Consideration should be given to the use of methotrexate to limit immunogenicity for selected anti-TNF agents.

Treating to Target

An evolving paradigm of RA treatment is that a combination of tight-control and treat-to-target strategies (seeing patients frequently and trying to achieve a quantitative target of low disease activity or remission) yields better long-term disease control and clinical, functional, and radiologic outcomes.[58,59] Although it has been assumed that a similar beneficial outcome would be seen in PsA,[60] this had not been studied formally until the recent TICOPA (TIght COntrol of Psoriatic Arthritis) trial.[61] When such a strategy was used in PsA, comparing a tight control arm aiming for minimal disease activity criteria,[62] there were significantly improved ACR and PASI response outcomes in the tight-control versus Standard-care arms.[61] However, there were more serious adverse events and greater financial costs caused by greater combination and biologic therapy use in the tight-control group.

Cost

Biologic therapy is expensive because of complex manufacturing processes and the cost of development. These therapies are out of reach for many people in the world because of high and increasing costs. In the future, forces that may bring cost down and make these agents affordable for more people globally include competition, as more products become available, and the introduction of biosimilar agents that closely mimic the pharmacokinetic properties of the innovator compound and that have been shown in clinical trials to yield results similar to the original innovator trials. It is important for these market forces, as well as humanitarian considerations, to make these therapies more affordable to address inequalities of access for patients in need in many parts of the world. Although rules of regulatory agencies are still evolving, it seems that, if a biosimilar agent is effective in a disease such as RA, then it will be approved, with some possible exceptions, for other indications for which the innovator is approved, including PsA.

SUMMARY

The treatment of PsA has been transformed in the last decade and a half by the introduction and use of biologic medications, therapeutic proteins that inhibit and modulate the effects of proinflammatory immune cells and cytokines. For most of this time, agents that inhibit the key cytokine TNFα have taken center stage because they consistently improve all key clinical domains of PsA, including arthritis, enthesitis, dactylitis, spondylitis, and skin and nail disease inhibit progressive joint damage; and improve function, quality of life, and fatigue. Serious side effects can occur, particularly infections, so balanced risk-benefit discussion with each patient is essential to minimize adverse events. As part of the discussion, note that the medicine may have no effect or may yield side effects that do not allow continuation of use, and, in a greater number, loss of efficacy occurs gradually with time. The reduction in efficacy may partly be caused by immunogenicity, which may require concomitant use of methotrexate or leflunomide. In the setting of nonresponse, either primary or secondary, the traditional approach is to cycle between agents; either to another anti-TNFα agent or to an emerging suite of biologics with a different mode of action, such as the IL-12/II-23 inhibitor, ustekinumab. More recently, the IL-17 inhibitors have shown significant promise in PsA in clinical trials. Although they are not yet approved for use in PsA, it is anticipated that such approvals will be forthcoming, and one agent, secukinumab, is approved for the treatment of psoriasis. As the understanding of the pathophysiology of PsA increases, it is clear that new targets of treatment will be revealed and new biologic strategies will be developed and added to the therapeutic armamentarium for PsA.

ACKNOWLEDGMENTS

The author thanks Catherine Loeffler, for assistance with article preparation.

REFERENCES

1. Mease PJ, Armstrong AW. Managing patients with psoriatic disease: the diagnosis and pharmacologic treatment of psoriatic arthritis in patients with psoriasis. Drugs 2014;74(4):423–41.
2. Acosta Felquer ML, Coates LC, Soriano ER, et al. Drug therapies for peripheral joint disease in psoriatic arthritis: a systematic review. J Rheumatol 2014;41(11): 2277–85.
3. Ritchlin CT, Kavanaugh A, Mease PJ, et al. Treatment recommendations for psoriatic arthritis. Ann Rheum Dis 2009;68(9):1387–94.
4. Gossec L, Smolen JS, Gaujoux-Viala C, et al. European league against rheumatism recommendations for the management of psoriatic arthritis with pharmacological therapies. Ann Rheum Dis 2012;71(1):4–12.
5. Mease PJ, Goffe BS, Metz J, et al. Etanercept in the treatment of psoriatic arthritis and psoriasis: a randomised trial. Lancet 2000;356(9227):385–90.
6. Mease PJ, Kivitz AJ, Burch FX, et al. Etanercept treatment of psoriatic arthritis: safety, efficacy, and effect on disease progression. Arthritis Rheum 2004;50(7): 2264–72.
7. Sterry W, Ortonne JP, Kirkham B, et al. Comparison of two etanercept regimens for treatment of psoriasis and psoriatic arthritis: PRESTA randomised double blind multicentre trial. BMJ 2010;340:c147.
8. Fagerli KM, Lie E, van der Heijde D, et al. The role of methotrexate co-medication in TNF-inhibitor treatment in patients with psoriatic arthritis: results from 440 patients included in the NOR-DMARD study. Ann Rheum Dis 2014;73(1):132–7.
9. Antoni C, Krueger GG, de Vlam K, et al. Infliximab improves signs and symptoms of psoriatic arthritis: results of the IMPACT 2 trial. Ann Rheum Dis 2005;64(8): 1150–7.
10. Mease PJ, Gladman DD, Ritchlin CT, et al. Adalimumab for the treatment of patients with moderately to severely active psoriatic arthritis: results of a double-blind, randomized, placebo-controlled trial. Arthritis Rheum 2005; 52(10):3279–89.
11. Mease PJ, Ory P, Sharp JT, et al. Adalimumab for long-term treatment of psoriatic arthritis: 2-year data from the Adalimumab Effectiveness in Psoriatic Arthritis Trial (ADEPT). Ann Rheum Dis 2009;68(5):702–9.
12. Vogelzang EH, Kneepkens EL, Nurmohamed MT, et al. Anti-adalimumab antibodies and adalimumab concentrations in psoriatic arthritis; an association

with disease activity at 28 and 52 weeks of follow-up. Ann Rheum Dis 2014; 73(12):2178–82.

13. Kavanaugh A, McInnes I, Mease P, et al. Golimumab, a new human tumor necrosis factor alpha antibody, administered every four weeks as a subcutaneous injection in psoriatic arthritis: Twenty-four-week efficacy and safety results of a randomized, placebo-controlled study. Arthritis Rheum 2009;60(4):976–86.

14. Kavanaugh A, van der Heijde D, Beutler A, et al. Patients with psoriatic arthritis who achieve minimal disease activity in response to golimumab therapy demonstrate less radiographic progression: Results through 5 years of the randomized, placebo-controlled, GO-REVEAL study. Arthritis Care Res (Hoboken) 2015. [Epub ahead of print].

15. Smolen JS, Kay J, Doyle MK, et al. Golimumab in Patients with Active Rheumatoid Arthritis After Treatment with Tumour Necrosis Factor Alpha Inhibitors (GO-AFTER study): a multicentre, randomised, double-blind, placebo-controlled, phase III trial. Lancet 2009;374(9685):210–21.

16. Mease PJ, Fleischmann R, Deodhar AA, et al. Effect of certolizumab pegol on signs and symptoms in patients with psoriatic arthritis: 24-week results of a phase 3 double-blind randomised placebo-controlled study (RAPID-PsA). Ann Rheum Dis 2014;73(1):48–55.

17. Mease P, Genovese MC, Gladstein G, et al. Abatacept in the treatment of patients with psoriatic arthritis: results of a six-month, multicenter, randomized, double-blind, placebo-controlled, phase II trial. Arthritis Rheum 2011;63(4): 939–48.

18. Fonseca JE, Santos MJ, Canhao H, et al. Interleukin-6 as a key player in systemic inflammation and joint destruction. Autoimmun Rev 2009;8(7):538–42.

19. Costa L, Caso F, Cantarini L, et al. Efficacy of tocilizumab in a patient with refractory psoriatic arthritis. Clin Rheumatol 2014;33(9):1355–7.

20. Mease P, Strand V, Shalamberidze L, et al. A phase II, double-blind, randomised, placebo-controlled study of BMS945429 (ALD518) in patients with rheumatoid arthritis with an inadequate response to methotrexate. Ann Rheum Dis 2012; 71(7):1183–9.

21. Mease PJ, Gottlieb A, Berman A, et al. A phase IIb, randomized, double-blind, placebo-controlled, dose-ranging, multicenter study to evaluate the efficacy and safety of clazakizumab, an anti-IL-6 monoclonal antibody, in adults with active psoriatic arthritis. Arthritis Rheum 2014;66(S10):S423 [abstract: 952].

22. Celis R, Planell N, Fernandez-Sueiro JL, et al. Synovial cytokine expression in psoriatic arthritis and associations with lymphoid neogenesis and clinical features. Arthritis Res Ther 2012;14(2):R93.

23. Mease PJ. Is there a role for rituximab in the treatment of spondyloarthritis and psoriatic arthritis? J Rheumatol 2012;39(12):2235–7.

24. Mease P, Kavanaugh A, Genovese M, et al. Rituximab in psoriatic arthritis provides modest clinical improvement and reduces expression of inflammatory biomarkers in skin lesions. Arthritis Rheum 2010;62(10 (Supp)):S818.

25. Rouvier E, Luciani MF, Mattei MG, et al. CTLA-8, cloned from an activated T cell, bearing AU-rich messenger RNA instability sequences, and homologous to a herpesvirus saimiri gene. J Immunol 1993;150(12):5445–56.

26. van den Berg WB, McInnes IB. Th17 cells and IL-17 a–focus on immunopathogenesis and immunotherapeutics. Semin Arthritis Rheum 2013;43(2): 158–70.

27. Miossec P, Korn T, Kuchroo VK. Interleukin-17 and type 17 helper T cells. N Engl J Med 2009;361(9):888–98.

28. Frleta M, Siebert S, McInnes IB. The interleukin-17 pathway in psoriasis and psoriatic arthritis: disease pathogenesis and possibilities of treatment. Curr Rheumatol Rep 2014;16(4):414.

29. Sherlock JP, Joyce-Shaikh B, Turner SP, et al. IL-23 induces spondyloarthropathy by acting on ROR-γt+ CD3+CD4-CD8- entheseal resident T cells. Nat Med 2012; 18(7):1069–76.

30. Lories RJ, McInnes IB. Primed for inflammation: enthesis-resident T cells. Nat Med 2012;18(7):1018–9.

31. Nestle FO, Kaplan DH, Barker J. Psoriasis. N Engl J Med 2009;361(5):496–509.

32. Raychaudhuri SP. Role of IL-17 in psoriasis and psoriatic arthritis. Clin Rev Allergy Immunol 2013;44(2):183–93.

33. Jandus C, Bioley G, Rivals JP, et al. Increased numbers of circulating polyfunctional Th17 memory cells in patients with seronegative spondylarthritides. Arthritis Rheum 2008;58(8):2307–17.

34. Suzuki E, Mellins ED, Gershwin ME, et al. The IL-23/IL-17 axis in psoriatic arthritis. Autoimmun Rev 2014;13(4–5):496–502.

35. Leonardi CL, Kimball AB, Papp KA, et al. Efficacy and safety of ustekinumab, a human interleukin-12/23 monoclonal antibody, in patients with psoriasis: 76-week results from a randomised, double-blind, placebo-controlled trial (PHOENIX 1). Lancet 2008;371(9625):1665–74.

36. Papp KA, Langley RG, Lebwohl M, et al. Efficacy and safety of ustekinumab, a human interleukin-12/23 monoclonal antibody, in patients with psoriasis: 52-week results from a randomised, double-blind, placebo-controlled trial (PHOENIX 2). Lancet 2008;371(9625):1675–84.

37. McInnes IB, Kavanaugh A, Gottlieb AB, et al. Efficacy and safety of ustekinumab in patients with active psoriatic arthritis: 1 year results of the phase 3, multicentre, double-blind, placebo-controlled PSUMMIT 1 trial. Lancet 2013;382(9894): 780–9.

38. Ritchlin C, Rahman P, Kavanaugh A, et al. Efficacy and safety of the anti-IL-12/23 p40 monoclonal antibody, ustekinumab, in patients with active psoriatic arthritis despite conventional non-biological and biological anti-tumour necrosis factor therapy: 6-month and 1-year results of the phase 3, multicentre, double-blind, placebo-controlled, randomised PSUMMIT 2 trial. Ann Rheum Dis 2014;73(6): 990–9.

39. Kavanaugh A, Ritchlin C, Rahman P, et al. Ustekinumab, an anti-IL-12/23 p40 monoclonal antibody, inhibits radiographic progression in patients with active psoriatic arthritis: results of an integrated analysis of radiographic data from the phase 3, multicentre, randomised, double-blind, placebo-controlled PSUMMIT-1 and PSUMMIT-2 trials. Ann Rheum Dis 2014;73(6):1000–6.

40. Podubbnyy D, Callhoff J, Listing J, et al. Ustekinumab for the treatment of patients with active ankylosing spondylitis: results of a 28-week, prospective, open-label, proof-of-concept study (TOPAS). Arthritis Rheum 2013;65(10 (Suppl)):S766.

41. Langley RG, Elewski BE, Lebwohl M, et al. Secukinumab in plaque psoriasis–results of two phase 3 trials. N Engl J Med 2014;371(4):326–38.

42. Mease P, McInnes I, Kirkham B, et al. Secukinumab, a human anti–interleukin-17A monoclonal antibody, improves active psoriatic arthritis and inhibits radiographic progression: efficacy and safety data from a phase 3 randomized, multicenter, double-blind, placebo-controlled study. Arthritis Rheum 2014;66(S10):S423.

43. van der Heijde D, Landewe R, Mease P, et al. Secukinumab, a monoclonal antibody to interleukin-17A, provides significant and sustained inhibition of joint

structural damage in active psoriatic arthritis regardless of prior TNF inhibitors or concomitant methotrexate: a phase 3 randomized, double-blind, placebo-controlled study. Arthritis Rheum 2014;66(S10):S424.

44. McInnes IB, Mease PJ, Kirkham B, et al. Secukinumab, a human anti-interleukin-17A monoclonal antibody, in patients with psoriatic arthritis (FUTURE 2): a randomised, double-blind, placebo-controlled, phase 3 trial. Lancet 2015. [Epub ahead of print].

45. Baeten D, Braun J, Baraliakos X, et al. Secukinumab, a monoclonal antibody to interleukin-17A, significantly improves signs and symptoms of active ankylosing spondylitis: results of a 52-week phase 3 randomized placebo-controlled trial with intravenous loading and subcutaneous maintenance dosing. Arthritis Rheum 2014;66(S10):S360.

46. Sieper J, Braun J, Baraliakos X, et al. Secukinumab, a monoclonal antibody to interleukin-17A, significantly improves signs and symptoms of active ankylosing spondylitis: results of a phase 3, randomized, placebo-controlled trial with subcutaneous loading and maintenance dosing. Arthritis Rheum 2014;66(10 (Suppl)): S232.

47. Leonardi C, Matheson R, Zachariae C, et al. Anti-interleukin-17 monoclonal antibody ixekizumab in chronic plaque psoriasis. N Engl J Med 2012;366(13): 1190-9.

48. Genovese MC, Greenwald M, Cho CS, et al. A phase II randomized study of subcutaneous ixekizumab, an anti-interleukin-17 monoclonal antibody, in rheumatoid arthritis patients who were naive to biologic agents or had an inadequate response to tumor necrosis factor inhibitors. Arthritis Rheum 2014;66(7): 1693-704.

49. Papp KA, Leonardi C, Menter A, et al. Brodalumab, an anti-interleukin-17-receptor antibody for psoriasis. N Engl J Med 2012;366(13):1181-9.

50. Mease PJ, Genovese MC, Greenwald MW, et al. Brodalumab, an anti-IL17RA monoclonal antibody, in psoriatic arthritis. N Engl J Med 2014;370(24):2295-306.

51. Martin DA, Churchill M, Flores-Suarez L, et al. A phase Ib multiple ascending dose study evaluating safety, pharmacokinetics, and early clinical response of brodalumab, a human anti-IL-17R antibody, in methotrexate-resistant rheumatoid arthritis. Arthritis Res Ther 2013;15(5):R164.

52. Pavelka K, Chon Y, Newmark R, et al. A randomized, double-blind, placebo-controlled, multiple-dose study to evaluate the safety, tolerability, and efficacy of brodalumab (AMG 827) in subjects with rheumatoid arthritis and an inadequate response to methotrexate. Arthritis Rheum 2012;64(S362) [abstract: 831].

53. Sofen H, Smith S, Matheson RT, et al. Guselkumab (an IL-23-specific mAb) demonstrates clinical and molecular response in patients with moderate-to-severe psoriasis. J Allergy Clin Immunol 2014;133(4):1032 40.

54. Tausend W, Downing C, Tyring S. Systematic review of interleukin-12, interleukin-17, and interleukin-23 pathway inhibitors for the treatment of moderate-to-severe chronic plaque psoriasis: ustekinumab, briakinumab, tildrakizumab, guselkumab, secukinumab, ixekizumab, and brodalumab. J Cutan Med Surg 2014; 18(3):156-69.

55. Leonardi CL, Gordon KB. New and emerging therapies in psoriasis. Semin Cutan Med Surg 2014;33(2 Suppl 2):S37-41.

56. Baranauskaite A, Raffayova H, Kungurov NV, et al. Infliximab plus methotrexate is superior to methotrexate alone in the treatment of psoriatic arthritis in methotrexate-naive patients: the RESPOND study. Ann Rheum Dis 2012; 71(4):541-8.

57. Mease P, Collier D, Karki N, et al. Persistence and predictors of biologic TNFi therapy among biologic naïve psoriatic arthritis patients in a US registry. Arthritis Rheum 2014;66(S10) [abstract: 1853].
58. Smolen JS, Steiner G. Therapeutic strategies for rheumatoid arthritis. Nat Rev Drug Discov 2003;2(6):473–88.
59. Smolen J, Breedveld F, Burmester G, et al. Extended report: treating rheumatoid arthritis to target: 2014 update of the recommendations of an international task force. Ann Rheum Dis 2015. [Epub ahead of print].
60. Smolen JS, Braun J, Dougados M, et al. Treating spondyloarthritis, including ankylosing spondylitis and psoriatic arthritis, to target: recommendations of an international task force. Ann Rheum Dis 2014;73(1):6–16.
61. Coates L, Moberley A, McParland L, et al. Results of a randomised, controlled trial comparing tight control of early psoriatic arthritis (TICOPA) with standard care: tight control improves outcome. Arthritis Rheum 2013;65(Supp 10):814.
62. Coates LC, Fransen J, Helliwell PS. Defining minimal disease activity in psoriatic arthritis: a proposed objective target for treatment. Ann Rheum Dis 2009; 69(1):48–53.

Novel Treatment Concepts in Psoriatic Arthritis

Tristan Boyd, MD[a],*, Arthur Kavanaugh, MD[b]

KEYWORDS

- Psoriatic arthritis • Treat-to-target • Tight control • Minimal disease activity criteria
- Comorbidities • Anti-TNF drugs • DMARDs (biologic) • Dose reduction

KEY POINTS

- Early diagnosis and implementation of highly effective therapies provides the possibility of achieving better outcome in PsA.
- Tight control with frequent adjustments to medications and a treat-to-target approach to maintain low disease activity has shown clinical benefit.
- Refractory patients pose a challenge, but strategies to overcome treatment failure exist (eg, switching TNF inhibitors or implementing alternative therapies). Evidence for these strategies is accumulating in clinical trials.
- Patients well controlled on treatment may be able to taper or discontinue therapy, although the long-term outcome of such an approach remains unknown.
- New and potentially effective therapies are currently in advanced stages of clinical development.

INTRODUCTION

Psoriatic arthritis (PsA) is a chronic inflammatory condition that affects approximately 0.3% of the general population and 20% to 30% of patients with psoriasis.[1] It is a heterogeneous condition with diverse clinical manifestations or domains, including peripheral arthritis, axial arthritis, enthesitis, dactylitis, skin and nail psoriasis, and other manifestations.[2] The severity of involvement varies widely within domains and among individual patients, often making determination of disease activity challenging.

There have been numerous advances in the understanding of and treatment approach to PsA in the last decade. Among these, increased experience with highly effective therapies, particularly tumor necrosis factor-α inhibitors (TNFi), has altered

Disclosure Statement: The authors have nothing to disclose.
[a] Division of Rheumatology, Western University, Schulich School of Medicine, St. Joseph's Health Care London, Room D2-161, 268 Grosvenor Street, London, ON N6A 4V2, Canada;
[b] Division of Rheumatology, Allergy and Immunology, University of California, San Diego, School of Medicine, 9500 Gilman Drive MC 0943, La Jolla, CA, 92093-0943, USA
* Corresponding author. Division of Rheumatology, Western University, Schulich School of Medicine, St. Joseph's Health Care London, Room D2-161, 268 Grosvenor Street, London, ON N6A 4V2, Canada.
E-mail address: tboyd9@uwo.ca

Rheum Dis Clin N Am 41 (2015) 739–754
http://dx.doi.org/10.1016/j.rdc.2015.07.011
0889-857X/15/$ – see front matter © 2015 Elsevier Inc. All rights reserved.

rheumatic.theclinics.com

expectations and revolutionized the approach to treatment. Several questions have been raised regarding the optimal use of these medications and other newer biologic therapies in PsA.

EARLY INTERVENTION

The importance of early intervention and initiation of therapy in PsA has become increasingly recognized (discussed elsewhere in this issue). This insight resulted mainly from the growing recognition that PsA is a more severe disease than previously thought, and the introduction of medications capable of altering the disease course in PsA. This section discusses early detection and diagnosis, early treatment, and highly effective therapy.

Early Detection and Diagnosis

The onset of skin disease precedes the onset of arthritis in greater than 80% of patients, often by more than a decade.[1] Consequently, there is a unique opportunity in PsA to identify patients with musculoskeletal manifestations early in the disease course (**Fig. 1**).[3] There are several challenges to the early detection and diagnosis of PsA, including who should be screened and how screening should be performed. In addition, patients may be asymptomatic or minimally symptomatic, and may fail to report symptoms. Time constraints may also hinder a comprehensive evaluation.

To overcome these obstacles, several screening tools have been devised to help identify musculoskeletal manifestations of PsA (**Table 1**).[4,5] These tools were developed to assist dermatologists and primary care physicians in making an appropriate referral to a rheumatologist when PsA is suspected to ultimately make the diagnosis.

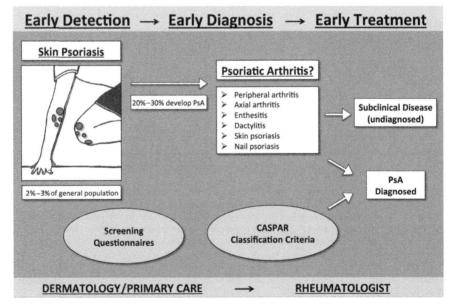

Fig. 1. Early intervention is recognized as the best strategy to achieve optimal outcome in PsA. Screening questionnaires help identify PsA in patients with skin psoriasis. The CASPAR classification criteria can be used to help make the diagnosis. Identifying subclinical disease remains a diagnostic challenge.

Table 1				
Screening tools developed and validated in dermatology and rheumatology cohorts				
	Screening Tools in Psoriatic Arthritis			
Screening	**Development Cohorts[4,5]**		**Clinical Practice[6]**	
Tool	Sensitivity (%)	Specificity (%)	Sensitivity (%)	Specificity (%)
PASE	82	73	74	38
ToPAS	87	93	77	30
PEST	92	78	77	37
PASQ	97	75	—	—
EARP	85	92	—	—
ToPAS2	96	99	—	—

A comparison of the performance of three screening tools in a study of patients recruited from dermatology clinics and subsequently assessed by a rheumatologist if a positive screening test was obtained.

Abbreviations: EARP, Early ARthritis for Psoriatic patients; PASE, Psoriatic Arthritis Screening and Evaluation; PASQ, Psoriatic Arthritis Screening Questionnaire; PEST, Psoriatic Epidemiology Screening Tool; ToPAS, Toronto Psoriatic Arthritis Screen.

Data from Refs.[2,4,6]

The target population includes patients with a history of skin psoriasis and those with a family history of psoriasis or PsA.

Although these screening questionnaires have demonstrated good and comparable sensitivity and specificity in development cohorts, a recent study suggests they do not perform as well in clinical settings.[6] This may be partly because patients can be asymptomatic, particularly in early stages of the disease.

Some limitations of currently available screening tests include potential for poor specificity. For example, it is often difficult to differentiate PsA from other musculoskeletal conditions that can accompany psoriasis, such as osteoarthritis and fibromyalgia. Moreover, recognition of patterns of PsA other than polyarticular disease can be challenging.[7] Refinement of available questionnaires is currently underway in hopes of improving performance in clinical practice.[8]

Following identification of a patient at risk for PsA, the next challenge is early diagnosis. Diagnosis, particularly in the early stages, requires differentiation from other rheumatic conditions at a time when many of the clinical features may not be present. Because the diagnosis of PsA at this stage is primarily clinical, with no pathognomonic serologic or imaging tests, the disease is frequently not identifed.[1] Also, the wide clinical spectrum, even at disease onset, poses challenges in diagnosis, particularly in patients who lack skin disease.

In 2006, the CASPAR (Classification of Psoriatic Arthritis) classification criteria were published (**Box 1**).[9] They include several features distinctive to PsA and have helped make study populations more uniform in clinical trials. The CASPAR criteria have been validated in early and long-standing disease and have become widely accepted and used.[10,11]

Advantages of the CASPAR criteria include accuracy in both family medicine and rheumatology clinics, ability to diagnose PsA in patients without psoriasis, and not excluding patients who are rheumatoid factor or anticitrullinated protein antibody positive.[12] The last point is important because, although most patients with PsA are seronegative for rheumatoid factor and anticitrullinated protein antibody, numerous studies have shown the prevalence of both rheumatoid factor and anticitrullinated protein antibody is greater among patients with PsA than in the general

---

Box 1

CASPAR criteria have high sensitivity and specificity for psoriatic arthritis (points scored are listed in parentheses)

Inflammatory articular disease (peripheral or axial arthritis, or enthesitis) PLUS greater than 3 points in the following five categories (validated in early and long-standing disease):

1. Psoriasis: current (2), personal history (1), family history (1)

2. Psoriatic nail dystrophy (1)

3. Dactylitis: current or previous (1)

4. Negative test for rheumatoid factor (1)

5. Radiograph evidence of new juxta-articular bone formation (1)

Sensitivity, 91.4%; specificity, 98.7%.
Adapted from Taylor W, Gladman D, Helliwell P, et al. Classification criteria for psoriatic arthritis: development of new criteria from a larger international study. Arthritis Rheum 2006;54:2665–73; with permission.

---

population.[13,14] The clinical relevance of this finding is still being elucidated. Excluding patients based solely on a positive test could lead to underdiagnosis.

In recent years, the potential severity of PsA has been increasingly recognized, particularly with regard to polyarticular peripheral arthritis, supporting the importance of early diagnosis and intervention.[15] The high sensitivity and specificity of the CASPAR criteria, in early and long-standing disease, suggest they may also be used as diagnostic criteria for PsA.[3]

Early Treatment

PsA was previously considered a mild form of arthritis, but is now recognized as an aggressive disease with the potential to cause significant joint damage and an impaired quality of life.[16] Approximately 40% to 60% of patients experience a severe, deforming arthritis with early radiographic changes.[17–19] In a prospective study of 129 patients with PsA treated with traditional disease-modifying antirheumatic drug (DMARD) therapy, erosive disease occurred in 47% of patients at 2 years, despite clinical improvement.[20] A delay as short as 6 months from symptom onset to first rheumatologic assessment has been associated with development of peripheral joint erosions and worse functional outcome in PsA.[21]

In the last decade, the availability of medications that can alter the disease course in PsA has generated new ideas concerning the optimal approach to managing early disease. It seems logical that ongoing joint inflammation would lead to subsequent damage and eventual loss of function.[22] This temporal relationship suggests that controlling inflammation may prevent downstream sequelae. Early treatment has been proven effective in rheumatoid arthritis (RA); however, the effectiveness of early aggressive therapy in the management of PsA has not been established.[23,24]

Evidence from McHugh and colleagues[17] confirmed that early treatment with disease-modifying therapy has a positive impact on long-term morbidity in PsA: disease progression was noted to be worse in patients presenting with established disease (duration >2 years), emphasizing the importance of early therapeutic intervention.[25] Hence, similar to RA, clinicians may have a "window of opportunity" in PsA, a period during which a more robust therapeutic response is observed compared with a less impressive response when the same agent is prescribed later in the disease course.

Highly Effective Therapy

Unlike traditional DMARDs, which do not prevent disease progression or decrease structural joint damage, TNFi effectively treats all domains of disease activity in PsA (**Fig. 2**).[1,26]

Currently, five TNFi are approved for use in many countries worldwide for the treatment of PsA. Although no head-to-head trials have been conducted, an indirect comparison meta-analysis demonstrated no significant difference in the effectiveness of TNFi.[27] Despite their proven efficacy, treatment recommendations suggest that use of TNFi be reserved for patients with moderate-to-severe disease.[28,29] In general, they are used only after inadequate response with anti-inflammatory drugs, corticosteroids, and traditional DMARDs, although they may be used as initial therapy in certain situations.

Aside from TNFi, the US Food and Drug Administration recently approved the use of two other highly effective medications for use in the treatment of PsA: ustekinumab (an interleukin [IL]-12/IL-23 inhibitor) and apremilast (a phosphodiesterase 4 inhibitor). Data from phase III clinical trials have shown significant improvement in PsA signs and symptoms, skin disease, enthesitis, dactylitis, and physical function for both medications.[30,31] Ustekinumab has also demonstrated efficacy in decreasing progression of radiographic damage.[32]

Finally, there are several IL-17 inhibitors (secukinumab, ixekizumab, and brodalumab) in advanced-phase clinical trials. Available data suggest significant improvement in skin psoriasis, and efficacy in treating peripheral and axial arthritis.[33]

DISEASE-SPECIFIC CONSIDERATIONS

Once likened to a mild form of seronegative RA, PsA is now recognized as a distinct clinical entity with unique features. One of the most striking differences is the

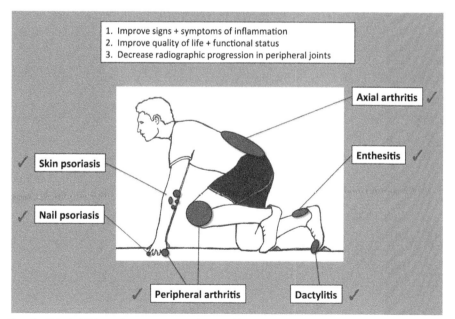

Fig. 2. TNF inhibitors in psoriatic arthritis effectively treat all signs and symptoms of inflammation, improve quality of life and functional status, and have been proven to decrease radiographic progression in peripheral joints.

significant heterogeneity that occurs in PsA. In addition to affecting multiple clinical domains, several associated extra-articular manifestations and comorbidities must also be taken into account when selecting therapy (**Fig. 3**). The term "psoriatic disease" was coined to encompass the diverse clinical spectrum, which occurs in variable degrees of severity and may influence treatment decisions.[34] This section discusses validated outcome measures, subclinical disease, prognostic markers, and comorbidities.

Validated Outcome Measures

Until recently, many outcome measures used in PsA have been extrapolated or borrowed from other conditions that share similar clinical features. Although many of these measures are validated in PsA, these borrowed disease activity indices do not cover all aspects of psoriatic disease and may, therefore, overlook disease activity in other domains.

The advent of therapies capable of altering disease outcome in PsA has been proven in numerous clinical trials. These trials highlighted the need for specific PsA outcome measures to quantify disease activity optimally. Currently validated instruments to measure all clinical manifestations seen in PsA were developed over the last several years (**Table 2**).[35] In addition, a core set of measures to be included in all clinical trials of patients with PsA was suggested; this change will allow meaningful comparisons across studies, an important step forward.[36]

Because of the heterogeneity of disease, and the importance of accounting for several domains of disease activity, composite outcome measures that provide a more complete clinical picture have gained considerable support in clinical practice and research trials.

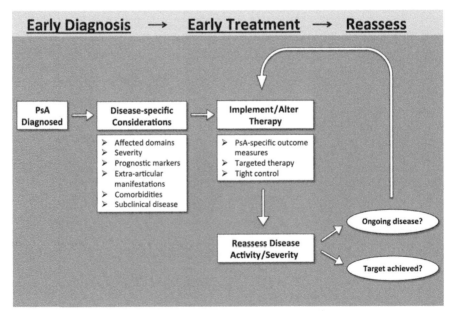

Fig. 3. After PsA is diagnosed, taking into account disease-specific considerations provides more comprehensive care and may influence treatment strategy. Highly effective therapies have changed the treatment paradigm in PsA with preliminary results of a treat-to-target approach showing benefit in clinical trials.

Table 2		
Outcome measures assess individual domains or a composite of several different domains		
Outcome Measures Arthritis[35]		
Individual domains		
Skin psoriasis	PASI	
Nail psoriasis	NAPSI, mNAPSI	
Axial arthritis	BASDAI	
Peripheral arthritis	TJC, SJC, ACR20/50/70, PsARC, PsAJAI	
Enthesitis	LEI, MEI, MASES	
Dactylitis	LDI	
Function/quality of life	PsAQoL, FACIT-F, DLQI	
Composite measures	DAPSA, CPDAI, GRACE index, PASDAS	

Core measures (six domains recommended to be included in all clinical trials)[36]: skin activity, peripheral joint activity, health-related quality of life, patient global assessment, physical function, and pain.

Abbreviations: ACR20/50/70, American College of Rheumatology response criteria >20%, >50%, >70%; BASDAI, Bath ankylosing spondylitis disease activity index; CPDAI, composite psoriatic disease activity index; DAPSA, disease activity in psoriatic arthritis; DLQI, dermatology life quality index; FACIT-F, functional assessment of chronic illness therapy fatigue scale; GRACE index, GRAPPA composite exercise index; LDI, Leeds dactylitis index; LEI, Leeds enthesitis index; MASES, Maastricht ankylosing spondylitis enthesitis score; MEI, Mander/Newcastle enthesitis index; mNAPSI, modified NAPSI; NAPSI, nail psoriasis severity index; PASDAS, psoriatic arthritis disease activity score; PASI, psoriasis area and severity index; PsAJAI, psoriatic arthritis joint activity index; PsAQoL, PsA-specific quality of life; PsARC, psoriatic arthritis response criteria; TJC/SJC, tender/swollen joint count.

Data from Refs.[9,35,36]

Subclinical Disease

One of the major challenges in treating PsA is the failure to detect patients with early or subtle disease. Patients may be asymptomatic or fail to recognize the potential consequences of their symptoms. Even after diagnosis, actively treated patients may have ongoing disease that remains undetected by the clinician. Two major challenges are associated with subclinical or occult disease: how to diagnose subclinical disease, and how to manage subclinical disease.

Asymptomatic PsA may represent the ideal population in which to initiate treatment, before accrual of joint damage and functional impairment.[37] First, the clinician must identify the presence of disease activity. Because current laboratory tests are not particularly useful in identifying asymptomatic PsA, there is ongoing investigation into the use of highly sensitive imaging and biomarkers of disease activity.

Imaging modalities proposed to detect subclinical disease in articular and periarticular tissues include musculoskeletal ultrasound, MRI, and others. These highly sensitive imaging techniques can detect evidence of inflammation even in the absence of clinical signs and symptoms.[38] They may also identify patients with more extensive disease than was detected on clinical examination. Discrepancies in the findings of clinical and imaging examinations suggest joint involvement in early PsA may be underappreciated and undertreated.[3]

Serologic biomarkers could potentially assist in the management of PsA by detecting early or subclinical disease. Several biomarkers have been identified that show potential in differentiating psoriasis from PsA.[39] Biomarkers could, therefore, have a role in screening patients with psoriasis for PsA. If a biomarker could reliably detect inflammation in the absence of clinical disease, it is possible that it may also help guide treatment strategies.[40]

Currently there are no data available on the progression of subclinical disease in PsA. There is also scant evidence to confirm that a lack of disease activity is required to prevent structural damage, particularly in domains other than peripheral arthritis.[38] Prospective studies are needed to determine the correct therapeutic approach to subclinical disease in PsA. It is currently believed that in the absence of other signs and symptoms, treatment should not be implemented solely based on subclinical disease.[37]

Prognostic Markers

Known predictors of disease progression and damage in peripheral joints in PsA include a high number of actively inflamed joints, loss of function, elevated inflammatory markers, prior damage, and poor response to therapy.[28] There has been increasing interest in identifying new prognostic markers, which may help guide therapy early in the disease course and potentially achieve better clinical outcomes.

The variable response to treatment (including to TNFi) in PsA can pose a challenge. It would be helpful to know in advance if a patient will or will not respond to a given therapy, because this may guide selection of therapy during this potentially critical phase of the disease. In established disease, prognostic markers may help determine appropriate candidates for tapering or withdrawal of therapy.

A recent study of patients with PsA treated with golimumab noted an association of several biomarkers with improvement in clinical response.[41] If biomarkers were able to help diagnose and predict response to specific treatments, they could hypothetically serve as prognostic markers in PsA, helping to facilitate early detection and predict disease severity.[42]

Comorbidities

Psoriatic disease is associated with an increased mortality risk and several medical comorbidities, including obesity, metabolic syndrome, cardiovascular disease, diabetes, and nonalcoholic fatty liver disease.[43] These comorbidities and extra-articular manifestations (eg, inflammatory eye disease and gastrointestinal tract involvement) are commonly seen in PsA, and may influence treatment decisions.

Unfortunately, published studies documenting the long-term benefits of treating comorbidities in PsA are limited. Likewise, the influence of uncontrolled disease on comorbidities remains poorly studied. Two reports, however, deserve mention. First, TNF-α inhibition may prevent the progression of subclinical atherosclerosis and reduce arterial stiffness in inflammatory arthritis.[44] Second, another study revealed the beneficial effects of weight loss in PsA: patients achieving loss greater than or equal to 5% from baseline weight were shown to have a higher likelihood of achieving minimal disease activity (MDA; odds ratio, 4.20; $P<.001$).[45]

It is important to identify and manage comorbidities because they may influence choice of therapy and may also have implications regarding response to treatment and prognosis. Patient education and a collaborative approach involving the patient, primary care physician, and rheumatologist are important in deciding which therapies are appropriate to use in PsA.

MODIFICATIONS TO THE TREATMENT PARADIGM

Newer and more effective therapies have changed the landscape for treating PsA. Once thought unattainable, remission and low disease activity are now considered realistic goals of therapy. This section discusses targeted therapy, treatment options in refractory disease, and treatment options in controlled disease.

Targeted Therapy

Until recently, one of the major challenges in PsA was the lack of a clearly defined, prespecified target on which to base treatment decisions, because no remission criteria have yet been validated for PsA. Recently, two major advances adopting a targeted approach to treatment in PsA were published.

First, criteria for MDA were developed (**Box 2**), which include measures of disease activity in several clinical domains, taking into account the heterogeneity seen in PsA.[46] The MDA criteria were validated in randomized controlled trials and observational cohorts, and showed prognostic value: patients achieving MDA for 12 months or more experienced a significant reduction in progression of joint damage.[47,48] The MDA criteria are commonly considered an acceptable therapeutic target.

Second, a European League Against Rheumatism (EULAR) task force published treat-to-target recommendations for spondyloarthritis, including PsA.[49] The major treatment target of these recommendations was remission or inactive disease in all musculoskeletal domains. Where remission was considered not possible, low disease activity was considered an appropriate alternative target. These recommendations highlight the importance of individualized treatment goals, incorporating extra-articular manifestations and comorbidities into selection of therapy.

Both the MDA criteria and the EULAR task force recommendations are consistent with the growing consensus that optimal treatment requires achieving the least amount of activity possible in all domains of psoriatic disease.[38] They stress the importance of having a prespecified treatment objective to guide adjustments to therapy accordingly.

Substantial evidence for the benefits of tight control has been demonstrated in RA, with improvement of function and quality of life, disease activity, and decreased radiographic progression using an intensive treatment strategy.[50] Until recently, the value of tight control in PsA was unknown. Preliminary results of the TICOPA (Tight Control of

---

Box 2
MDA Criteria – GRAPPA

The MDA criteria include several clinical domains, taking into account the heterogeneity seen in psoriatic arthritis. A patient is classified as having MDA if they satisfy five out of seven of the following criteria (validated in clinical trials):

1. Tender joint count ≤ 1

2. Swollen joint count ≤ 1

3. PASI ≤ 1 or BSA $\leq 3\%$

4. Patient pain, VAS ≤ 15 mm

5. Patient global disease activity, VAS ≤ 20 mm

6. HAQ score ≤ 0.5

7. Tender enthesitis points ≤ 1

Abbreviations: BSA, body surface area; HAQ, health assessment questionnaire; PASI, Psoriasis Activity and Severity Index; VAS, Visual Analogue Scale.
  Data from Coates LC, Fransen J, Helliwell PS. Defining minimal disease activity in psoriatic arthritis: a proposed objective for treatment. Ann Rheum Dis 2010;69:48–53.

Psoriatic Arthritis) trial, however, suggest improved outcomes with intensive treatment in newly diagnosed PsA: those treated using a tight control strategy achieved significantly better clinical outcomes in American College of Rheumatology (ACR) 20/50/70 responses (61.8%/51.2%/38.4% vs 44.6%/25.0%/17.4%, respectively), Psoriasis Activity and Severity Index 75 (58.7% vs 33.4%, respectively), and patient-reported outcomes at Week 48 compared with those in the standard care group.[22,51]

Although the patients in the tight control group showed improved treatment response, they also experienced more adverse effects (eg, nausea, liver function test abnormalities, and infections) than the standard care group. Because it has not been established if the absence of disease activity is necessary to prevent the progression of joint damage in PsA, aiming for this goal could result in overtreatment.[38] One possibility to overcome this problem is to permit low levels of disease activity in some disease domains in select patients.

Treatment Options in Refractory Disease

TNFi are effective in PsA with most patients achieving a prompt and sustained response; nevertheless, some patients have clinical manifestations that either do not respond to TNFi or achieve less of a clinical response than desired. These "TNFi failures" can be classified as either primary failures (ie, lack of initial response) or secondary failures (ie, loss of effect over time). There are several strategies available to deal with patients who have an inadequate response to a first TNFi (**Fig. 4**).

Switching to another tumor necrosis factor inhibitor

Switching from one TNFi to another is a concept that has been established in RA. Although the data in PsA are more limited, despite fewer effective treatment options,

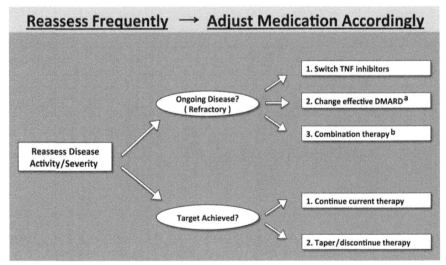

Fig. 4. Strategies to deal with the challenges of active or refractory disease are developing alongside the growing knowledge base with highly effective therapies. The possibility of tapering or discontinuing therapy in patients achieving remission or low disease activity state is also being addressed. [a]Consider IL-12/IL-23 inhibitor or phosphodiesterase 4 inhibitor (and potentially IL-17 inhibitors in future). [b]Consider additional DMARD, which may have synergistic effect. In the future, bispecific biologic therapy may become a therapeutic option.

some evidence supports switching to another TNFi. Clinical trial data for certolizumab in the RAPID-PsA study showed comparable outcomes for patients previously exposed to TNFi and those who were TNFi-naive.[52]

Data from the Norwegian DMARD (NOR-DMARD) registry found that 20% to 40% of patients respond to a second TNFi, although the durability of remaining on the second TNFi was shorter.[53] Data from the Danish nationwide registry of biologic therapies (DANBIO) also revealed that switching TNFi can result in clinical improvement: after 2 years, 47% of patients who had switched TNFi achieved an ACR20 response. Response rates and drug survival were both lower in patients who had switched TNFi.[54] Because a significant proportion of patients achieve a good clinical response, switching TNFi should always be considered in PsA.[55]

Changing to another class of therapy

Another possibility is changing to a medication with an alternative mechanism of action. The recent approval of ustekinumab and apremilast for treatment of PsA has provided alternatives to TNFi in patients who either fail to respond or have contraindications to their use. IL-17 inhibitors, which are in advanced stages of clinical trials in PsA, and have received approval for skin psoriasis, may also be an option.

Evidence for ustekinumab The P-SUMMIT 2 trial included patients with PsA who had previously received treatment with TNFi. Improvements were noted in skin and joint activity, although the magnitude of clinical response was less than in TNF-naive patients.[56]

Evidence for apremilast In the PALACE 1 trial, approximately 24% of patients had previously received biologic therapy, and 9.3% were considered treatment failures.[31] Higher ACR20 response rates were observed in patients who were biologic-naive compared with those who had previous biologic exposure or treatment failure; however, all groups demonstrated significant improvement of PsA signs and symptoms by Week 16. Overall, the efficacy profile of apremilast was found to be modest in comparison with other biologic therapies. Nevertheless, apremilast may offer an effective option in patients with less severe skin and joint manifestations, particularly in light of its favorable safety profile.

Combination therapy

Cotherapy with methotrexate In RA, the combination of methotrexate (MTX) and anti-TNF therapy has demonstrated synergistic efficacy in clinical trials.[57] In contrast, whether patients with PsA might have improved outcomes with concomitant use of MTX with TNFi has not been systematically studied.

A study of patients with PsA treated with TNFi from the NOR-DMARD registry compared patients receiving TNFi monotherapy with those receiving concomitant MTX. Similar clinical outcomes were observed in both groups; however, increased drug survival was seen in patients receiving combination therapy.[58] A review of 14 studies examining the use of MTX in combination with TNFi noted no improvement of clinical symptoms beyond those attained by monotherapy with the anti-TNF agent.[59] However, these studies were not specifically designed to compare efficacy between patients treated with TNFi monotherapy and concomitant MTX.

Bispecific biologic therapies Current therapies in PsA are based on inhibition of a single cytokine (eg, TNF-α). Recently, the effects of combined inhibition of TNF-α and IL-17 on suppression of inflammation in RA were investigated in a mouse model.[60] The effects of combined blockade were more effective than single blockade in preventing inflammation and also damage of cartilage and bone.

These bispecific antibodies may treat inflammatory arthritis more effectively than single cytokine blockade, and may help overcome some of the challenges faced in patients with poor response to therapy. Whether these results will prove effective in human trials and can be extrapolated to PsA remains unknown.

Treatment Options in Controlled Disease

In contrast with patients who have active or refractory disease, patients with PsA achieving low disease activity or remission may not require ongoing maintenance therapy at the same levels required to induce remission. This is an emerging concept in rheumatology that has been studied extensively in RA with some notable success, particularly in patients treated early in the disease course.[61] Potential benefits of dose reduction include reduced risk of adverse events and decreased financial burden. Two strategies of dose reduction are discussed here: tapering and discontinuation of therapy (see **Fig. 4**).

Tapering therapy

Tapering or withdrawing therapy can be performed either by reducing the dose of the agent given, or increasing the interval of administration. There is some evidence to support tapering biologic therapy in PsA: in a prospective study of patients with PsA who had previously had a complete response to adalimumab therapy, 86.6% of patients remained in remission when the interval of administration was increased from every 2 to 4.4 weeks.[62]

Success with reducing the dose of TNFi has also been observed in axial spondyloarthropathy and peripheral spondyloarthropathy.[63] Patients tapering anti-TNF therapy often remain on traditional DMARDs; nevertheless, this strategy may be beneficial with respect to safety concerns and economic burden of therapies with high costs.

Discontinuation

Although many studies have examined clinical outcome after discontinuation of biologic therapy in RA, they have been small in size and lacked uniformity in their assessment.[64] Recently published data from RA suggests that discontinuation of TNFi may be associated with sustained clinical benefit, with approximately 50% of patients maintaining clinical response up to 20 months after discontinuation.[65]

Clinical outcome after discontinuation of TNFi in patients with PsA who have achieved remission is uncertain. In a prospective study of patients with peripheral PsA, those receiving TNFi achieved remission (defined according to ACR remission criteria) for longer periods after discontinuation of therapy than patients treated with traditional DMARDs.[66] It should be noted that relapses occurred in 49% of these patients within 12 ± 2.4 months after discontinuing treatment.

Despite relapse in a significant proportion of patients with PsA, they remained in remission for prolonged periods of time after discontinuation of their TNFi therapy. It is possible that patients may benefit from intermittent treatment, with periods of temporary discontinuation followed by reinitiating therapy if disease recurs.[67]

Further study is required to assess the impact of dose reduction in domains other than peripheral arthritis, and whether certain patient characteristics can predict clinical response to lower doses of therapy.

SUMMARY

Therapeutic options for patients with PsA have increased substantially over the last decade. Nevertheless, the high variability and potential severity of clinical manifestations and comorbidities along with the combination of domain involvement in a single patient confronts the clinician with a range of challenges. Further studies are needed to provide evidence that the aforementioned strategies are effective, not only in peripheral arthritis and skin disease, but also in other domains of PsA.

Disease-specific definitions and criteria (eg, diagnostic criteria, remission, and gradations of disease activity) will be beneficial in influencing therapeutic choices in the future. In addition, predictors of disease progression are needed to help guide therapy, particularly with patients in low disease activity states or remission who may be able to taper or discontinue therapy.

REFERENCES

1. Huynh DH, Kavanaugh A. Psoriatic arthritis: current therapy and future approaches. Rheumatology (Oxford) 2015;54:20–8.
2. Gladman D, Antoni C, Mease P, et al. Psoriatic arthritis: epidemiology, clinical features, course, and outcome. Ann Rheum Dis 2005;64(Suppl 2):ii14–7.
3. Anandarajah AP, Ritchlin CT. The diagnosis and treatment of early psoriatic arthritis. Nat Rev Rheumatol 2009;5:634–41.
4. Gladman DD, Helliwell PS, Khraishi M, et al. Dermatology screening tools: project update from the GRAPPA 2012 annual meeting. J Rheumatol 2013;40:1425–7.
5. Tinazzi I, Adami S, Zanolin EM, et al. The early psoriatic arthritis screening questionnaire: a simple and fast method for the identification of arthritis in patients with psoriasis. Rheumatology 2012;51:2058–63.
6. Coates LC, Aslam T, Al Balushi F, et al. Comparison of three screening tools to detect psoriatic arthritis in patients with psoriasis (CONTEST study). Br J Dermatol 2013;168:802–7.
7. Haroon M, Kirby B, FitzGerald O. High prevalence of psoriatic arthritis patients with severe psoriasis with suboptimal performance of screening questionnaires. Ann Rheum Dis 2013;72:736–40.
8. Coates LC, Walsh J, Haroon M, et al. Development and testing of new candidate psoriatic arthritis screening questionnaires combining optimal questions from existing tools. Arthritis Care Res 2014;66:1410–6.
9. Taylor W, Gladman D, Helliwell P, et al. Classification criteria for psoriatic arthritis: development of new criteria from a larger international study. Arthritis Rheum 2006;54:2665–73.
10. Chandran V, Schentag CT, Gladman DD. Sensitivity of the classification of psoriatic arthritis criteria in early psoriatic arthritis. Arthritis Rheum 2007;57:1560–3.
11. Coates LC, Conaghan PG, Emery P, et al. Sensitivity and specificity of the classification criteria of psoriatic arthritis criteria in early psoriatic arthritis. Arthritis Rheum 2012;64:3150–5.
12. Chandran V, Schentag CT, Gladman DD. CASPAR criteria are sensitive in early psoriatic arthritis (PsA) and are accurate when applied to patients attending a family practice clinic. Ann Rheum Dis 2007;66(Suppl II):415.
13. Vander CB, Hoffman IE, Zmierczak H, et al. Anti-citrullinated peptide antibodies may occur in patients with psoriatic arthritis. Ann Rheum Dis 2005;64:1145–9.
14. Inanc N, Dalkilic E, Kamali S, et al. Anti-CCP antibodies in rheumatoid arthritis and psoriatic arthritis. Clin Rheumatol 2007;26:17–23.
15. Kavanaugh A. Defining remission in psoriatic arthritis. Clin Exp Rheumatol 2006; 24(Suppl 43):S83–7.
16. Gladman DD. Can we identify psoriatic arthritis early? Curr Rheumatol Rep 2008; 10:419–21.

17. McHugh NJ, Balachrishnan C, Jones SM. Progression of peripheral joint disease in psoriatic arthritis. Rheumatology (Oxford) 2003;42:778–83.
18. Gladman DD, Stafford-Brady F, Chang CH, et al. Longitudinal study of clinical and radiological progression in psoriatic arthritis. J Rheumatol 1990;17:809–12.
19. Sokoll KB, Helliwell PS. Comparison of disability and quality of life in rheumatoid and psoriatic arthritis. Rheumatology (Oxford) 2003;42:778–83.
20. Kane D, Stafford L, Bresnihan B, et al. A prospective, clinical and radiological study of early psoriatic arthritis: an early synovitis clinic experience. Rheumatology 2003;42:1460–8.
21. Haroon M, Gallagher P, FitzGerald O. Diagnostic delay of more than 6 months contributes to poor radiographic and functional outcome in psoriatic arthritis. Ann Rheum Dis 2015;74(6):1045–50.
22. Coates LC. Treating to target in psoriatic arthritis. Curr Opin Rheumatol 2015;27: 107–10.
23. Nell VP, Machold KP, Eberl G, et al. Benefit of very early referral and very early therapy with disease-modifying anti-rheumatic drugs in patients with early rheumatoid arthritis. Rheumatology 2004;43:906–14.
24. Olivieri I, D'Angelo S, Palazzi C, et al. Advances in the management of psoriatic arthritis. Nat Rev Rheumatol 2014;10:531–42.
25. Gladman DD, Thavaneswaran A, Chandran V, et al. Do patients with psoriatic arthritis who present early fare better than those presenting later in the disease? Ann Rheum Dis 2011;70:2152–4.
26. Mease P. Management of psoriatic arthritis: the therapeutic interface between rheumatology and dermatology. Curr Rheumatol Rep 2006;8:348–54.
27. Thorlund K, Druyts E, Avina-Zubieta JA, et al. Anti-tumor necrosis factor (TNF) drugs for the treatment of psoriatic arthritis: an indirect comparison meta-analysis. Biologics 2012;6:417–27.
28. Ritchlin CT, Kavanaugh A, Gladman DD, et al. Treatment recommendations for psoriatic arthritis. Ann Rheum Dis 2009;68:1387–94.
29. Gossec L, Smolen JS, Gaujoux-Viala C, et al. European League Against Rheumatism recommendations for the management of psoriatic arthritis with pharmacologic therapies. Ann Rheum Dis 2012;71:4–12.
30. McInnes IB, Kavanaugh A, Gottlieb AB, et al. Efficacy and safety of ustekinumab in patients with active psoriatic arthritis: 1 year results of the phase 3, multicenter, double-blind, placebo-controlled PSUMMIT 1 trial. Lancet 2013;382:780–9.
31. Kavanaugh A, Mease PJ, Gomez-Reino JJ, et al. Treatment of psoriatic arthritis in a phase 3 randomised, placebo-controlled trial with apremilast, an oral phosphodiesterase 4 inhibitor. Ann Rheum Dis 2014;73:1020–6.
32. Kavanaugh A, Ritchlin C, Rahman P, et al. Ustekinumab, an anti-IL-12/23 p40 monoclonal antibody, inhibits radiographic progression in patients with active psoriatic arthritis: results of an integrated analysis of radiographic data from the phase 3, multicenter, randomized, double-blind, placebo-controlled PSUMMIT-1 and PSUMMIT-2 trials. Ann Rheum Dis 2014;73:1000–6.
33. Mease P. Inhibition of interleukin-17, interleukin-23 and the TH17 cell pathway in the treatment of psoriatic arthritis and psoriasis. Curr Opin Rheumatol 2015;27:127–33.
34. Scarpa R, Ayala F, Caporaso N, et al. Psoriasis, psoriatic arthritis, or psoriatic disease? J Rheumatol 2006;33:210–2.
35. Mease PJ. Measures of psoriatic arthritis. Arthritis Care Res (Hoboken) 2011; 63(Suppl 11):S64–85.
36. Gladman DD, Mease PJ, Strand V, et al. Consensus on a core set of domains for psoriatic arthritis. J Rheumatol 2007;34:1167–70.

37. Palazzi C, Lubrano E, D'Angelo S, et al. Beyond early diagnosis: occult psoriatic arthritis. J Rheumatol 2010;37:1556–8.
38. Kavanaugh A. Psoriatic arthritis: treat-to-target. Clin Exp Rheumatol 2012; 30(Suppl 73):S123–5.
39. Chandran V. Soluble biomarkers may differentiate psoriasis from psoriatic arthritis. J Rheumatol 2012;39(Suppl 89):65–6.
40. Van Kuijk AW, Gerlag DM, Vos K, et al. A prospective, randomized, placebo-controlled study to identify biomarkers associated with active treatment in psoriatic arthritis: effects of adalimumab treatment on synovial tissue. Ann Rheum Dis 2009;68:1303–9.
41. Wagner CL, Visvanathan S, Elashoff M, et al. Markers of inflammation and bone remodeling associated with improvement in clinical response measures in psoriatic arthritis patients treated with golimumab. Ann Rheum Dis 2013;72:83–8.
42. Chandran V, Gladman DD. Update on biomarkers in psoriatic arthritis. Curr Rheumatol Rep 2010;12:288–94.
43. Ogdie A, Schwartzman S, Husni ME. Recognizing and managing comorbidities in psoriatic arthritis. Curr Opin Rheumatol 2015;27:118–26.
44. Tam LS, Kitas GD, Gonzalez-Gay MA. Can suppression of inflammation by anti-TNF prevent progression of subclinical atherosclerosis in inflammatory arthritis? Rheumatology 2014;53:1108–19.
45. Di Minno MN, Peluso R, Iervolino S, et al. Weight loss and achievement of minimal disease activity in patients with psoriatic arthritis starting treatment with tumor necrosis factor alpha blockers. Ann Rheum Dis 2014;73:1157–62.
46. Coates LC, Fransen J, Helliwell PS. Defining minimal disease activity in psoriatic arthritis: a proposed objective for treatment. Ann Rheum Dis 2010;69:48–53.
47. Coates LC, Helliwell PS. Validation of minimal disease activity for psoriatic arthritis using interventional trial data. Arthritis Care Res 2010;62:965–9.
48. Coates LC, Cook R, Lee KA, et al. Frequency, predictors, and prognosis of sustained minimal disease activity in an observational psoriatic arthritis cohort. Arthritis Care Res 2010;62:970–6.
49. Smolen JS, Braun J, Dougados M, et al. Treating spondyloarthritis, including ankylosing spondylitis and psoriatic arthritis, to target: recommendations of an international task force. Ann Rheum Dis 2014;73:6–16.
50. Grigor C, Capell H, Stirling A, et al. Effect of a treatment strategy of tight control for rheumatoid arthritis (the TICORA study): a single-blind randomized controlled trial. Lancet 2004;364:263–9.
51. Coates LC, Moverly A, McParland L, et al. Results of a randomized control trial comparing tight control of psoriatic arthritis (TICOPA) with standard care: tight control improves outcome. San Diego (CA): ACR meeting; 2013 [abstract: 814].
52. Mease PJ, Fleischmann R, Deadhar AA, et al. Effect of certolizumab pegol on signs and symptoms in patients with psoriatic arthritis: 24-week results of a phase 3 double-blind randomized placebo-controlled study (RAPID-PsA). Ann Rheum Dis 2014;73:48–55.
53. Fagerli K, Lie E, van der Heijde D, et al. Switching between TNF inhibitors in psoriatic arthritis: data from the NOR-DMARD study. Ann Rheum Dis 2013;72: 1840–4.
54. Glintborg B, Ostergaard M, Krogh NS, et al. Clinical response, drug survival, and predictors thereof among 548 patients with psoriatic arthritis who switched tumor necrosis factor α inhibitor therapy: results from the Danish Nationwide DANBIO registry. Arthritis Rheum 2013;65:1213–23.

55. Coates LC, Cawkwell LS, Ng NWF, et al. Sustained response to long-term biologics and switching in psoriatic arthritis: results from real life experience. Ann Rheum Dis 2008;67:717–9.

56. Ritchlin C, Gottlieb A, McInnes I, et al. Ustekinumab in active psoriatic arthritis including patients previously treated with anti-TNF agents: results of a phase III, multicenter double-blind, placebo controlled study. Washington, DC: ACR; 2012 [abstract: 2557].

57. Kavanaugh A, Cohen S, Cush J. The evolving use of TNF inhibitors in rheumatoid arthritis. J Rheumatol 2004;31:1881–4.

58. Fagerli KM, Lie E, van der Heijde D, et al. The role of methotrexate co-medication in TNF-inhibitor treatment in patients with psoriatic arthritis: results from 440 patients included in the NOR-DMARD study. Ann Rheum Dis 2014;73:132–7.

59. Daly M, Alikhan A, Armstrong AW. Combination systemic therapies in psoriatic arthritis. J Dermatolog Treat 2011;22:276–84.

60. Fischer JAA, Hueber AJ, Wilson S, et al. Combined inhibition of tumor necrosis factor α and interleukin-17 as a therapeutic opportunity in rheumatoid arthritis: development and characterization of a novel bispecific antibody. Arthritis Rheumatol 2015;67:51–62.

61. Emery P, Hammoudeh M, FitzGerald O, et al. Sustained remission with etanercept tapering in early rheumatoid arthritis. N Engl J Med 2014;371:1781–92.

62. Cantini F, Niccoli L, Cassara E, et al. Sustained maintenance of clinical remission after adalimumab dose reduction in patients with early psoriatic arthritis: a long-term follow-up study. Biologics 2012;6:201–6.

63. Olivieri I, D'Angelo S, Padula A, et al. Can we reduce the dosage of biologics in spondyloarthritis? Autoimmun Rev 2013;12:691–3.

64. Yoshida K, Sung YK, Kavanaugh A, et al. Biologic discontinuation studies: a systematic review of methods. Ann Rheum Dis 2014;73:595–9.

65. Kavanaugh A, Lee S, Curtis JR, et al. Discontinuation of tumour necrosis factor inhibitors in patients with rheumatoid arthritis in low-disease activity: persistent benefits. Data from the Corrona registry. Ann Rheum Dis 2015;74(6):1150–5.

66. Cantini F, Niccoli L, Nannini C, et al. Frequency and duration of clinical remission in patients with peripheral psoriatic arthritis requiring second-line drugs. Rheumatology (Oxford) 2008;47:872–6.

67. Tanaka Y. Intensive treatment and treatment holiday of TNF-inhibitors in rheumatoid arthritis. Curr Opin Rheumatol 2012;24:319–26.

Index

Note: Page numbers of article titles are in **boldface** type.

A

ABIN-1 gene, 627
Acetretin, 671
Acquired immune response, 628–631
Acro-osteolysis, 652
Actinobacterium, 645–646
Adalimumab, 632–633, 724–725, 750
    for inflammatory bowel disease, 686
    for ophthalmic disease, 685
Adalimumab Effectiveness in Psoriatic Arthritis Trial (ADEPT), 705, 725
Adaptive immunity, 667–668
ADEPT (Adalimumab Effectiveness in Psoriatic Arthritis Trial), 705, 725
Adhesion molecules, 669
Adipocytes and adipokines, 646
American College of Rheumatology, 701
Aminosalicylates, for inflammatory bowel disease, 686
Amphiregulin, 656
Andersson lesion, 604
Angiogenesis, 669
Ankyloses, 652
Ankylosing spondylitis, 584
Anticitrullinated peptide antibodies, 584–585
Antigen presentation, 628–629
Anxiety, 680, 683, 685–686
Apremilast, 655, 686, 713, 717–718
    in early stages, 743
    switching to, 749
Armor criteria, for PsA, 547–548
Arthritis mutilans, 547, 549, 570–571, 583, 652
Arthritis, psoriatic. *See* Psoriatic arthritis.
AS disease activity score (ASDAS), 703
ASDAS (AS disease activity score), 703
Assessment of Spondyloarthritis International Society criteria, 547–548
Atherosclerosis, 585, 672, 678–679, 681
Autoimmune disorders, ophthalmic, 684–685
Axial PsA, 572–573, 595–596
    as outcome measure domain, 703, 706
    clinical features of, 572–573
    computed tomography for, 597
    MRI for, 604–606
    radiography for, 595–596
Axial spondyloarthropathy, 547–548

Rheum Dis Clin N Am 41 (2015) 755–767
http://dx.doi.org/10.1016/S0889-857X(15)00086-1
0889-857X/15/$ – see front matter © 2015 Elsevier Inc. All rights reserved.

rheumatic.theclinics.com

United States Postal Service

Statement of Ownership, Management, and Circulation
(All Periodicals Publications Except Requestor Publications)

1. Publication Title	2. Publication Number	3. Filing Date
Rheumatic Disease Clinics of North America	0 0 6 - 2 7 2 2	9/18/15

4. Issue Frequency	5. Number of Issues Published Annually	6. Annual Subscription Price
Feb, May, Aug, Nov	4	$610.00

7. Complete Mailing Address of Known Office of Publication (Not printer) (Street, city, county, state, and ZIP+4®)

Elsevier Inc.
360 Park Avenue South
New York, NY 10010-1710

Contact Person
Stephen R. Bushing

Telephone (Include area code)
215-239-3688

8. Complete Mailing Address of Headquarters or General Business Office of Publisher (Not printer)

Elsevier Inc., 360 Park Avenue South, New York, NY 10010-1710

9. Full Names and Complete Mailing Addresses of Publisher, Editor, and Managing Editor (Do not leave blank)

Publisher (Name and complete mailing address)

Linda Belfus, Elsevier Inc., 1600 John F. Kennedy Blvd., Suite 1800, Philadelphia, PA 19103

Editor (Name and complete mailing address)

Jennifer Flynn-Briggs, Elsevier Inc., 1600 John F. Kennedy Blvd., Suite 1800, Philadelphia, PA 19103-2899

Managing Editor (Name and complete mailing address)

Adrianne Brigido, Elsevier Inc., 1600 John F. Kennedy Blvd., Suite 1800, Philadelphia, PA 19103-2899

10. Owner (Do not leave blank. If the publication is owned by a corporation, give the name and address of the corporation immediately followed by the names and addresses of all stockholders owning or holding 1 percent or more of the total amount of stock. If not owned by a corporation, give the names and addresses of the individual owners. If owned by a partnership or other unincorporated firm, give its name and address as well as those of each individual owner. If the publication is published by a nonprofit organization, give its name and address.)

Full Name	Complete Mailing Address
Wholly owned subsidiary of	1600 John F. Kennedy Blvd, Ste. 1800
Reed/Elsevier, US holdings	Philadelphia, PA 19103-2899

11. Known Bondholders, Mortgagees, and Other Security Holders Owning or Holding 1 Percent or More of Total Amount of Bonds, Mortgages, or Other Securities. If none, check box ☐ None

Full Name	Complete Mailing Address
N/A	

12. Tax Status (For completion by nonprofit organizations authorized to mail at nonprofit rates) (Check one)
The purpose, function, and nonprofit status of this organization and the exempt status for federal income tax purposes:
☐ Has Not Changed During Preceding 12 Months
☐ Has Changed During Preceding 12 Months (Publisher must submit explanation of change with this statement)

PS Form 3526, July 2014 (Page 1 of 3 [Instructions Page 3]) PSN 7530-01-000-9931 PRIVACY NOTICE: See our Privacy policy in www.usps.com

---

13. Publication Title	14. Issue Date for Circulation Data Below
Rheumatic Disease Clinics of North America	August 2015

15. Extent and Nature of Circulation		Average No. Copies Each Issue During Preceding 12 Months	No. Copies of Single Issue Published Nearest to Filing Date
a. Total Number of Copies (Net press run)		553	443
b. Legitimate Paid and/or Requested Distribution (By Mail and Outside the Mail)	(1) Mailed Outside County Paid/Requested Mail Subscriptions stated on PS Form 3541. (Include paid distribution above nominal rate, advertiser's proof copies, and exchange copies)	235	173
	(2) Mailed In-County Paid/Requested Mail Subscriptions stated on PS Form 3541. (Include paid distribution above nominal rate, advertiser's proof copies, and exchange copies)		
	(3) Paid Distribution Outside the Mails Including Sales Through Dealers And Carriers, Street Vendors, Counter Sales, and Other Paid Distribution Outside USPS®	123	140
	(4) Paid Distribution by Other Classes of Mail Through the USPS (e.g. First-Class Mail®)		
c. Total Paid and or Requested Circulation (Sum of 15b (1), (2), (3), and (4))	▶	358	313
d. Free or Nominal Rate Distribution (By Mail and Outside the Mail)	(1) Free or Nominal Rate Outside-County Copies included on PS Form 3541	52	37
	(2) Free or Nominal Rate In-County Copies included on PS Form 3541		
	(3) Free or Nominal Rate Copies mailed at Other classes Through the USPS (e.g. First-Class Mail®)		
	(4) Free or Nominal Rate Distribution Outside the Mail (Carriers or Other means)		
e. Total Nonrequested Distribution (Sum of 15d (1), (2), (3) and (4))	▶	52	37
f. Total Distribution (Sum of 15c and 15e)	▶	410	350
g. Copies not Distributed (See Instructions to publishers #4 (page #3))	▶	143	93
h. Total (Sum of 15f and g)	▶	553	443
i. Percent Paid and/or Requested Circulation (15c divided by 15f times 100)		87.32%	89.43%

* If you are claiming electronic copies go to line 16 on page 3. If you are not claiming Electronic copies, skip to line 17 on page 3.

16. Electronic Copy Circulation	Average No. Copies Each Issue During Preceding 12 Months	No. Copies of Single Issue Published Nearest to Filing Date
a. Paid Electronic Copies		
b. Total paid Print Copies (Line 15c) + Paid Electronic copies (Line 16a)		
c. Total Print Distribution (Line 15f) + Paid Electronic Copies (Line 16a)		
d. Percent Paid (Both Print & Electronic copies) (16b divided by 16c X 100)		

☐ I certify that 50% of all my distributed copies (electronic and print) are paid above a nominal price

17. Publication of Statement of Ownership
If the publication is a general publication, publication of this statement is required. Will be printed in the __November 2015__ issue of this publication.

18. Signature and Title of Editor, Publisher, Business Manager, or Owner		Date
Stephen R. Bushing		September 18, 2015
Stephen R. Bushing – Inventory Distribution Coordinator		

I certify that all information furnished on this form is true and complete. I understand that anyone who furnishes false or misleading information on this form or who omits material or information requested on the form may be subject to criminal sanctions (including fines and imprisonment) and/or civil sanctions (including civil penalties).

PS Form 3526, July 2014 (Page 3 of 3)

Printed and bound by CPI Group (UK) Ltd, Croydon, CR0 4YY

03/10/2024

01040494-0005